Hypercalcemia

Editors

CLAUDIO MARCOCCI
FILOMENA CETANI

ENDOCRINOLOGY AND METABOLISM CLINICS OF NORTH AMERICA

www.endo.theclinics.com

Consulting Editor
ADRIANA G. IOACHIMESCU

December 2021 • Volume 50 • Number 4

ELSEVIER

1600 John F. Kennedy Boulevard • Suite 1800 • Philadelphia, Pennsylvania, 19103-2899

http://www.theclinics.com

ENDOCRINOLOGY AND METABOLISM CLINICS OF NORTH AMERICA Volume 50, Number 4
December 2021 ISSN 0889-8529, ISBN 13: 978-0-323-81325-9

Editor: Katerina Heidhausen
Developmental Editor: Jessica Cañaberal

Endocrinology and Metabolism Clinics of North America (ISSN 0889-8529) is published quarterly by Elsevier Inc., 360 Park Avenue South, New York, NY 10010-1710. Months of issue are March, June, September, and December. Periodicals postage paid at New York, NY and additional mailing offices. Subscription prices are USD 383.00 per year for US individuals, USD 1037.00 per year for US institutions, USD 100.00 per year for US students and residents, USD 454.00 per year for Canadian individuals, USD 1089.00 per year for Canadian institutions, USD 497.00 per year for international individuals, USD 1089.00 per year for international institutions, USD 100.00 per year for Canadian students/residents, and USD 245.00 per year for international students/residents. To receive student/resident rate, orders must be accompanied by name of affiliated institution, date of term, and the signature of program/residency coordinator on institution letterhead. Orders will be billed at individual rate until proof of status is received. Foreign air speed delivery is included in all *Clinics* subscription prices. All prices are subject to change without notice. **POSTMASTER:** Send address changes to *Endocrinology and Metabolism Clinics of North America*, Elsevier Health Sciences Division, Subscription Customer Service, 3251 Riverport Lane, Maryland Heights, MO 63043. **Customer Service: Telephone: 1-800-654-2452** (U.S. and Canada); **1-314-447-8871** (outside U.S. and Canada). **Fax: 1-314-447-8029. E-mail: journalscustomerservice-u-sa@elsevier.com (for print support); journalsonlinesupport-usa@elsevier.com (for online support).**

Reprints. For copies of 100 or more, of articles in this publication, please contact the Commercial Rights Department, Elsevier Inc., 360 Park Avenue South, New York, NY 10010-1710; phone: +1-212-633-3874; fax: +1-212-633-3820; E-mail: reprints@elsevier.com.

Endocrinology and Metabolism Clinics of North America is covered in *MEDLINE/PubMed (Index Medicus)*, *EMBASE/Excerpta Medica*, *Current Contents/Clinical Medicine*, *Current Contents/Life Sciences*, *Science Citation Index*, *ISI/BIOMED*, *BIOSIS*, and *Chemical Abstracts*.

Contributors

CONSULTING EDITOR

ADRIANA G. IOACHIMESCU, MD, PhD
Emory University School of Medicine, Atlanta, Georgia, USA

EDITORS

CLAUDIO MARCOCCI, MD
Full Professor, Department of Clinical and Experimental Medicine, University of Pisa, and Endocrine Unit 2, University Hospital of Pisa, Pisa, Italy

FILOMENA CETANI, MD, PhD
Endocrine Unit 2, University Hospital of Pisa, Pisa, Italy

AUTHORS

CARLO ALFIERI, MD
Department of Nephrology, Dialysis and Renal Transplantation, Fondazione IRCCS Ca' Granda Ospedale Policlinico, Department of Clinical Sciences and Community Health, University of Milan, Milan, Italy

DALAL S. ALI, MD, FRCPI
Division of Endocrinology and Metabolism, McMaster University, Bone Research and Education Centre, Oakville, Ontario, Canada

ANNE BLANCHARD, MD, PhD
Assistance Publique-Hôpitaux de Paris (AP-HP), Hôpital Européen Georges Pompidou, Centre d'Investigations Cliniques 1418, Paris, France

FILOMENA CETANI, MD, PhD
Endocrine Unit 2, University Hospital of Pisa, Pisa, Italy

MARLENE CHAKHTOURA, MD, MSc
Calcium Metabolism and Osteoporosis Program, Division of Endocrinology, WHO Collaborating Center for Metabolic Bone Disorders, American University of Beirut, Beirut, Lebanon

KAREL DANDURAND, MD, FRCPC
Division of Endocrinology and Metabolism, McMaster University, Bone Research and Education Centre, Oakville, Ontario, Canada

GHADA EL-HAJJ FULEIHAN, MD, MPH, FRCP
Calcium Metabolism and Osteoporosis Program, Division of Endocrinology, WHO Collaborating Center for Metabolic Bone Disorders, American University of Beirut, Beirut, Lebanon

DAVID GOLTZMAN, MD
Calcium Research Laboratory, Senior Scientist, Professor, Department of Medicine and Physiology, McGill University, Research Institute of the McGill University Health Centre, Montreal, Quebec, Canada

MIMI I. HU, MD
Professor, Department of Endocrine Neoplasia & Hormonal Disorders, Professor, The University of Texas MD Anderson Cancer Center, Houston, Texas, USA

PETER KAMENICKÝ, MD, PhD
Professor, Assistance Publique-Hôpitaux de Paris (AP-HP), Hôpital de Bicêtre, Service d'Endocrinologie et des Maladies de la Reproduction, Centre de Référence des Maladies Rares du Métabolisme du Calcium et du Phosphate, Filière OSCAR; Université Paris-Saclay, Inserm, Physiologie et Physiopathologie Endocriniennes, Le Kremlin-Bicêtre, France

ALIYA A. KHAN, MD, FRCPC, FACP, FACE
Division of Endocrinology and Metabolism, McMaster University, Bone Research and Education Centre, Oakville, Ontario, Canada

STEPHANIE J. KIM, MD, MPH
Assistant Clinical Professor, Division of Endocrinology and Metabolism, University of California, San Francisco, California, USA

ANNE-LISE LECOQ, MD, PhD
Assistance Publique-Hôpitaux de Paris (AP-HP), Hôpital de Bicêtre, Service d'Endocrinologie et des Maladies de la Reproduction, Centre de Référence des Maladies Rares du Métabolisme du Calcium et du Phosphate, Filière OSCAR, Le Kremlin Bicêtre, France

MARINE LIVROZET, MD, PhD
Assistance Publique-Hôpitaux de Paris (AP-HP), Hôpital Européen Georges Pompidou, Centre d'Investigations Cliniques 1418, Paris, France

CLAUDIO MARCOCCI, MD
Full Professor, Department of Clinical and Experimental Medicine, University of Pisa, and Endocrine Unit 2, University Hospital of Pisa, Pisa, Italy

NIINA MATIKAINEN, MD, PhD
Endocrinology, Abdominal Center, Helsinki University Hospital and University of Helsinki, Helsinki, Finland

DEBORAH MATTINZOLI
Renal Research Laboratory Fondazione IRCCS Ca' Granda Ospedale Policlinico, Milan, Italy

PIERGIORGIO MESSA, MD
Professor, Department of Nephrology, Dialysis and Renal Transplantation, Fondazione IRCCS Ca' Granda Ospedale Policlinico, Department of Clinical Sciences and Community Health, University of Milan, Milan, Italy

PAUL J. NEWEY, MBChB (Hons), DPhil, FRCP
Senior Lecturer, Division of Molecular and Clinical Medicine, Ninewells Hospital and Medical School, Jacqui Wood Cancer Centre, Dundee, Scotland, United Kingdom

ELENA PARDI, MS, PhD
Department of Clinical and Experimental Medicine, University of Pisa, Pisa, Italy

TUULA PEKKARINEN, MD, PhD
Endocrinology, Abdominal Center, Helsinki University Hospital and University of Helsinki, Helsinki, Finland

LARS REJNMARK, PhD, DMSc
Clinical Professor, Chief Physician, Department of Endocrinology and Internal Medicine, Aarhus University Hospital, Aarhus N, Denmark

EEVA M. RYHÄNEN, MD, PhD
Endocrinology, Abdominal Center, Helsinki University Hospital and University of Helsinki, Helsinki, Finland

FEDERICA SAPONARO, MD, PhD
Department of Surgical, Medical, and Molecular Pathology and Critical Care Medicine, University of Pisa, Pisa, Italy

CAMILLA SCHALIN-JÄNTTI, MD, PhD
Endocrinology, Abdominal Center, Helsinki University Hospital and University of Helsinki, Helsinki, Finland

KARL PETER SCHLINGMANN, MD
Department of General Pediatrics, University Children's Hospital, Münster, Germany

DOLORES M. SHOBACK, MD
Endocrine Research Unit - 111N, San Francisco Department of Veterans Affairs Medical Center, Professor of Medicine, Division of Endocrinology and Metabolism, San Francisco VA Medical Center, University of California, San Francisco, California, USA

SHONNI J. SILVERBERG, MD
Professor of Medicine, Division of Endocrinology, Department of Medicine, Columbia University, Columbia University Irving Medical Center, New York, New York, USA

JO KROGSGAARD SIMONSEN, MD
Department of Endocrinology and Internal Medicine, Aarhus University Hospital, Aarhus N, Denmark

MARCELLA WALKER, MD, MS
Associate Professor of Medicine, Division of Endocrinology, Department of Medicine, Columbia University Irving Medical Center, New York, New York, USA

Contents

Calcium plays a key role in skeletal mineralization and several intracellular and extracellular homeostatic networks. It is an essential element that is only available to the body through dietary sources. Daily acquisition of calcium depends, in addition to the actual intake, on the hormonally regulated state of calcium homeostasis through three main mechanisms: bone turnover, intestinal absorption, and renal reabsorption. These procedures are regulated by a group of interacting circulating hormones and their key receptors. This includes parathyroid hormone (PTH), PTH-related peptide, 1,25-dihydroxyvitamin D, calcitonin, fibroblast growth factor 23, the prevailing calcium concentration itself, the calcium-sensing receptor, as well as local processes in the bones, gut, and kidneys.

Extracellular calcium is normally tightly regulated by parathyroid hormone (PTH), 1,25-dihydroxyvitamin D, as well as by calcium ion (Ca^{++}) itself. Dysregulated PTH production leading to hypercalcemia occurs most commonly in sporadic primary hyperparathryoidism (PHPT) but may also result from select genetic mutations in familial disorders. Parathyroid hormone-related protein shares molecular mechanisms of action with PTH and is the most common cause of hypercalcemia of malignancy. Other cytokines and mediators may also cause resorptive hypercalcemia once bone metastases have occurred. Less commonly, extrarenal production of calcitriol can occur in malignancies and in infectious and noninfectious inflammatory conditions and can cause hypercalcemia.

Sporadic primary hyperparathyroidism is a common endocrinopathy, particularly afflicting postmenopausal women and both African American men and women. Although classic signs and symptoms of the disease are well appreciated and described, because of the ease and availability and low threshold for screening, the disorder often is diagnosed in patients who are minimally symptomatic or asymptomatic. Surgery conducted by experienced endocrine surgeons has a high cure rate, particularly if guided by concordant imaging. In patients who cannot safely undergo surgery or who fail to be cured, medical therapy with the oral calcimimetic cinacalcet is a validated option for controlling serum calcium levels.

Nontraditional aspects of primary hyperparathyroidism refer to the condition's rheumatic, gastrointestinal, cardiovascular, and neuropsychological effects. Although gastrointestinal and rheumatic symptomatology were features of classical primary hyperparathyroidism, they do not seem to be a part of the modern presentation of primary hyperparathyroidism. In contrast, neuropsychological symptoms such as altered mood and cognition, as well as cardiovascular disease, have been associated with the form of primary hyperparathyroidism seen today, but the relationship is not clearly causal. Evidence does not support reversibility after parathyroidectomy and therefore none of the nontraditional manifestations are considered sole indications for recommending surgery at this time.

Patients who have undergone kidney transplantation (KTx) (KTxps) are a distinctive population characterized by the persistence of some metabolic anomalies present during end-stage renal disease. Mineral metabolism (MM) parameters are frequently altered after KTx. These alterations involve calcium, phosphorus, vitamin D, and parathormone (PTH) disarrangements. At present, there is little consensus about the correct monitoring and management of PTH disorders in KTxps. This article presents the prevalence and epidemiologic and clinical impact of post-KTx hyper-PTH. The principal biochemical and instrumental investigations and the therapeutic options for these conditions are also reported.

Primary hyperparathyroidism (PHPT) is a commonly encountered clinical problem and occurs as part of an inherited disorder in ~10% of patients. Several features may alert the clinician to the possibility of a hereditary PHPT disorder (eg, young age of disease onset) whilst establishing any relevant family history is essential to the clinical evaluation and will help inform the diagnosis. Genetic testing should be offered to patients at risk of a hereditary PHPT disorder, as this may improve management and allow the identification and investigation of other family members who may also be at risk of disease.

The most common causes of hypercalcemia are primary hyperparathyroidism (PHPT) and malignancy. Parathyroid carcinoma (PC), causing a severe PHPT, is the rarest parathyroid tumor. A diagnosis of PC is challenging because the clinical profile overlaps with that of benign counterpart. Surgery is the mainstay treatment. CDC73 mutations have been detected in up to 80% of sporadic PCs. Ectopic production of parathyroid hormone (PTH) by malignant nonparathyroid tumors is a rare condition accounting for less than 1% of hypercalcemia of malignancy. PTH secretion can be considered an aberration in the tissue specificity of gene expression and may involve heterogeneous molecular mechanisms.

The most common causes of hypercalcemia are primary hyperparathyroidism and malignancy, constituting 80% to 90% of all cases. Although less common, several nonparathyroid endocrine disorders are associated with hypercalcemia. The most well described is hyperthyroidism, although the reported prevalence of hypercalcemia in hyperthyroid patients varies depending on applied method for measuring serum calcium levels. Also, adrenal insufficiency, pheochromocytoma, and vasoactive intestinal polypeptide are associated with hypercalcemia. These are differential diagnoses when assessing the hypercalcemic patient for whom common causes have been excluded. Further investigation is needed regarding hypothyroidism; acromegaly, hyperprolactinemia, gonadal dysfunction, and diabetes are not associated with hyperthyroidism.

Hypercalcemia of malignancy (HCM) is considered an oncologic emergency associated with significant symptom burden and increased comorbid conditions and mortality. Underlying pathologic processes most often stimulate osteoclast-mediated bone resorption. Although long-term control of HCM depends on effective management of the underlying cancer, temporizing management strategies for acute and/or symptomatic HCM include hydration and antiresorptive bone-modifying agents. Although most patients respond well to the antiresorptive therapies available, further investigation into other agents for those who are refractory to both bisphosphonates and denosumab is needed.

Vitamin D metabolism represents a well-integrated, hormonally regulated endocrine unit interlinking calcium and phosphate metabolism. Pathophysiologic processes disturbing vitamin D metabolism comprise classic defects of vitamin D activation and action presenting as different forms of vitamin D–dependent rickets as well as disorders with increased vitamin D activity. The latter may result in hypercalcemia, hypercalciuria, and renal calcifications. Acquired and hereditary disorders causing hypervitaminosis D are discussed, including vitamin D intoxication, granulomatous disease, and idiopathic infantile hypercalcemia that may be caused by either a defective vitamin D degradation or by a primary defect in phosphate conservation.

This review focuses on the commonly prescribed medicaments that can be responsible for hypercalcemia, considering the prevalence, the predominant pathophysiological mechanisms, and the optimal medical management of each drug-induced hypercalcemia. Vitamin D supplements and 1α-hydroxylated vitamin D analogues increase intestinal calcium absorption, renal calcium reabsorption as well as bone resorption. In patients with hypoparathyroidism receiving recombinant human PTH, transient hypercalcemia can occur because of overtreatment, usually during acute illness. Thiazide-induced hypercalcemia is mainly explained by enhanced renal proximal calcium reabsorption, changing preexistent asymptomatic normocalcemic or intermittently hypercalcemic hyperparathyroidism into the classic hypercalcemic hyperparathyroidism. Lithium causes hypercalcemia mainly by drug-induced hyperparathyroidism.

Hypercalcemic disorders are rare in pregnant women and are usually due to primary hyperparathyroidism. Clinical manifestations of hypercalcemia are nonspecific and can be masked by the physiologic changes of pregnancy. Furthermore, routine antenatal screening does not include serum calcium measurement and a hypercalcemia diagnosis may therefore be delayed until term or even after delivery. Timely recognition and appropriate interventions are essential to decrease maternal and fetal complications. Conservative measures are appropriate in the presence of mild hypercalcemia. Parathyroidectomy remains the mainstay of treatment for primary hyperparathyroidism with significant hypercalcemia not responding to conservative measures.

This article discusses rare causes of hypercalcemia. Hypercalcemia can rarely be associated with immobilization, genetic diseases in children such as Williams-Beuren syndrome, Hypophosphatasia, Jansen Metaphyseal Chondrodysplasia (JMC), cosmetic injection, milk-alkali syndrome (MAS), calcium sulfate beads administration, manganese intoxication, postacute kidney failure recovery, and Paget's disease.

The treatment of hypercalcemia of malignancy (HCM) consists of enhancing renal calcium excretion, mostly through hydration with isotonic fluids and the use of antiresorptive therapies. Intravenous zoledronic acid is currently the first-line treatment. Subcutaneous denosumab is used for bisphosphonate-refractory hypercalcemia and in patients with renal failure. There is no evidence that bisphosphonates prevent the occurrence of HCM. Conversely, denosumab, compared with zoledronic acid, is associated with a lower risk of HCM, both first episode and recurrence, in patients with breast cancer and multiple myeloma.

ENDOCRINOLOGY AND METABOLISM CLINICS OF NORTH AMERICA

SERIES OF RELATED INTEREST

Medical Clinics
https://www.medical.theclinics.com
Primary Care: Clinics in Office Practice
https://www.primarycare.theclinics.com/

VISIT THE CLINICS ONLINE!
Access your subscription at:
www.theclinics.com

Foreword

Hypercalcemia and its Multiple Facets

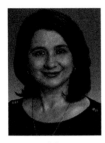

Adriana G. Ioachimescu, MD, PhD
Consulting Editor

It is my great pleasure to introduce the Hypercalcemia issue of the *Endocrinology and Metabolism Clinics of North America* to our readers. The guest editors, Dr Claudio Marcocci and Dr Filomena Cetani from University of Pisa in Italy, are well-known experts in the field.

Hypercalcemia is a common laboratory finding with multiple possible causes and can be sporadic or genetically inherited. A good understanding of the pathophysiology of calcium regulation is necessary for a correct diagnosis and treatment. In hospitalized patients, severe hypercalcemia is a medical emergency requiring immediate intervention. Therefore, this collection of review articles pertains to a wide spectrum of specialties, including primary care, internal medicine, critical care, emergency medicine, nephrology, endocrinology, and genetics.

Calcium homeostasis is thoroughly addressed by Dr Camilla Schalin-Jäntti and colleagues, who emphasize main regulators, including the parathyroid hormone (PTH), PTH-related protein, 1,25-dihydroxyvitamin D, calcitonin, and FGF-23. The mechanisms to maintain the narrow calcium normal range during physiologic circumstances entail specific processes at the level of the intestine, bone, and kidney.

Pathophysiology of hypercalcemia is unveiled by Dr Goltzman, who provides insight into PTH-dependent and independent mechanisms.

PTH-dependent hypercalcemia is the most common cause of hypercalcemia. Sporadic primary hyperparathyroidism is presented by Drs Stephanie Kim and Dolores Shoback, who emphasize its wide array of symptoms and current standards of management. While in the past this diagnosis was made in advanced stages with end-organ complications, currently it also pertains to many asymptomatic patients who undergo screening biochemical tests. The nontraditional aspects of sporadic primary hyperparathyroidism are addressed by Drs Marcella Walker and Shonni Silverberg, who emphasize cardiovascular and neuropsychological manifestations

Endocrinol Metab Clin N Am 50 (2021) xiii–xiv
https://doi.org/10.1016/j.ecl.2021.09.002
0889-8529/21/© 2021 Published by Elsevier Inc.

and their course after treatment of hypercalcemia. Hereditary primary hyperparathyroidism is less prevalent and includes familial isolated hyperparathyroidism, multiple tumor syndromes, familial hypocalciuric hypercalcemia, and neonatal hypercalcemia; these entities are unveiled by Dr Paul Newey. Tertiary and postrenal transplantation hyperparathyroidism are presented by Dr Piergiorgio Messa and colleagues, who emphasize the prevalence, clinical implications, and therapeutic challenges in this patient population. Parathyroid carcinoma and ectopic secretion of PTH are rare entities that require expert care; their genetic fingerprints, presentation, and management are unveiled by Dr Filomena Cetani and colleagues.

PTH-independent hypercalcemia has many facets, which are explored by Drs J.K. Simonsen and L. Rejnmark. These include predominantly malignant disorders, as well as nonparathyroid endocrine conditions, such as hyperthyroidism, adrenal insufficiency, pheochromocytoma, and VIPoma. A closer look at hypercalcemia of malignancy is offered by Dr Mimi Hu; this entity is an important aspect of cancer patient care, representing the most common paraneoplastic syndrome. Treatment of hypercalcemia of malignancy is detailed in the section by Dr Ghada El-Hajj Fuleihan. Vitamin D–dependent hypercalcemia includes a heterogeneous spectrum of genetic and acquired disorders affecting infants or adults, which are explained by Dr Karl Peter Schlingmann.

Drug-induced hypercalcemia is not rare; the main culprits are over-the-counter vitamin D supplements, thiazides, lithium, and medications used to treat hypocalcemia, secondary hyperparathyroidism, or cancer. The pathophysiologic and management implications are presented by Dr Peter Kamenický and colleagues.

Hypercalcemia of pregnancy is presented by Dr Aliya Khan and colleagues, who underline its main causes and current standards of management. Although a small proportion of women exhibits hypercalcemia during gestation, the challenges are multiple, including how to distinguish clinical manifestations from those of pregnancy, how to make a correct diagnosis, and how to treat clinically significant or severe hypercalcemia.

Rare causes of hypercalcemia, such as immobilization, heritable diseases in young children, cosmetic injections, and milk-alkali syndrome, are important for clinician to consider; these are presented by Dr Federica Saponaro.

I hope you will find this issue of the *Endocrinology and Metabolism Clinics of North America* informative and helpful in your practice. I thank Dr Marcocci and Dr Cetani for guest-editing this important collection of articles and the authors for their excellent contributions. I would like to take this opportunity to thank the Elsevier editorial staff for their outstanding work.

Adriana G. Ioachimescu, MD, PhD
Emory University School of Medicine
1365 B Clifton Road, Northeast, B6209
Atlanta, GA 30322, USA

E-mail address:
aioachi@emory.edu

Preface

Hypercalcemia

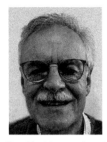 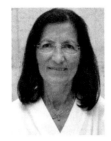

Claudio Marcocci, MD   Filomena Cetani, MD, PhD
Editors

Total serum calcium concentration has three components: (i) ionized serum calcium (about 50%), (ii) serum calcium complexed to anions (about 3%), and (iii) protein-bound (mostly albumin) serum calcium (about 47%).

Hypercalcemia is defined as a serum calcium concentration greater than 2 standard deviations above the normal mean in a reference laboratory and is usually distinct according to serum calcium concentration in mild when below 12 mg/dL, moderate when between 12 and 14 mg/dL, and severe when greater than 14 mg/dL.

Calcium homeostasis is tightly regulated and maintained by the equilibrium among renal excretion, bone resorption, and intestinal absorption of calcium. In 1979, Parfitt proposed three different pathophysiologic mechanisms of hypercalcemia: (i) "Equilibrium" hypercalcemia, characterized by an average serum calcium above the upper normal, which is maintained at the same levels with few fluctuations. This pattern typically occurs in patients with mild to moderate primary hyperparathyroidism (PHPT) and is caused by an increased calcium bone resorption, which is balanced by an increased renal tubular excretion; (ii) "Disequilibrium" hypercalcemia, characterized by a rapid increase in serum calcium, due to a marked increase of bone resorption associated with the inability of the kidney to excrete the increased calcium overload. It may occur when precipitating conditions beake the equilibrium in patients with "equilibrium" hypercalcemia or can arise in the beginning, where a major disturbance of the bone remodeling system occurs; (iii) Hyperabsorption hypercalcemia, due to increased intestinal calcium absorption and positive calcium balance, as in vitamin D intoxication. Hypercalciuria is the first biochemical abnormality in all types of hypercalcemia unless renal function is markedly deteriorated.

Hypercalcemia is rather common in the general population with a prevalence of about 1% and is often incidentally discovered in diagnostic workup for unrelated disorders, particularly since the widespread availability of multichannel biochemistry autoanalyzers. The prevalence increases in emergency departments and hospitalized

Endocrinol Metab Clin N Am 50 (2021) xv–xvi
https://doi.org/10.1016/j.ecl.2021.07.011
endo.theclinics.com

subjects, up to 3% to 7% according to different series and causes. The principal challenge in clinical practice is to distinguish parathyroid hormone (PTH) -related hypercalcemia from other forms hypercalcemia due to different causes, which require a more complex diagnostic approach and different treatments.

PHPT is the most common cause of hypercalcemia in free-living individuals, followed by hypercalcemia of malignancy, which is the most common form in hospitalized patients. The clinical manifestations vary according to the severity of hypercalcemia. Severe hypercalcemia is an emergency and requires urgent evaluation and treatment.

We are very grateful to all the authors who contributed to this initiative, which sums up recent accomplishments in the field of hypercalcemia and provides guidance on diagnosis and treatment.

The first part of the issue deals with the physiology of calcium homeostasis and the pathophysiology of hypercalcemia. A large amount of space is dedicated to the different forms of PTH-dependent hypercalcemia with particular emphasis on recent advances in our understanding of target organ involvement and management. The following sections address the PTH-independent forms of hypercalcemia, including other endocrine disorders, hypercalcemia of malignancy, vitamin D–dependent hypercalcemia, drug-related hypercalcemia, and most rare forms of hypercalcemia. A specific article is devoted to hypercalcemia in pregnancy, which offers specific diagnostic and treatments challenges. The last part is dedicated to the epidemiology of hypercalcemia, its clinical assessment, and management.

We hope that this issue provides useful information to the readers and guidance for the diagnosis and management of hypercalcemia.

Claudio Marcocci, MD
Department of Clinical and
Experimental Medicine
University of Pisa, and Endocrine Unit 2
University Hospital of Pisa
Via Paradisa
56124 Pisa, Italy

Filomena Cetani, MD, PhD
Endocrine Unit 2
University Hospital of Pisa
Via Paradisa
56124 Pisa, Italy

E-mail addresses:
claudio.marcocci@unipi.it (C. Marcocci)
cetani@endoc.med.unipi.it (F. Cetani)

Physiology of Calcium Homeostasis: An Overview

Niina Matikainen, MD, PhD, Tuula Pekkarinen, MD, PhD,
Eeva M. Ryhänen, MD, PhD, Camilla Schalin-Jäntti, MD, PhD*

KEYWORDS

- Bone metabolism • Calcium • Calcium homeostasis • Calcium-sensing receptor
- Parathyroid hormone • Parathyroid hormone related protein • Phosphorus
- Vitamin D

KEY POINTS

- The concentration of calcium in the blood and total body balance of calcium ions are maintained within narrow limits by powerful, interactive homeostatic mechanisms.
- Vital regulators of calcium homeostasis include prevailing plasma calcium concentration, parathyroid hormone, 1,25-dihydroxyvitamin D, calcitonin, and fibroblast growth factor 23.
- The adaptation of calcium metabolism during physiologic challenges relies on flexibility of absorption in the gut, excretion through kidney, and buffering properties of bone.

INTRODUCTION

Calcium is an essential trace element and a vital contributor to numerous reactions in virtually every human cell. To ensure normal physiologic functions, intracellular and extracellular calcium concentrations are tightly controlled by intestinal absorption, renal reabsorption, and exchange from bone. This dynamic homeostasis is regulated by several hormones, pH, and other extracellular fluid (ECF) ions such as phosphorus. This review focuses on body calcium homeostasis and the key mechanisms in the gut, kidneys, and bones involved in the regulation of calcium balance in healthy adults.

Funding: The data collection and drafting of the article was financed by independent research grants from Finska Läkaresällskapet (to C. Schalin-Jäntti) and the Helsinki University Hospital Research Funds (TYH2018223 and TYH2019254 to C. Schalin-Jäntti) and (TYH2020402 and M1021YLI31 to N. Matikainen).
Endocrinology, Abdominal Center, Helsinki University Hospital and University of Helsinki, PB 340, 00029 HUS, Helsinki, Finland
* Corresponding author.
E-mail address: camilla.schalin-jantti@hus.fi

endo.theclinics.com

BASIC ASPECTS OF CALCIUM HOMEOSTASIS
Distribution and Biochemistry of Total Body Calcium

A healthy adult body contains around 1 kg of calcium, 99% of which is deposited in bone and teeth, while only 1% of the total body calcium is found in blood, ECF, and soft tissues. Calcium is present in two fractions, either in an inactive, bound form or as a highly reactive divalent cation, Ca2+. Calcium is measured in the blood from serum or plasma, as total calcium concentration, total albumin-corrected calcium concentration (common reference interval $\sim$ 2.15–2.51 mmol/L), or in its active ionized form (reference interval $\sim$ 1.16–1.31 mmol/L).

Ionized calcium comprises about 47% of plasma calcium. Of the bound calcium, 8% to 10% is complexed to organic and inorganic acids (eg, citrate, sulfate, and phosphate), and approximately 40% is protein-bound, primarily to albumin (80%) but also to globulins (20%).[1] The protein-bound fraction of calcium provides a readily available reserve should the need for Ca2+ acutely increase. Concentrations of binding proteins, especially albumin, affect the measurement of total calcium concentration. This is particularly important in patients with acid-base and electrolyte disorders or disturbances in plasma protein concentrations. Therefore, physiologically relevant measure of calcium is best obtained by determination of the Ca2+ concentration. One commonly used algorithm estimates that total plasma calcium declines by approximately 0.8 mg/dL (0.2 mmol/L) for each 1 g/dL (10 g/L) decrease in albumin concentration. The following formulas can be used to calculate albumin-corrected calcium: (a) 0.8 * (normal albumin concentration − the patient's albumin concentration) + serum Ca (in mg/dl); and (b) 0.02 * (normal albumin concentration − the patient's albumin concentration) + serum Ca (in mmol/l), respectively.[2–4]

The concentrations of extracellular calcium and phosphate are tightly regulated, as they together are close to the point of precipitation and mineralization of soft tissues. An increase or decrease in the ECF phosphate concentration is reflected as opposite changes in the ECF Ca2+ concentration. Most (85%) of the body phosphorus is in the mineral phase in bone, 15% is intracellular, and less than 1% is extracellular or found in plasma.[5] Yet poorly understood mechanisms allow controlled deposition of calcium phosphate in bone but not in other tissues.[6,7] In bone, calcium and phosphorus form hydroxyapatite, the main inorganic component that accounts for its rigidity, strength, and elasticity.[8] This also allows for normal movement of the body and exercise. Other bone minerals include calcium carbonate and calcium citrate. Magnesium is the fourth most abundant cation in the body. Half of the body magnesium is found in bone.[5]

Intracellular and Extracellular Functions of Calcium in the Body

Calcium is an essential contributor to numerous reactions in virtually every human cell. These can be divided into intracellular and extracellular homeostatic reactions, tightly bound to intact regulation of local calcium concentration.[9] Free calcium in the ECF is one of the most rapidly regulated ions because of a negative feedback loop that allows minute-to-minute corrections of its concentration. Blood calcium concentration shows only minor circadian rhythmicity with reduced concentrations across the night which is independent of timing of sleep and only scarcely affected by food intake.[10,11]

In addition to its crucial functions in the skeleton, intracellular calcium, maintained at a 1000-fold lower concentration (10^{-7} mol/L) than plasma calcium (10^{-3} mol/L), is a key regulator of most physiologic processes in the body, including muscle contraction, hormone secretion, nerve conduction, cell proliferation and differentiation, adenosine triphosphate (ATP) metabolism, and blood coagulation.[9] Extracellular calcium is the physiologic ligand of the calcium-sensing receptor (CaSR) and thus serves as a hormone.[12,13] CaSRs are expressed on the membranes of parathyroid, bone, renal tubule, and thyroid C cells and in many other tissues throughout the body. **Fig. 1** demonstrates the distribution of CaSRs in various target tissues and main hormone-like actions of calcium.

Dietary Calcium

Humans are dependent on daily dietary intake of calcium. The balance of bone formation, resorption, and losses through urine and other compartments determine the daily requirements of dietary calcium (**Fig. 2**). These are especially high during growth, pregnancy, and lactation.

Milk, other dairy products, and calcium-fortified foods comprise the main sources of calcium intake. Variable amounts of calcium are found in fish and fish products, pulses, nuts, seeds, and green vegetables. Recommended daily calcium allowance for adolescents and adults[14,15] and population reference for calcium intake[16] are given in **Table 1**. Excessive intake of calcium supplements can be harmful and increase the risk for nephrolithiasis, nephrocalcinosis, dyspepsia, constipation, and, possibly, vascular calcifications.[17] The daily tolerable upper limit of calcium intake varies between 2500 mg for children older than 1 year to 3000 mg for adults.[15]

Local factors in the intestine are important determinants of dietary calcium intake.[18] Phosphate binders such as aluminum hydroxide increase calcium absorption. On the other hand, if the bioavailability of dietary calcium is reduced by calcium-binding

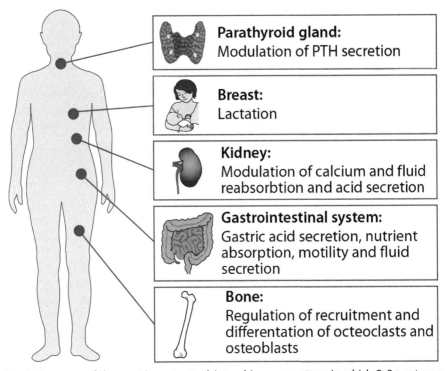

Parathyroid gland:
Modulation of PTH secretion

Breast:
Lactation

Kidney:
Modulation of calcium and fluid
reabsorbtion and acid secretion

Gastrointestinal system:
Gastric acid secretion, nutrient
absorption, motility and fluid
secretion

Bone:
Regulation of recruitment and
differentation of octeoclasts and
osteoblasts

Fig. 1. Summary of the most important calciotrophic organ systems in which Ca2+ acts as a physiologic hormone-like ligand of the calcium-sensing receptor (CaSR). Although CaSR is expressed in a wide range of cell types, its expression in these organs affects the body calcium homeostasis.

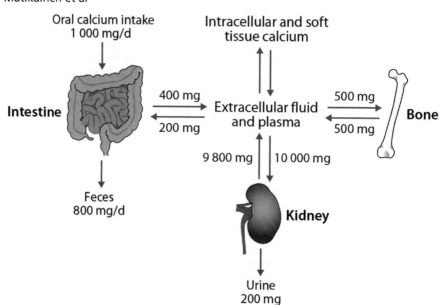

Fig. 2. In the adult, about 1 g of elemental Ca (Ca2+) is ingested in the diet daily, and approximately 800 mg is excreted in the feces and 200 mg in the urine. About 400 mg of calcium of the 1 g is absorbed by the intestine, and calcium is lost into the intestinal secretions about 200 mg daily.

agents such as cellulose, phosphate, and oxalate, calcium absorption decreases.[13] Recent studies highlight the importance of the gut microbiome as a modulator of intestinal calcium availability and absorption.[19]

Regulation of Calcium Concentrations

Body calcium balance must adapt to alterations caused by growth, pregnancy, lactation, menopause, and aging. The principal components determining ECF (plasma)

Table 1
Recommended daily allowance (RDA)[a] for calcium according to Institute of Medicine (IOM[14]) and population reference intake (PRI)[b] for calcium according to European Food Safety Authority (ESFA[16])

Population	Life-stage Group	RDA, IOM 2010 (mg/d)	Life-stage Group	PRI, EFSA 2017 (mg/d)
Children	1–3 y	700	1–3 y	450
	4–8 y	1000	4–10 y	800
	9–18 y	1300	11–17 y	1150
Adults	19–50 y	1000	18–24 y	1000
	51–70-y, m/f	1000/1200	Over 24 y	950
	Over 70 y	1200		
	Pregnant/lactating over 18 y	1000	Pregnant/lactating women 18–24 y	1000
			Pregnant/lactating women over 24 y	950

Abbreviations: f, females; m, males; y, years of age.
[a] Derived from the estimated average requirement and meets or exceeds the requirement for 97.5% of the population.
[b] The level of nutrient intake that is adequate for virtually all people in a population.

Ca2+ concentration consist of dietary calcium intake, intestinal absorption, retention and release of calcium from bone, excretion in the urine, and, finally, the balance between bound and free fractions.[5] The gut, bones, and kidneys dynamically interact to maintain calcium homeostasis through the effects of 1,25-dihydroxyvitamin D $(1,25(OH)_2D)$, parathyroid hormone (PTH), and fibroblast growth factor 23 (FGF23). The three key organ receptors of the calcium-regulating system are highlighted in **Fig. 3**. The CaSRs on the surface of different cell types sense perturbations in plasma and ECF calcium concentrations and mediate the changes to the key hormone-producing cells and key organs, as indicated in **Fig. 1**. PTH acts through PTH receptors which are vital mediators of calcium homeostasis in the bones and kidneys. The third seminal receptor is the vitamin D receptor (VDR) found in the bones and intestine.[20]

Several other hormones such as sex steroids, glucocorticoids, and growth and thyroid hormones, as well as changes in ion concentrations and pH, also affect calcium balance. Increased anion (ie, phosphate, bicarbonate, citrate) concentrations chelate calcium and thereby decrease Ca2+. Similarly, a shift toward alkaline pH reduces the concentration of Ca2+, as the affinity of albumin for calcium increases. By contrast, acidosis decreases the binding of calcium to albumin and increases plasma Ca2+ concentrations. Systemic acidosis can also increase urinary calcium loss and activate

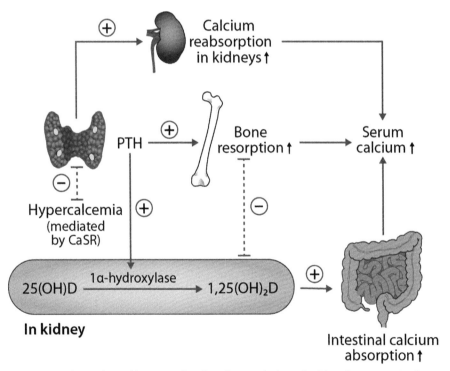

Fig. 3. Role of parathyroid hormone (PTH) in the regulation of calcium homeostasis. The increase or fall in extracellular fluid (ECF) calcium concentrations is censored by the calcium-sensing receptor (CaSR) in the parathyroid cells. Hypercalcemia inhibits PTH secretion from the parathyroid gland but during hypocalcemia, rapid release of PTH enhances bone resorption and improves calcium retention in the kidneys to prevent urinary losses. Increase in vitamin D activation to 1,25-dihydroxyvitamin D ($1,25(OH)_2D$, calcitriol) directly increases absorption of dietary calcium in the intestine and further releases bone calcium through actions of vitamin D receptor (VDR).

osteoclastic bone resorption, which provides "bone buffering" for the maintenance of plasma calcium concentration.

ENDOCRINE CONTROL OF CALCIUM HOMEOSTASIS
Parathyroid Hormone

Physiology of parathyroid hormone
PTH is synthesized by the parathyroid chief cells, stored in vesicles, and released through exocytosis into the blood stream. First, pre-pro-PTH, a 115-amino acid polypeptide, is cleaved within the cell to form pro-PTH and thereafter full-length, intact PTH, comprising 84 amino acids. The N-terminal PTH fragment (1–34) serves as the functional domain. PTH secretion is extremely sensitive to changes in Ca2+, which are mediated by the CaSRs on the parathyroid cells. A decrease in Ca2+ promotes PTH secretion, while increased Ca2+ concentration inhibits PTH release.[21] The transcription activity of the PTH gene, located on chromosome 11, also regulates long-term secretion of PTH and is repressed by calcitriol.[12,22]

The half-life of PTH is 2 minutes, and it is degraded by the liver and kidneys. The rapid response mechanisms of PTH secretion, the minute-to-minute regulation of blood Ca2+ by CaSRs, and the negative feedback loop including the short half-life of PTH maintain the plasma calcium concentration in a narrow range (see **Fig. 3**).

In clinical practice, it is essential to use assays that measure intact PTH to detect the true quantity of the active PTH.[23]

Parathyroid hormone in the control of calcium balance
PTH increases calcium concentrations by different actions in bone (calcium release), kidneys (calcium reabsorption), and the intestine (calcium absorption) (see **Fig. 3**). In bone and the kidneys, the effect is mediated through PTH1 receptors highly expressed in these organs.[24] PTH also acts on the PTH2 receptor in other organs, and these effects are not related to calcium homeostasis.

In the kidneys, PTH can rapidly reduce urinary calcium concentration by increasing calcium and magnesium reabsorption in the distal nephron, including cortical thick ascending limbs (TAL) of the loop of Henle and distal convoluted tubules (DCTs). In the TAL, binding of PTH to the PTH1 receptor leads to increased Na/K/2Cl-transporter activity and enhanced the reabsorption of calcium, sodium, chloride, and magnesium. PTH inhibits reabsorption of phosphate in the proximal tubule.[25] PTH also stimulates 1-alpha-hydroxylase activity in the kidneys[26] (**Fig. 4**).

In bones, the PTH1 receptor-mediated effects of PTH on the osteoblast cell lineage are both catabolic and anabolic. PTH has only indirect effects on osteoclasts, which lack PTH1 receptors. PTH promotes the production of cytokines in osteoblast cells favoring osteoclast formation and bone resorption.[27,28] PTH can improve bone formation in trabecular bone by its actions on osteoblastic cells. These are partly mediated by effects on Wnt-signaling and reductions in sclerostin expression in osteocytes.[29] The mode of PTH administration determines the net effect on bone, with intermittent administration enhancing bone formation and continuous administration leading to bone resorption. These dynamic properties explain why bone loss is a hallmark of chronic hypersecretion of PTH.[30]

Parathyroid Hormone–Related Protein

PTH-related protein (PTHrP) was first discovered in patients with malignancy and humoral hypercalcemia.[31] PTHrP may thus be ectopically secreted by malignant tumors and cause paraneoplastic hypercalcemia. PTHrP is expressed in many tissues where

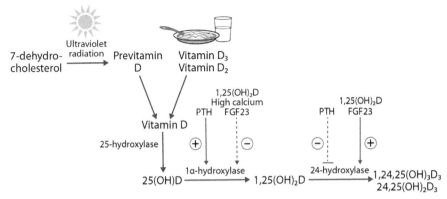

Fig. 4. Metabolism and role of vitamin D in calcium homeostasis. 25(OH)D is produced in the liver from its precursors. In the kidneys, it is activated by 1-alpha-hydroxylase to the active form, 1,25-dihydroxyvitamin D (1,25(OH)$_2$D, calcitriol). 1,25(OH)$_2$D increases calcium absorption in the intestine. Mitochondrial 1-alpha-hydroxylase is present in multiple cell types. 1,25(OH)$_2$D produced in these cells plays important roles in regulation of immunologic and nervous systems. DBP = vitamin D–binding protein.

it acts as a paracrine regulator.[5] The amino-terminal end of PTHrP shares homology with PTH and binds to the PTH1 receptor.

PTHrP plays an important physiologic role in pregnancy, during which it is secreted by placenta to regulate maternal-to-fetal calcium transport and ensure sufficient calcium availability for fetal bone development.[32] PTHrP is also produced in the breast tissue during lactation. PTHrP acts as a growth factor for bone and other organs in fetal and early life.[33] According to studies in mouse model, PTHrP is expressed by a population of chondrocytes and regulate their maturation.[34]

Vitamin D and Calcitriol

Vitamin D affects not only bone growth, osteoblasts, and osteoclasts but also muscle cells, cell proliferation, and the immune and nervous systems.[35,36] 1,25(OH)$_2$D (calcitriol), the active metabolite of vitamin D, enhances intestinal and renal absorption of calcium and phosphate and the bone mineralization (see **Fig. 3**). 1,25(OH)$_2$D acts through the VDR.

Vitamin D3 (cholecalciferol) can be synthesized in the epidermal layer of the skin from 7-dehydrocholesterol under the ultraviolet B radiation. Prehormones of vitamin D in the diet (see **Fig. 4**) are vitamin D2 (ergocalciferol), derived from plant source foods, and vitamin D3, obtained from animal source foods. Dietary D2 and D3 are absorbed in the small intestine and transported in chylomicrons to the liver. These precursors are metabolized to 25(OH)D, which is then bound to vitamin D–binding protein (DBP) and secreted into the blood. DBP binds vitamin D and all its metabolites. The half-life of 25(OH)D is 3 weeks.

Finally, 25(OH)D must be hydroxylated by 1-alpha-hydroxylase to 1,25(OH)$_2$D in the kidneys. The proteins cubilin and megalin, expressed on the surface of the renal proximal tubules, facilitate uptake of 25(OH)D. 1-alpha-hydroxylase is also expressed in extrarenal sites, such as the gastrointestinal tract, skin, osteoblasts, and osteoclasts.[5,37,38] The last hydroxylation step is tightly controlled by PTH[26] and FGF23.[39] 1,25(OH)$_2$D is degraded by 24-hydroxylase in the proximal convoluted tubule cells and in all target cells expressing VDR.[37,38] The balance between these two hydroxylases regulates the $1,25(OH)_2D$ concentration. $1,25(OH)_2D$ inhibits PTH production and parathyroid cell proliferation but stimulates 24-hydroxylase. PTH inhibits 24-hydroxylase. FGF23, on the contrary, inhibits 1-alpha-hydroxylase and increases 24-hydroxylase activity.

Fibroblast Growth Factor 23

FGF23 is an important regulator of phosphate homeostasis that indirectly effects calcium homeostasis by decreasing $1,25(OH)_2D$ production and thus reducing intestinal calcium absorption[39] (see **Fig. 4**). It is a 231-amino acid protein produced by the mature osteoblasts and osteocytes in bone. After cleavage of the 24-amino acid terminus, the active form of FGF23 binds to its receptor together with klotho, an essential coprotein.[40,41] FGF23 secretion increases in response to hyperphosphatemia. Consequently, the amount of sodium-phosphate cotransporters 2a and 2c decreases leading to reduced renal phosphate reabsorption. Intestinal phosphate and calcium absorption decrease, as FGF23 also reduces $1,25(OH)_2D$ production. PTH also increases FGF23 release from osteocytes.

Calcitonin

Calcitonin (CT) is a 32-amino acid protein produced by the thyroid C cells. The physiologic role of CT is still uncertain in humans more than 50 years after its discovery.[42] Hypercalcemia increases CT secretion. This is mediated by CaSR expression in the C cells. CT increases $1,25(OH)_2D$ production in the proximal tubules of the kidneys, and $1,25(OH)_2D$ suppresses CT secretion. During pregnancy and lactation, both CT and $1,25(OH)_2D$ increase, which may help maintain maternal bone mass.[5] CT has a rapid, short-term effect on osteoclast activity, reducing calcium and phosphate release from bone.

RECEPTOR-MEDIATED REGULATION OF CALCIUM BALANCE IN TARGET TISSUE
Calcium-Sensing Receptor

CaSRs detect even very small changes in blood calcium and modulate the production of the hormones involved in calcium metabolism. They are G-protein-coupled receptors with a wide tissue distribution. CaSRs regulate PTH secretion, urinary Ca2+ secretion, bone metabolism, and lactation (see **Fig. 1**).[21] CaSRs also have noncalciotropic roles in many processes such as gastrointestinal nutrient sensing and motility, vascular contractility, and wound healing.[20,22]

Ca2+ serves as the ligand, and binding leads to conformational change of the CaSR. The CaSR acts together with several protein partners in mediating intracellular calcium signaling. In the parathyroid, this also results in inhibition of the release of preformed PTH. If ECF calcium concentration decreases, CaSR remains inactivated, and PTH secretion continues (see **Fig. 3**).

In bones, CaSRs activated by calcium stimulate bone formation. In the kidneys, CaSR regulates Ca2+ reabsorption independent of PTH.[43] CaSR is highly expressed in the basolateral membrane of TAL where the interaction with claudin-14 protein permits paracellular Ca2+ reabsorption. CaSR is expressed also in the proximal tubule, where it regulates 1-alpha-hydroxylase activity. In the DCT, CaSR promotes calcium reabsorption via transient receptor potential vanilloid member (TRPV) 5 channel.[44] In the collecting ducts, it enhances urinary acidification and water excretion. CaSR is also found along the gastrointestinal system where it mediates nutrient sensing, gastric acid secretion, and fluid movement during normal digestion.[45,46]

PTH1 Receptor

The amino-terminal region of PTH binds to PTH1 (or PTH/PTHrP) receptor, which is a classic G-protein-coupled receptor. PTHrP binds to this same receptor. PTH1R is highly expressed on osteoblasts and osteocytes in bones and on tubular cells in the kidneys, in which the major ligand seems to be the circulating PTH. PTH1 receptors are also expressed in many other tissues where the ligand seems to be PTHrP in auto-crine/paracrine manner. The binding of PTH to PTH1R activates the adenylate cyclase/cAMP/protein kinase A and phospholipase/protein kinase C signaling path-ways which mediate the effects of PTH.[24,47]

Vitamin D Receptor

The action of $1,25(OH)_2D$ is mediated by VDR. VDR is a nuclear receptor and affects gene transcription after forming a heterodimer with the retinoid X receptor.[48] The VDR is found in most cell types.[38] In addition to its role in calcium metabolism, $1,25(OH)_2D$ and VDR have effects on the immune and nervous systems. $1,25(OH)_2D$ and VDR con-trol expression of genes associated to cell proliferation and differentiation. There is ongoing research to clarify whether vitamin D protects against chronic diseases such as cardiovascular diseases, cancer, and diabetes.[38,49]

THE GASTROINTESTINAL-BONE-RENAL AXIS
Role of the Intestine

Absorption of dietary calcium from the intestine maintains a neutral calcium balance, that is, compensates for losses caused by calcium excretion. Intestinal calcium ab-sorption adapts to dietary calcium availability and is substantially increased during growth, lactation, and other situations of increased body calcium needs. Of the rec-ommended normal daily calcium intake of 1 g, approximately 400 mg is absorbed by the intestine, 200 mg is lost with intestinal secretion, and net daily absorption equals about 200 mg, that is, close to 20% of the ingested calcium. A normal glomer-ular filtration rate of 170 L per day filters about 10 g of calcium through the kidneys, with 100 to 300 mg calcium lost in the urine.[18,50] In a balanced state, bone excretes and absorbs about 500 mg calcium daily (see **Fig. 2**).

Calcium is absorbed through the whole intestine, but mainly in duodenum and jejunum. The proportion of calcium absorbed also depends on the amount of daily cal-cium intake, with increased absorption when long-term calcium intake is low. Efficacy of intestinal calcium absorption rate increases up to 60% if the calcium demand in-creases, as during growth, pregnancy, and lactation.[51] Intestinal absorption de-creases with aging. In children and adolescents, calcium retention in the body increases linearly with calcium intake.[52,53] This is attributable to increased absorption of calcium, combined with decreased bone resorption.[54]

The absorption process of calcium involves two central mechanisms: (1) transcellu-lar active transport in the duodenum and jejunum and (2) paracellular transport by the entire small intestine[55,56] (**Fig. 5**). The former mechanism is of special importance at low-calcium-intake stages. Instead, passive diffusion dominates at times of high cal-cium intake, but this pathway usually accounts for only about 8% to 23% of the total calcium absorption.[57,58] In duodenum, where VDRs are abundant, active calcium transport is dependent on upregulation of the VDR and calcium transport protein genes. $1,25(OH)_2D$ mainly controls active calcium absorption, but also paracellular transport.[59]

The *active calcium transport* pathway is transcellular and involves three steps. The first step is luminal calcium entry into the intestinal cell via the apical calcium channel

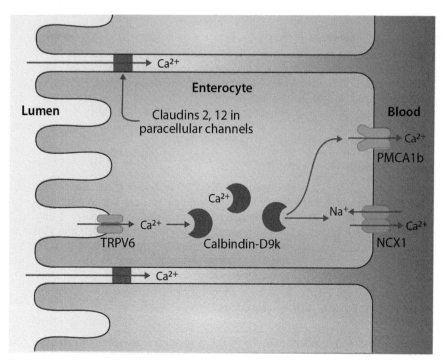

Fig. 5. Transcellular and paracellular calcium absorption in the intestine. The transcellular absorption is via transient receptor potential vanilloid family member 6 (TRPV6), intracellular calcium transport by calbindin-D9k, and basolateral calcium extrusion via Na+/Ca2+ exchanger 1 (NCX) and plasma membrane Ca2+-ATPase 1b (PMCA1b).

of the transient receptor potential TRPV6. After this, calcium (mainly bound to calbindin-D_{9k} and, to a lesser extent, to other proteins such as calmodulin) is transported across the cell. The final step is basolateral extrusion of calcium via plasma membrane Ca2+⁻ATPase 1b and the Na$^+$/Ca2+ exchanger 1 (NCX1).[44,60] Reduction in dietary calcium intake increases PTH production and thus renal 1,25(OH)$_2$D production. This increases the synthesis of calbindin and enhances calcium absorption, thus compensating for low calcium intake.[61]

Both passive and active *paracellular routes* for calcium absorption exist. The passive transport is driven by the high calcium concentration gradient between lumen and plasma.[55] During high calcium intake, passive transport mainly accounts for calcium absorption, while 1,25(OH)$_2$D is suppressed. Active paracellular transport is mediated by solvent drag, induced by sodium efflux by Na+/K + -ATPase which creates a hyperosmotic environment. This further induces diffusion of water to the plasma, dragging along small molecules such as calcium. 1,25(OH)$_2$D regulates claudin 2 and claudin 12, which form paracellular calcium channels. 1,25(OH)$_2$D also reroutes calcium through paracellular epithelial cell junctions and render them more permeable to calcium.[56,62]

Bone Turnover and Calcium Balance

The mineralized skeleton is essential for bone rigidity, strength, and elasticity.[8] In addition, the skeletal remodeling process provides a dynamic pool of minerals, mainly calcium, phosphorus, and magnesium and alkali and is thus critical for overall mineral and acid-base homeostasis.[6,14] Bone tissue consists of the mineralized and nonmineralized matrix (osteoid) and three principal cellular components; the bone-forming osteoblasts, some of which are embedded within the osteoid and become terminally differentiated osteocytes, and the bone-resorbing osteoclasts. The communication between these cells determines the balance between bone formation and resorption that releases and deposits about 500 mg of calcium daily in a healthy adult (see **Fig. 2**).

The predominant mechanism for skeletal Ca2+ mobilization acutely and chronically is the interaction of PTH with the PTHR1 in bone.[24] Increases in levels of PTH and 1,25(OH)$_2$D during low calcium levels activate osteoclastic bone resorption indirectly, through the stimulation of osteoblasts.[47] Osteoblasts, that arise from mesenchymal-derived cells, produce and deposit the osteoid as a template for hydroxyapatite mineral deposition. Osteoblasts are in close contact with matrix-embedded osteocytes through gap junctions. The osteocytes also regulate the mineralization of the bone matrix through their production of dentin matrix protein-1 (DMP-1), matrix extracellular phosphoglycoprotein (MEPE), and sclerostin.[63,64] Osteoblasts and osteocytes produce FGF23 in response to the interactive effects of plasma calcium, phosphorus, 1,25(OH)$_2$D, and possibly PTH concentrations[65] (see **Fig. 3**). Lining cells that are apparently dormant osteoblasts participating in the calcium exchange between the mineralized matrix and the bone marrow compartment can be reactivated within a few hours in response to PTH to contribute to local bone formation processes.[66] Osteoblast lineage cells control the differentiation of osteoclasts through their production of receptor activator of NF-KB ligand (RANKL), osteoprotegerin (OPG), and macrophage colony-stimulating factor. The RANK-RANKL interaction enhances the differentiation and activation of osteoclasts[27] leading to bone resorption.[27,28] Bone resorption releases substances that in turn enhance osteoblast activity and, thus, couple the formation and resorption of bone. The main factor in controlling osteoclast activation and bone resorption is the ratio between OPG and RANKL levels.[28,67,68]

Elevated Ca2+ concentrations inhibit resorption and enhance bone formation. The effect is mediated through CaSR in osteoblasts and osteoclasts (see **Fig. 1**). CaSR participates in the defense against hypercalcemia and regulation of bone cell maturation.[69–71] In addition, PTH acts on bone to increase FGF23 expression and thus completes a bone-parathyroid endocrine feedback loop.[72]

Role of the Kidney

The kidney is a central regulator of calcium homeostasis through several calcium reabsorption mechanisms. As described previously, 10 g of calcium is filtered daily to the primary urine solute, but ultimately, only about 100 to 300 mg of urinary calcium losses occur (see **Fig. 2**). Renal calcium reabsorption occurs via paracellular and transcellular pathways similar to the reabsorption in the intestine. Most filtered calcium is reabsorbed in the proximal tubule (about 60%–70%) and in the TAL (about 15%–20%) mainly by paracellular transport. In the proximal tubule calcium, sodium and water reabsorption occurs down the electrochemical gradient or through solvent drag. This way is influenced by sodium, chloride, bicarbonate, and potassium availability.

As illustrated in **Fig. 5**, the reabsorption of calcium in the TAL is mediated by claudins 14, 16, and 19 by altering the permeability of the tight junction.[73] Claudins 16 and 19 form a cation-permeable pore in the tight junctions, whereas claudin 14 normally binds to and inhibits claudins 16 and 19 leading to decreased reabsorption of cations such as calcium.

CaSR, expressed at the basolateral membrane of the TAL, modulates this claudin network. Inhibition of the CaSR increases the permeability to calcium of the paracellular pathway.[74] Increased blood calcium stimulates the CaSR, and finally claudin 14 protein expression is inhibited, and paracellular calcium reabsorption diminishes. The details of this transport are reviewed elsewhere.[75]

About 10% to 15% of filtered calcium reabsorption occurs in the distal nephron. Transport is active transcellular against chemical and electrical gradients. Calcium enters tubular cells via TRPV5 channels, binds to calbindin-D_{28k} protein inside the cell, and finally extrudes into the blood through the NCX1 (3Na/Ca exchanger) and plasma membrane Ca2+-ATPase 1b channels.[76] 1,25(OH)$_2$D, downstream of PTH, increases active calcium reabsorption via transcriptional regulation.[44,60] PTH, independent of 1,25(OH)$_2$D, increases transcription of TRPV5, Calbindin-D28k, and NCX and directly increases the probability of opening of the TRPV5 channel, thus increasing calcium reabsorption.[25,77]

SUMMARY

The maintenance of stable plasma Ca2+ concentrations requires timely alterations of calcium transport across renal or intestinal epithelia, bone resorption, or concerted action of these all. There is, however, a limit to the efficiency of these defense mechanisms. Although ECF calcium concentrations may remain normal, the extended consequences of stressed homeostatic mechanisms are harmful to the cardiovascular system, kidney function, and bones in the long run. Hypercalcemia or hypocalcemia may still occur regardless of maximal activation of these mechanisms, or due to failure of one or more of its elements, and indicate major disturbances of calcium homeostasis but do not, however, reveal the status of body calcium stores on their own.[20,78]

CLINICS CARE POINTS

- A healthy adult body contains around 1 kg of calcium, 99% of which is deposited in bone and teeth, while only 1% of the total body calcium is found in blood, extracellular fluid, and soft tissues.

- Calcium contributes to numerous reactions in our cells and is only available to the body through dietary sources. Calcium requirements are especially high during growth, pregnancy, and lactation.

- Calcium concentration is maintained within narrow limits and tightly regulated.

- Hypercalcemia or hypocalcemia only occur when maximal adaptive mechanisms fail to maintain stable calcium concentrations.

DISCLOSURE

The authors have nothing to disclose.

REFERENCES

1. Walser M. Ion association. VI. interactions between calcium, magnesium, inorganic phosphate, citrate and protein in normal human plasma. J Clin Invest 1961;40:723–30.
2. McLean FC, Hastings AB. The state of calcium in the fluids of the body. J Biol Chem 1934;105:285–322.
3. Robertson WG, Marshall RW, Walser M. Calcium measurements in serum and plasma—total and ionized. CRC Crit Rev Clin Lab Sci 1979;11(3):271–304.

4. Payne RB, Little AJ, Williams RB, et al. Interpretation of serum calcium in patients with abnormal serum proteins. Br Med J 1973;4(5893):643–6.
5. Bringhurst FR, Demay MB, Kronenberg HM. Hormones and disorders of mineral metabolism. In: Melmed S, Polonsky KS, Larsen PR, et al, editors. Williams Textbook of Endocrinology. 13th edition. Philadelphia: Elsevier; 2020. p. 1254-322.
6. Murshed M, Harmey D, Millan JL, et al. Unique coexpression in osteoblasts of broadly expressed genes accounts for the spatial restriction of ECM mineralization to bone. Genes Dev 2005;19(9):1093–104.
7. Evrard S, Delanaye P, Kamel S, et al. Vascular calcification: From pathophysiology to biomarkers. Clinica Chim Acta 2015;438:401–14.
8. Gao H, Ji B, JÃ¤ger IL, et al. Materials become insensitive to flaws at nanoscale: Lessons from nature. Proc Natl Acad Sci U S A 2003;100(10):5597–600.
9. Berridge MJ, Bootman MD, Roderick HL. Calcium signalling: Dynamics, homeostasis and remodelling. Nat Rev Mol Cel Biol 2003;4(7):517–29.
10. Wills M. The effect of diurnal variation on total plasma calcium concentration in normal subjects. J Clin Pathol 1970;23(9):772–7.
11. Ridefelt P, Axelsson J, Larsson A. Diurnal variability of total calcium during normal sleep and after an acute shift of sleep. Clin Chem Lab Med 2012;50(1):147–51.
12. Brown EM, Gamba G, Riccardi D, et al. Cloning and characterization of an extracellular Ca2 -sensing receptor from bovine parathyroid. Nature 1993;366(6455):575–80.
13. Brown EM. Clinical lessons from the calcium-sensing receptor. Nat Clin Pract Endocrinol Metab 2007;3(2):122–33.
14. Ross AC, Manson JE, Abrams SA, et al. The 2011 report on dietary reference intakes for calcium and vitamin D from the institute of medicine: What clinicians need to know. J Clin Endocrinol Metab 2011;96(1):53–8.
15. Institute of Medicine (US) Committee to Review Dietary Reference Intakes for Vitamin D and Calcium; Ross AC, Taylor CL, Yaktine AL, et al, editors. Dietary Reference Intakes for Calcium and Vitamin D. Washington (DC): National Academies Press (US); 2011. Available at: https://www.ncbi.nlm.nih.gov/books/NBK56070/doi:10.17226/13050.
16. European Food Safety Authority. Dietary reference values for nutrients summary report. EFSA Supporting Publications 2017;14(12):e15121E.
17. Harvey NC, Biver E, Kaufman J, et al. The role of calcium supplementation in healthy musculoskeletal ageing. Osteoporos Int 2017;28(2):447–62.
18. Nordin B, Peacock M. Role of kidney in regulation of plasma-calcium. Lancet 1969;2:1280–3.
19. McCabe L, Britton RA, Parameswaran N. Prebiotic and probiotic regulation of bone health: Role of the intestine and its microbiome. Curr Osteoporos Rep 2015;13(6):363–71.
20. Brown EM. Role of the calcium-sensing receptor in extracellular calcium homeostasis. Best Pract Res Clin Endocrinol Metab 2013;27(3):333–43.
21. Shoback DM, Membreno LA, McGhee JG. High calcium and other divalent cations increase inositol trisphosphate in bovine parathyroid cells. Endocrinology 1988;123(1):382–9.
22. Hannan FM, Kallay E, Chang W, et al. The calcium-sensing receptor in physiology and in calcitropic and noncalcitropic diseases. Nat Rev Endocrinol 2019;15(1):33–51.
23. Endres DB, Villanueva R, Sharp CF Jr, et al. Measurement of parathyroid hormone. Endocrinol Metab Clin North Am 1989;18(3):611–30.

24. Juppner H, Abou-Samra AB, Freeman M, et al. A G protein-linked receptor for parathyroid hormone and parathyroid hormone-related peptide. Science 1991; 254(5034):1024–6.

25. Van Abel M, Hoenderop JG, van der Kemp, et al. Coordinated control of renal Ca2 transport proteins by parathyroid hormone. Kidney Int 2005;68(4):1708–21.

26. Brenza HL, Kimmel-Jehan C, Jehan F, et al. Parathyroid hormone activation of the 25-hydroxyvitamin D3-1alpha-hydroxylase gene promoter. Proc Natl Acad Sci U S A 1998;95(4):1387–91.

27. Lee S, Lorenzo JA. Parathyroid hormone stimulates TRANCE and inhibits osteoprotegerin messenger ribonucleic acid expression in murine bone marrow cultures: Correlation with osteoclast-like cell formation. Endocrinology 1999;140(8): 3552–61.

28. Huang JC, Sakata T, Pfleger LL, et al. PTH differentially regulates expression of RANKL and OPG. J Bone Miner Res 2004;19(2):235–44.

29. Bellido T, Ali A, Gubrij I, et al. Chronic elevation of parathyroid hormone in mice reduces expression of sclerostin by osteocytes: A novel mechanism for hormonal control of osteoblastogenesis. Endocrinology 2005;146(11):4577–83.

30. Silva BC, Bilezikian JP. Parathyroid hormone: Anabolic and catabolic actions on the skeleton. Curr Opin Pharmacol 2015;22:41–50.

31. Suva LJ, Winslow GA, Wettenhall RE, et al. A parathyroid hormone-related protein implicated in malignant hypercalcemia: Cloning and expression. Science 1987; 237(4817):893–6.

32. Kovacs CS. Bone development and mineral homeostasis in the fetus and neonate: Roles of the calciotropic and phosphotropic hormones. Physiol Rev 2014;94(4):1143–218.

33. McCauley LK, Martin TJ. Twenty-five years of PTHrP progress: From cancer hormone to multifunctional cytokine. J Bone Miner Res 2012;27(6):1231–9.

34. Chung UI, Lanske B, Lee K, et al. The parathyroid hormone/parathyroid hormone-related peptide receptor coordinates endochondral bone development by directly controlling chondrocyte differentiation. Proc Natl Acad Sci U S A 1998; 95(22):13030–5.

35. Holick MF, MacLaughlin JA, Clark MB, et al. Photosynthesis of previtamin D3 in human skin and the physiologic consequences. Science 1980;210(4466):203–5.

36. Holick MF. Vitamin D deficiency. N Engl J Med 2007;357(3):266–81.

37. Haussler MR, Jurutka PW, Mizwicki M, et al. Vitamin D receptor (VDR)-mediated actions of 1α, 25 (OH) 2vitamin D3: Genomic and non-genomic mechanisms. Best Pract Res Clin Endocrinol Metab 2011;25(4):543–59.

38. Bouillon R, Marcocci C, Carmeliet G, et al. Skeletal and extraskeletal actions of vitamin D: Current evidence and outstanding questions. Endocr Rev 2019; 40(4):1109–51.

39. Shimada T, Kakitani M, Yamazaki Y, et al. Targeted ablation of Fgf23 demonstrates an essential physiological role of FGF23 in phosphate and vitamin D metabolism. J Clin Invest 2004;113(4):561–8.

40. Shimada T, Mizutani S, Muto T, et al. Cloning and characterization of FGF23 as a causative factor of tumor-induced osteomalacia. Proc Natl Acad Sci U S A 2001; 98(11):6500–5.

41. Goetz R, Beenken A, Ibrahimi OA, et al. Molecular insights into the klotho-dependent, endocrine mode of action of fibroblast growth factor 19 subfamily members. Mol Cell Biol 2007;27(9):3417–28.

42. Copp DH, Cheney B. Calcitonin—a hormone from the parathyroid which lowers the calcium-level of the blood. Nature 1962;193(4813):381–2.

43. Hebert SC. Extracellular calcium-sensing receptor: Implications for calcium and magnesium handling in the kidney. Kidney Int 1996;50(6):2129–39.

44. Dimke H, Hoenderop JG, Bindels RJ. Molecular basis of epithelial Ca2 and Mg2 transport: Insights from the TRP channel family. J Physiol (Lond) 2011;589(7): 1535–42.

45. Cheng I, Qureshi I, Chattopadhyay N, et al. Expression of an extracellular calcium-sensing receptor in rat stomach. Gastroenterology 1999;116(1):118–26.

46. Geibel J, Sritharan K, Geibel R, et al. Calcium-sensing receptor abrogates secretagogue- induced increases in intestinal net fluid secretion by enhancing cyclic nucleotide destruction. Proc Natl Acad Sci U S A 2006;103(25):9390–7.

47. Fermor B, Skerry TM. PTH/PTHrP receptor expression on osteoblasts and osteocytes but not resorbing bone surfaces in growing rats. J Bone Miner Res 1995; 10(12):1935–43.

48. Brumbaugh PF, Haussler MR. 1 alpha,25-dihydroxycholecalciferol receptors in intestine. I. association of 1 alpha,25-dihydroxycholecalciferol with intestinal mucosa chromatin. J Biol Chem 1974;249(4):1251–7.

49. Giustina A, Adler RA, Binkley N, et al. Controversies in vitamin D: Summary statement from an international conference. J Clin Endocrinol Metab 2019;104(2): 234–40.

50. Johnson JA, Kumar R. Renal and intestinal calcium transport: Roles of vitamin D and vitamin D-dependent calcium binding proteins. Semin Nephrol 1994;14(2): 119–28.

51. Winter EM, Ireland A, Butterfield NC, et al. Pregnancy and lactation, a challenge for the skeleton. Endocr Connections 2020;9(6):R143–57.

52. Matkovic V, Heaney RP. Calcium balance during human growth: Evidence for threshold behavior. Am J Clin Nutr 1992;55(5):992–6.

53. Jackman LA, Millane SS, Martin BR, et al. Calcium retention in relation to calcium intake and postmenarcheal age in adolescent females. Am J Clin Nutr 1997; 66(2):327–33.

54. Wastney M, Martin B, Peacock M, et al. Changes in calcium kinetics in adolescent girls induced by high calcium intake. J Clin Endocrinol Metab 2000; 85(12):4470–5.

55. Bronner F, Pansu D, Stein WD. An analysis of intestinal calcium transport across the rat intestine. Am J Physiol 1986;250(5 Pt 1):G561–9.

56. Fujita H, Sugimoto K, Inatomi S, et al. Tight junction proteins claudin-2 and-12 are critical for vitamin D-dependent Ca2 absorption between enterocytes. Mol Biol Cell 2008;19(5):1912–21.

57. Sheikh MS, Ramirez A, Emmett M, et al. Role of vitamin D-dependent and vitamin D-independent mechanisms in absorption of food calcium. J Clin Invest 1988; 81(1):126–32.

58. McCormick CC. Passive diffusion does not play a major role in the absorption of dietary calcium in normal adults. J Nutr 2002;132(11):3428–30.

59. Christakos S, Li S, De La Cruz J, et al. Vitamin D and the intestine: Review and update. J Steroid Biochem Mol Biol 2020;196:105501.

60. Hoenderop JG, Nilius B, Bindels RJ. Calcium absorption across epithelia. Physiol Rev 2005;85(1):373–422.

61. Lieben L, Benn B, Ajibade D, et al. Trpv6 mediates intestinal calcium absorption during calcium restriction and contributes to bone homeostasis. Bone 2010; 47(2):301–8.

62. Kutuzova GD, DeLuca HF. Gene expression profiles in rat intestine identify pathways for 1, 25-dihydroxyvitamin D3 stimulated calcium absorption and clarify its immunomodulatory properties. Arch Biochem Biophys 2004;432(2):152–66.

63. Ecarot-Charrier B, Glorieux FH, van der Rest M, et al. Osteoblasts isolated from mouse calvaria initiate matrix mineralization in culture. J Cell Biol 1983;96(3): 639–43.

64. Vrahnas C, Sims NA. Basic aspects of osteoblast function. In: Leder BZ, Wein MN, editors. Osteoporosis: Pathophysiology and Clinical Management. Cham, Switzerland: Springer Nature Switzerland AG; 2020. p. 1–16.

65. David V, Dai B, Martin A, et al. Calcium regulates FGF-23 expression in bone. Endocrinology 2013;154(12):4469–82.

66. Dobnig H, Turner RT. Evidence that intermittent treatment with parathyroid hormone increases bone formation in adult rats by activation of bone lining cells. Endocrinology 1995;136(8):3632–8.

67. Simonet W, Lacey D, Dunstan C, et al. Osteoprotegerin: A novel secreted protein involved in the regulation of bone density. Cell 1997;89(2):309–19.

68. Anderson DM, Maraskovsky E, Billingsley WL, et al. A homologue of the TNF receptor and its ligand enhance T-cell growth and dendritic-cell function. Nature 1997;390(6656):175–9.

69. Kameda T, Mano H, Yamada Y, et al. Calcium-sensing receptor in mature osteoclasts, which are bone resorbing cells. Biochem Biophys Res Commun 1998; 245(2):419–22.

70. Yamaguchi T, Chattopadhyay N, Kifor O, et al. Extracellular calcium (Ca2 o)-sensing receptor in a murine bone marrow-derived stromal cell line (ST2): Potential mediator of the actions of Ca2 o on the function of ST2 cells. Endocrinology 1998;139(8):3561–8.

71. Yamaguchi T, Chattopadhyay N, Kifor O, et al. Expression of extracellular calcium-sensing receptor in human osteoblastic MG-63 cell line. Am J Physiol Cell Physiol 2001;280(2):C382–93.

72. Lavi-Moshayoff V, Wasserman G, Meir T, et al. PTH increases FGF23 gene expression and mediates the high-FGF23 levels of experimental kidney failure: A bone parathyroid feedback loop. Am J Physiol Renal Physiol 2010;299(4): F882–9.

73. Yu AS. Claudins and the kidney. J Am Soc Nephrol 2015;26(1):11–9.

74. Loupy A, Ramakrishnan SK, Wootla B, et al. PTH-independent regulation of blood calcium concentration by the calcium-sensing receptor. J Clin Invest 2012; 122(9):3355–67.

75. Moor MB, Bonny O. Ways of calcium reabsorption in the kidney. Am J Physiol Renal Physiol 2016;310(11):F1337–50.

76. Lambers T, Bindels R, Hoenderop J. Coordinated control of renal Ca2 handling. Kidney Int 2006;69(4):650–4.

77. Kopic S, Geibel JP. Gastric acid, calcium absorption, and their impact on bone health. Physiol Rev 2013;93(1):189–268.

78. Peacock M. Calcium metabolism in health and disease. Clin J Am Soc Nephrol 2010;5(Suppl 1):S23–30.

Pathophysiology of Hypercalcemia

David Goltzman, MD

KEYWORDS

- Hypercalcemia • Parathyroid hormone • Parathyroid hormone-related protein
- Vitamin D

KEY POINTS

- Parathyroid hormone (PTH) is a key regulator of normal calcium homeostasis; its dysregulation can occur sporadically or as a familial, hereditary abnormality.
- Parathyroid hormone-related protein (PTHrP) is a genetic relative of PTH; the 2 proteins use common molecular pathways via a shared G protein-coupled receptor.
- PTHrP may be produced in excess by malignancies before and after metastasizing to the skeleton.
- Extrarenal production of excess 1,25-dihydroxyvitamin D can produce absorptive and resorptive hypercalcemia.

INTRODUCTION AND PHYSIOLOGIC REGULATION OF EXTRACELLULAR CALCIUM

Circulating calcium is transported partly bound to plasma protein, notably albumin (about 45%); partly complexed with anions such as phosphate, bicarbonate, and citrate (about 10%); and partly in the free or ionized state (about 45%). Hypercalcemia can be defined as serum calcium greater than 2 SDs more than the normal mean in a reference laboratory. The ionized calcium (Ca^{++}) is the biologically active moiety that can cross plasma membranes and enter into cells to activate cellular processes. Because of its critical importance in several physiologic processes, Ca^{++} is maintained within a tight range by the action of several hormones, including parathyroid hormone (PTH), the active form of vitamin D [calcitriol or $1,25(OH)_2D$], fibroblast growth factor 23 (FGF23), as well as by Ca^{++} itself.[1]

PTH can enhance renal Ca^{++} reabsorption by augmenting basolateral Na^+/Ca^{++} (NCX1) exchanger activity in the distal convoluted tubule (DCT), thus increasing extrusion of Ca^{++} from the cell into the blood, and by increasing the Na-K-2Cl cotransporter (SLC12A1) activity in the cortical thick ascending limb (TAL) of the loop of

Calcium Research Laboratory, Department of Medicine and Physiology, McGill University, Research Institute of the McGill University Health Centre, Glen Site, 1001 Decarie Boulevard, Room EM1.3220, Montreal, Quebec H4A 3J1, Canada
E-mail address: david.goltzman@mcgill.ca

Endocrinol Metab Clin N Am 50 (2021) 591–607
https://doi.org/10.1016/j.ecl.2021.07.008

Henle, thus stimulating paracellular Ca^{++} and magnesium reabsorption.[2] PTH can also act on the proximal renal tubule to stimulate transcription of the enzyme CYP27B1 (25-hydroxyvitamin D-1α-hydroxylase or 1(OH)ase) and thus increase conversion of the inactive precursor of vitamin D, 25-hydroxyvitamin D [25(OH)D], to active 1,25(OH)$_2$D.[3] 1,25(OH)$_2$D can enhance intestinal absorption by stimulating both active and passive intestinal Ca^{++} transport.[4] Both PTH[5] and 1,25(OH)$_2$D,[6] when present in high and relatively sustained circulating concentrations, can increase bone turnover, leading to osteoclast-mediated bone resorption, and release of Ca^{++} into the circulation (**Fig. 1**).

The principal regulator of PTH release from the parathyroid cell is Ca^{++} itself, acting via a G protein-coupled receptor (GPCR), the calcium-sensing receptor (CaSR)[7] (**Fig. 2**). When Ca^{++} binds to the extracellular domain of CaSR, it induces homodimerization and a conformational change in the intracellular domain, resulting in second messenger signaling. Thus CaSR activation by elevated Ca^{++} leads to activation of Gqα11[8] and downstream signaling via the inositol triphosphate pathway and the adaptor-protein 2 sigma (AP2s) subunit that, with other subunits, plays a central role in clathrin-mediated endocytosis of plasma membrane constituents, such as GPCRs.[9] Ca^{++} signaling via CaSR can then reduce PTH production by inhibiting PTH biosynthesis and enhancing intracellular PTH degradation, and can inhibit

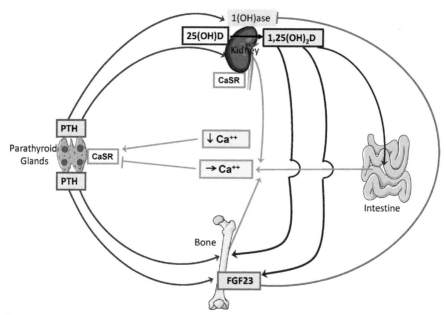

Fig. 1. Hormonal regulation of Ca^{++} homeostasis. A decrease ($\downarrow$) in ionized Ca (Ca^{++}) reduces inhibition of PTH release by calcium-sensing receptor (CaSR) facilitating increased PTH secretion. Increased circulating PTH can augment Ca^{++} reabsorption from the kidney. In addition, with decreased Ca^{++}, CaSR is not activated to cause calciuria. PTH can also stimulate the renal 1(OH)ase enzyme to increase conversion of 25(OH)D to 1,25(OH)2D. The 1,25(OH)$_2$D produced can increase intestinal absorption of Ca^{++}. PTH and 1,25(OH)$_2$D can increase bone resorption and mobilize Ca^{++} release from bone. The overall result is normalization ($\rightarrow$) of Ca^{++} and inhibition ( ) of further PTH release. 1,25(OH)$_2$D can also stimulate FGF23 release from bone, which in turn can inhibit further renal 1,25(OH)$_2$D production from 25(OH)D. PTH may also stimulate FGF23 release.

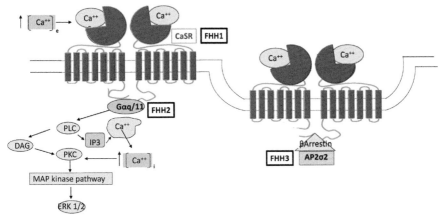

Fig. 2. Model of the action of CaSR and of genetic alterations resulting in FHH1, FHH2, and FHH3. In the presence of increased extracellular calcium ($[Ca^{++}]_e$), CaSR homodimerizes, and via Gq/11 action, increases phospholipase C (PLC) activity; this results in increased inositol triphosphate (IP3), which can mobilize intracellular calcium ($[Ca^{++}]i$) from cell organelles. In addition, diacylglycerol (DAG) produced activates phosphokinase C (PKC), which can activate the mitogen-activated protein (MAP) kinase pathway and extracellular signal-regulated kinase (ERK). FHH1 is due to loss-of-function mutations in CaSR, FHH2 is due to loss-of-function mutations in the Gα protein subunit q11 (Gαq/11), and FHH3 is due to loss-of-function mutations of the adaptor-related protein complex 2, sigma 2 subunit (AP2σ2), which, with β arrestin, plays a central role in clathrin-mediated endocytosis of plasma membrane constituents such as GPCRs.

bioactive PTH secretion. Elevated Ca^{++} may also inhibit parathyroid cell proliferation. CaSR is also located in the basolateral membrane of the TAL, and its activation leads to suppression of the Na-K-2Cl symporter, resulting in decreased sodium and Ca^{++} reabsorption.[10] Elevated Ca^{++} may therefore increase calciuria partly via its action to reduce PTH secretion and partly via a direct action on the kidney.

An important regulator of the calcium-regulating hormones as well as of phosphate homeostasis is the hormone FGF23. FGF23 is an important phosphaturic factor that inhibits luminal phosphate transport in the proximal renal tubule by reducing sodium/phosphate transporter (Npt2a and Npt2c) activity (analogous to the action of PTH), thus promoting phosphaturia and hypophosphatemia. Elevated $1,25(OH)_2D$,[11] as well as an increased serum calcium/phosphate ratio,[12] can enhance FGF23 release from osteocytes in bone, whereas FGF23 can inhibit $1,25(OH)_2D$ production in the proximal renal tubule. FGF23 has also been reported to inhibit PTH release (see **Fig. 1**).

Hypercalcemia occurs when these calcium homeostatic processes fail; this may occur due to inappropriately increased PTH production and secretion from the parathyroid glands; malignancy with increased PTHrP, PTH, $1,25(OH)_2D$, or other mediators; or due to vitamin D-mediated hypercalcemia in the absence of neoplasia. Less commonly, hypercalcemia may result from excess actions of PTH and/or PTH-related protein (PTHrP) in the absence of increased circulating PTH/PTHrP, from other endocrine abnormalities such as thyrotoxicosis, from ion abnormalities such as aluminum intoxication, or from certain medication or vitamins such as vitamin A (**Box 1**).

Box 1
Classification of causes of hypercalcemia

1. Inappropriately increased PTH production
   a. Sporadic PHPT
   b. PHPT associated with lithium
   c. PHPT associated with thiazides
   d. Tertiary hyperparathyroidism
      i. Following chronic secondary hyperparathyroidism
      ii. Following renal transplantation
   e. Familial PHPT
      i. MEN syndromes
         1. MEN1
         2. MEN2 (MEN2A)
         3. MEN4
      ii. HPT-JT syndrome
      iii. FIHP
      iv. FHH
         1. FHH1
         2. FHH2
         3. FHH3

2. Excess PTH/PTHrP actions in the absence of increased circulating PTH/PTHrP

3. Malignancy and hypercalcemia
   a. Excess circulating PTHrP in the absence of skeletal metastases
   b. Local osteolytic hypercalcemia with skeletal metastases
   c. Ectopic PTH secretion
   d. Excess production of extrarenal 1,25-dihydroxyvitamin D [1,25(OH)2D] in malignancy

4. Vitamin D-mediated hypercalcemia in the absence of neoplasia
   a. Extrarenal 1,25-dihydroxyvitamin D production
   b. Calcidiol or vitamin D intoxication
   c. Poorly monitored therapy with alfacalcidol or calcitriol
   d. Reduced 1,25(OH)2D metabolism: IIH

5. Other endocrine abnormalities
   a. Thyrotoxicosis
   b. Hypoadrenalism

6. Ion abnormalities
   a. Milk-alkali syndrome
   b. Aluminum intoxication

7. Other medication and vitamins
   a. Aminophylline/theophylline
   b. Vitamin A

8. Immobilization

Abbreviations: FHH, familial hypocalciuric hypercalcemia; FIHP, familial isolated hyperparathyroidism; HPT-JT, hyperparathyroidism-jaw tumor; IIH, idiopathic infantile hypercalcemia; MEN, multiple endocrine neoplasia; PHPT, primary hyperparathyroidism.

PATHOPHYSIOLOGY OF HYPERCALCEMIA IN CLINICAL DISORDERS
Alterations of Parathyroid Hormome Production

Hyperparathyroidism (HPT) results from dysregulation of PTH production and secretion, by one or more parathyroid glands.

Sporadic primary hyperparathyroidism
Sporadic primary hyperparathyroidism (PHPT) is the most common cause of hypercalcemia. Most patients with PHPT have single parathyroid adenomas (80%) or multiple

hyperplastic glands (15% to 20%), although multiglandular disease may also be due to 2 or, rarely, 3 adenomas. Parathyroid carcinoma is a rare event.[13] In parathyroid carcinomas, genomic alterations have been identified, consisting mainly of loss-of-function mutations in the *CDC73* gene, encoding the protein parafibromin. Whole-exome sequencing has, however, identified mutations in other genes, including *mTOR, KMT2D, CDKN2C, THRAP3, PIK3CA,* and *EZH2,* and amplification of the *CCND1* gene.[14]

In PHPT, typically, the PTH level is frankly elevated, but it can also be within the normal range. Symptomatic PHPT can be due to severe (>12 mg/dL) or rapid-onset hypercalcemia, or due to skeletal, renal, or gastrointestinal manifestations. Thus skeletal manifestations, due to the action of PTH to increase bone turnover and to accelerate osteoclastic resorption relative to formation, has classically included osteitis fibrosa cystica[15] but more recently is characterized by fragility fractures, skeletal deformities, and bone pain or only low bone mass or osteoporosis.[16] Renal manifestations may occur when the filtered load of calcium (due to increased bone resorption and increased gut absorption of calcium) exceeds the capacity of elevated PTH to enhance renal calcium reabsorption and the elevated circulating Ca^{++} enhances calciuria due to stimulation of renal CaSR; this may be characterized by hypercalciuria, nephrolithiasis, nephrocalcinosis,[17] and/or reduced renal function. Normocalcemic PHPT may manifest only inappropriately elevated PTH and may be symptomatic or asymptomatic. In fact, with widespread biochemical screening for serum calcium and PTH, asymptomatic PHPT has become the main clinical presentation.[18]

Lithium intoxication

Lithium (Li) may initially induce acute and potentially reversible hypercalcemia as a result of its action on the CaSR pathway, giving rise to a biochemical picture similar to that seen in familial hypocalciuric hypercalcemia (FHH). Chronic Li therapy may unmask PHPT in patients with a subclinical parathyroid adenoma, or possibly may initiate multiglandular HPT.[19]

Thiazides

Sustained hypercalcemia in association with intake of thiazide diuretics may occur due to inhibition of the Na/Ca exchanger in the renal tubule and may unmask underlying PHPT; the hypercalcemia may or may not be reversed when the diuretic is stopped.[20]

Tertiary hyperparathyroidism

1. Tertiary HPT (THPT) can occur following long-standing secondary HPT when advancement to an autonomous state of parathyroid function occurs leading to uncontrolled PTH release despite hypercalcemia. This condition may typically occur in chronic kidney disease (CKD) or in phosphate treatment of hypophosphatemic rickets/osteomalacia.[21]
2. After renal transplantation for end-stage CKD, preexisting parathyroid gland hyperplasia associated with pretransplant CKD may persist for months to years. This persistent HPT, in the presence of normalized renal $1,25(OH)_2D$ production and normalized phosphate balance, may lead to transient or prolonged hypercalcemia and a state of THPT.[22] .

Familial primary hyperparathryoidism

In approximately 10% of patients, the possibility of a genetic basis for PHPT is suggested by occurrence before 45 years of age, a family history of PHPT, and/or the presence of a multigland endocrine syndrome.[23] Genetic disorders producing PHPT include the following.

Multiple endocrine neoplasia syndromes. Multiple endocrine neoplasia (MEN) syndromes associated with PHPT are autosomal dominant disorders, each characterized by the occurrence of specific tumors.

MEN type 1 (MEN1) is caused by germline heterozygous inactivating mutations of the *MEN1* gene encoding menin, a tumor suppressor, and is associated with parathyroid, gastroenteropancreatic, and anterior pituitary gland tumors; less commonly with tumors of the adrenal cortical gland, thymus, and bronchi; and, in some patients, with other nonendocrine tumors.[24]

MEN type 2A (MEN2A) is caused by germline missense mutations of the rearranged during transfection (*RET*) proto-oncogene. These alter the conserved cysteine codons adjacent to the transmembrane domain of the encoded tyrosine kinase receptor RET. MEN2 is associated with parathyroid tumors, medullary thyroid carcinoma, and pheochromocytoma.

MEN type 4 (MEN4) is caused by heterozygous inactivating mutations of cyclin-dependent kinase inhibitor 1B (*CDNK1B*) encoding p27Kip1 that acts as a negative regulator of cell cycle progression[24] and is associated with parathyroid and anterior pituitary tumors, in possible association with tumors of the adrenals, kidneys, and reproductive organs.

Hyperparathyroidism-jaw tumor syndrome. Hyperparathyroidism-jaw tumor (HPT-JT) syndrome is caused by mutations in the cell division cycle 73 (*CDC73/HRPT2*) gene, which encodes parafibromin, a tumor suppressor gene, and is characterized by the occurrence of PHPT and ossifying fibroma of the maxilla and/or mandible, associated with an increased risk of parathyroid carcinoma.[25] Occurrence of renal cysts or tumors, multiple uterine polyps, and thyroid tumors has also been reported.

Familial isolated hyperparathyroidism. Familial isolated hyperparathyroidism (FIHP) is an autosomal disorder characterized by PHPT due to single or multiple parathyroid tumors in at least 2 first-degree relatives in the absence of evidence of other endocrine disorders or tumors. Unique activating mutations of glial cells missing 2 (GCM2), a parathyroid-specific transcription factor, have been reported in about 20% of these patients[26]; incomplete expression of MEN1, FHH, and HPT-JT genes can also lead to the FIHP phenotype (**Fig. 3**).

Familial hypocalciuric hypercalcemia. Genetic disorders of calcium metabolism in which the set point for serum calcium concentration is elevated include the heterozygous disorder FHH and its homozygous counterpart neonatal severe hyperparathyroidism (NSHPT). FHH is an autosomal dominant, genetically heterogeneous disorder usually due to an inactivating mutation of the CaSR gene leading to lifelong and usually asymptomatic elevation of serum Ca^{++} with normal or slightly elevated PTH levels and decreased urinary calcium excretion. In FHH, the 24-hour urinary calcium excretion is generally very low (<100 mg) and the calcium clearance/creatinine clearance ratio is <0.01 Because of the calcium-conserving action of PTH on the kidney, however, low urinary calcium excretion may also occur in sporadic PHPT, especially in patients whose vitamin D status or dietary calcium intake is low.[27,28]

There are 3 clinically indistinguishable variants of FHH (FHH1 to FHH3) due to loss-of-function mutations of *CaSR* or of downstream intracellular signaling mediators (see **Fig. 3**). FHH1 comprises about 65% of patients with FHH and is due to loss-of-function mutations of *CaSR* per se. NSHPT is an autosomal recessive disorder caused

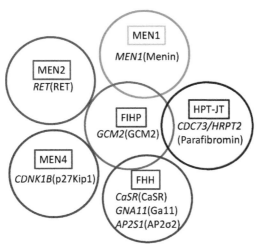

Fig. 3. Venn diagram of familial forms of hyperparathyroidism. Mutations in the *MEN1* gene encoding menin occur in MEN1 syndrome, mutations in the Ret gene that encodes the Ret proto-oncogene occur in the MEN2A syndrome, and mutations in *CDNK1B* encoding p27Kip1 occur in the MEN4 syndrome. In HPT-JT, mutations in *CDC73/HRPT2* encoding parafibromin occur, and in FHH 1, 2, and 3, respective mutations are in *CaSR* encoding CaSR, in *GNA11* encoding Ga11, and in *AP2S1* encoding AP2σ2. In FIHP, some patients have been found to have mutations in GCM2. Some FIHP overlap occurs with MEN1, HPT-JT, and FHH where genes causing, MEN1, HPT-JT, and FHH have been found in patients lacking syndromal features of these entities and seem to represent incomplete expression of MEN1, HPT-JT, and FHH.

by a homozygous inactivating mutation in the *CaSR* gene.[29] FHH2 comprises less than 5% of all patients with FHH and is due to loss-of-function mutations of *GNA11*, which encodes G-protein subunit α-11 (Ga11).[8] FHH3 may occur in about 20% of patients with FHH without CaSR mutations[10] and is due to loss-of-function mutations of the *AP2S1* gene encoding adaptor-related protein complex 2, sigma 2 subunit (AP2σ2).[30]

Identification of mutated genes in PHPT has diagnostic, prognostic, and therapeutic implications for clinical patient management and may also shed light on the molecular mechanisms giving rise to nonhereditary PHPT.

Excess Actions of Parathyroid Hormone/Parathyroid Hormone-Related Protein in the Absence of Increased Circulating Parathyroid Hormone/Parathyroid Hormone-Related Protein

Jansen syndrome (excess PTH1R activation)
Jansen metaphyseal chondrodysplasia is an autosomal dominant disease associated with heterozygous mutations of PTH1R, the common GPCR for PTH and PTHrP (**Fig. 4**), causing constitutive ligand-independent activation.[31] Circulating PTH and PTHrP concentrations are normal or undetectable. PTHrP is a genetic relative of PTH, and as a result of sequence homology in the amino-terminal domains of the 2 proteins they both interact at PTH1R and can carry out similar actions in modulating ion homeostasis.[32] In contrast to PTH, whose expression is limited mainly to parathyroid cells, PTHrP is widely expressed in many fetal and adult tissues.[33] In addition to mimicking many effects of PTH on calcium homeostasis, the physiologic effects of PTHrP can be considered as those relating to smooth muscle relaxation[34] and those

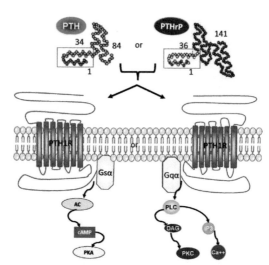

Fig. 4. PTH and PTHrP bind to and signal via a common G-protein-coupled receptor, PTH1R. The amino-terminal domains of PTH and PTHrP, designated as 1 to 34 and 1 to 36, can bind to PTH1R, which then can activate adenylyl cyclase (AC) via the G protein alpha subunit, Gsα, and generate cyclic AMP, which then stimulates protein kinase A (PKA). Alternatively, bound PTH1R can activate PLC via Gqα, which can generate DAG and IP3. DAG can activate PKC, and IP3 can activate intracellular Ca^{++} as subsequent intracellular messengers.

associated with cell growth, differentiation, and apoptosis in several tissues.[35] PTHrP regulates chondrocyte differentiation and is critical for normal endochondral bone formation[36]; it also functions in other tissues including the placenta, lactating breast, vascular smooth muscle, skin, hair follicles, hematopoiesis, teeth, and brain. Most of the physiologic effects of PTHrP seem to occur by short-range, that is, paracrine/autocrine and intracrine, mechanisms rather than long-range, that is, endocrine, mechanisms used by PTH. In addition to severe hypercalcemia and hypercalciuria, Jansen syndrome is characterized by short-limbed dwarfism and a variety of other skeletal abnormalities, which seem to reflect the overactivity of PTH and PTHrP during development and growth and in the adult skeleton.

Malignancy and Hypercalcemia

Hypercalcemia of malignancy, the most common cause of severe hypercalcemia, can occur in up to 20% of all cases of carcinoma[37] and is usually due to increased osteoclastic bone resorption.

Excess circulating parathyroid hormone-related protein in the absence of skeletal metastases

Humoral hypercalcemia of malignancy (HHM), also called malignancy-associated hypercalcemia (MAH), accounts for approximately 80% of hypercalcemia in patients with cancer [38] and usually results from the oversecretion of PTHrP[39] in the absence of bone metastases. PTHrP-induced hypercalcemia commonly occurs in squamous cell carcinomas (head and neck, lung esophageal, and cervical) and breast, kidney, colon, bladder, endometrial, and ovarian cancers. This condition occurs more rarely in pancreatic neuroendocrine tumors such as VIPomas[40] and in Hodgkin and non-Hodgkin lymphomas.[41] Excess PTHrP secretion has also been associated with hypercalcemia due to pheochromocytoma, in which case serum PTHrP concentrations may be reduced by alpha-adrenergic blockers.[42] The parathyroid hormone-like hormone

(*PTHLH*) gene, which encodes PTHrP, is a single-copy gene located on the short arm of chromosome 12, whereas the gene encoding PTH is found on chromosome 11. These 2 chromosomes encode many similar genes and are believed to have arisen by an ancient duplication event. The PTHrP and PTH genes seem to be members of a single gene family.[43] The human *PTHLH* gene is driven by at least three promoters, contains at least 7 exons, shows several patterns of alternative splicing, and is considerably more complex than the *PTH* gene. Each gene encodes a leader or "pre" sequence, a "pro" sequence, and a mature form. In the case of human PTH, the mature form is 84 amino acids. In the case of human PTHrP, 3 isoforms of 139, 141, and 173 residues can occur by alternate splicing. The biologically active amino-terminal ends of secreted PTH and PTHrP are highly homologous, with 8 of the first 13 amino acid residues being identical; the 2 proteins share a similar secondary structure over the next 21 amino acids.[44] Consequently, the amino-terminal domains, 1 to 34 and 1 to 36, respectively, of both PTH and PTHrP, both bind to PTH1R, activating similar second messengers such as cyclic adenosine monophosphate (cAMP), protein kinase A and C, phospholipase C, and inositol triphosphate (see **Fig. 4**).

Patients with HHM due to PTHrP production may manifest biochemical features compatible with PTH hypersecretion including elevated renal excretion of nephrogenous cAMP, increased calcium reabsorption in the ascending limb of loop of Henle and DCT of the kidney, and inhibition of phosphate reabsorption in the proximal convoluted tubule leading to hypophosphatemia and phosphaturia. PTHrP and PTH have similar capacities to increase $1,25(OH)_2D$ levels.[45] Nevertheless, serum $1,25(OH)_2D$ concentrations, which are generally high or high normal with PTH excess, are frequently low or low normal in HHM, possibly reflecting the higher levels of ambient calcium observed in HHM, which may directly inhibit the renal 1a(OH)ase enzyme. The major mechanism for PTHrP in causing hypercalcemia in malignancy, however, is accelerated bone resorption. Thus, PTHrP can increase the expression, in osteoblasts, of receptor activator of nuclear factor-κB ligand (RANKL), which then activates the receptor activator of nuclear factor-κB (RANK) on osteoclast precursors and osteoclasts. PTHrP uncouples bone resorption from formation favoring osteoclast activation and osteoblast suppression, thus leading to marked calcium efflux from bone into circulation.[46] This effect is in part mediated by cytokines such as tumor necrosis factor (TNF), prostaglandin E, lymphotoxin, and interleukin-1 (IL-1) that stimulate osteoclasts and bone resorption. Such enhanced osteoclastic bone resorption increases efflux of skeletal calcium and phosphate into the circulation.

Local osteolytic hypercalcemia with skeletal metastases
Osteolytic metastases leading to excess calcium release from bone accounts for approximately 20% of cases of hypercalcemia of malignancy. The most common causes of such metastases are metastatic breast cancer and multiple myeloma, followed by leukemia and lymphoma.[47] Local cytokines released from the tumor can stimulate the local production of PTHrP, which in turn induces RANKL/RANK interaction[48] resulting in excessive osteoclast activation, increased bone resorption, and hypercalcemia (**Fig. 5**). The major humoral factors/cytokines associated with increased bone remodeling and hypercalcemia include the cytokines, IL-1, IL-3, IL-6, TNFα, transforming growth factor α and β (TGFα, TGFβ), lymphotoxin, and prostaglandins of the E series.[49] Macrophage inflammatory protein 1alpha (MIP1α) induces osteoclastogenesis in human bone marrow cells, inhibits the differentiation of marrow stromal cells into osteoblasts, and plays an important role in hypercalcemia associated with multiple myeloma.[50]

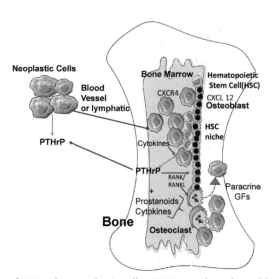

Fig. 5. Production of PTHrP by neoplastic cells. PTHrP may be released by neoplastic cells, which have not yet invaded bone, and cause HHM. When neoplastic cells travel to bone via blood vessels and/or lymphatics, CXCR4 expressing tumor cells interact with CXCL 12-positive osteoblasts and colonize the hematopoietic stem cell (HSC) niche. Neoplastic cells can subsequently be released from dormancy and secrete osteoclast- and osteoblast-stimulating factors, including PTHrP, prostanoids, and cytokines. PTHrP may then enter the circulation after release from bone metastases. In bone, the osteoblast- and osteoclast-stimulating factors, including PTHrP, further stimulate osteoclastic bone resorption; this can release paracrine growth factors from the bone matrix, which further enhances neoplastic cell proliferation.

Ectopic secretion of parathyroid hormone

True ectopic PTH production by malignant cells is very rare. Ectopic PTH production has been described in cancers of the neck/head, lung,[51] and ovary[52] and in neuroendocrine tumors.[53]

Excess production of extrarenal 1,25-dihydroxyvitamin D in malignancy

Approximately 1% of all cases of hypercalcemia of malignancy is due to increased production of the active metabolite, $1,25(OH)_2D$. In $1,25(OH)_2D$-induced hypercalcemia, cancer cells recruit adjacent macrophages to express CYP27B1[1(OH)ase] and convert endogenous $25(OH)D$ to $1,25(OH)_2D$; this generally occurs in both Hodgkin and non-Hodgkin lymphomas, and more commonly in large diffuse B-cell lymphomas, particularly of the nongerminal cell subtype.[54] The $1,25(OH)_2D$ produced can bind to the vitamin D receptor (VDR) in the gut and bone and, respectively, enhance gut absorption of calcium and, to a lesser extent, resorb bone. $1,25(OH)_2D$ may also serve as a marker of high-grade lymphoma or of its transformation. These mechanisms have also been reported, although rarely, in ovarian dysgerminoma.[55]

Vitamin D-Mediated Hypercalcemia in the Absence of Neoplasia

Extrarenal 1,25-dihydroxyvitamin D production

$1,25(OH)_2D$-induced hypercalcemia has been reported in various nonmalignant granulomatous diseases, including noninfectious diseases such as sarcoidosis and Wegener granulomatosis and infectious diseases such as tuberculosis, as well as in other inflammatory conditions.[56] Most cases of hypercalcemia in these cases are explained by the overproduction of $1,25(OH)_2D$ by activated macrophages. Studies in patients with tuberculosis revealed that macrophages activated by Toll-like receptor (TLR) 2/1 present increased expression of 1(OH)ase and VDR. Other cytokines may also contribute to increased 1(OH)ase stimulation. Increased expression of the receptor TREM-2 has been found in pulmonary sarcoidosis on myeloid cells, and $1,25(OH)_2D$ may increase the total numbers and percentages of TREM2-positive cells in bronchoalveolar lavage fluid. TREM-2 plays an important role in cell fusion and granuloma formation, and expression of VDRs has only been found in the alveolar lymphocytes of subjects with sarcoidosis. Therefore, most cases involving hypercalcemia in the setting of sarcoidosis are explained by the overproduction of $1,25(OH)_2D$ by activated macrophages, and $1,25(OH)_2D$ itself promotes granuloma formation.[57] Although increased gut absorption of calcium may be the major source of hypercalcemia in sarcoidosis, and a decrease in bone mineral density has not been reported, an increased incidence of vertebral deformities has been found.

Sequestration of macrophages in inflammatory tissues of infectious disorders, for example, in viral disorders such as HIV and cytomegalovirus, bacterial disorders such as cat scratch fever and leprosy, and fungal disorders including coccidiomycosis, histoplasmosis, and *Pneumocystis jirovecii* pneumonia, can all cause dysregulated production of $1,25(OH)_2D$ resulting in hypercalcemia.

Vitamin D or calcidiol intoxication
In vitamin D and in calcidiol [25(OH)D] toxicity, 25(OH)D level is elevated but $1,25(OH)_2D$ level is usually normal, suggesting that the hypercalcemia is not due to the actions of $1,25(OH)_2D$. It has been reported that elevated 25(OH)D can directly bind to VDR and increase serum calcium levels in mice devoid of $1,25(OH)_2D$ by binding directly to the VDR.[58]

Poorly monitored therapy with alfacalcidol or calcitriol
Hypercalcemia can result from the excess use of active forms of vitamin D, that is, calcitriol or alfacalcidol, in disorders such as hypoparathyroidism, CKD, or hypophosphatemic rickets.

Reduced 1,25(OH)₂D metabolism: idiopathic infantile hypercalcemia
Idiopathic infantile hypercalcemia (IIH) is an autosomal recessive disorder caused by inactivating mutations in the *CYP24A1* gene that encodes the vitamin D 24-hydroxylase, which catabolizes $1,25(OH)_2D$ to 1,24,25 $(OH)_3D$; this reduced catabolism results in elevated serum levels of $1,25(OH)_2D$.[59] Individuals with biallelic disease, that is, homozygous or compound heterozygous mutations, are usually symptomatic, whereas heterozygous patients with monoallelic mutations can be only mildly symptomatic.[60]

Other Endocrine Abnormalities

Thyrotoxicosis
In thyrotoxicosis with hypercalcemia, bone turnover and resorption are increased due to direct effects of increased triiodothyronine on bone.[61] The liberated calcium seems to suppress PTH release, and renal calcium reabsorption is diminished; $1,25(OH)_2D$ levels are also reduced. Treatment with a beta-adrenergic antagonist may reduce the hypercalcemia, and therapy for the hyperthyroidism reverses the hypercalcemia.

Hypoadrenalism

Both primary and secondary hypoadrenalism have been associated with hypercalcemia[62]; the underlying cause is unclear, although volume depletion and decreased glomerular filtration in addition to increased calcium mobilization from bone have been suggested. PTH and 1,25(OH)$_2$D levels are suppressed. The hypercalcemia is usually reversed by volume expansion and glucocorticoids.

Ion Abnormalities

Milk-alkali syndrome

Consumption of large quantities of calcium carbonate (at least 3 g/d), often with milk or other dairy products, may cause hypercalcemia accompanied by alkalosis.[63] The alkali may enhance precipitation of calcium in renal tissue, causing nephrocalcinosis and ultimately renal failure.

Aluminum intoxication

Aluminum intoxication was observed when large amounts of aluminum-containing phosphate-binding agents were prescribed to patients with CKD to control hyperphosphatemia. Clustered outbreaks of aluminum intoxication occurred when inadequately purified water was used for dialysis or for total parenteral nutrition.[64] Aluminum intoxication can inhibit bone turnover in patients with CKD, and hypercalcemia can occur possibly due to insufficient calcium deposition in bone. Reduced use of aluminum-containing medications has decreased the frequency of this disorder.

Other Medication and Vitamins

Aminophylline/theophylline

Hypercalcemia has been reported with theophylline usage for chronic obstructive pulmonary disease or asthma and seems to be reversible with cessation of therapy, or amenable to treatment with beta-adrenergic antagonists.[65]

Vitamin A

Retinoic acid receptors are located on both osteoclasts and osteoblasts. In vitro, retinoic acid suppresses osteoblast activity and increases osteoclast activity, resulting in increased bone resorption and decreased bone formation. Vitamin A has also been shown to stimulate PTH secretion. High doses of vitamin A and its analogues cis-retinoic acid and all-trans-retinoic acid have all been associated with enhanced bone resorption, which may manifest as osteopenia and fractures[66] as well as hypercalcemia.

Immobilization

Immobilization-induced hypercalcemia occurs due to lack of mechanical stimulation.[67] This condition causes uncoupling of bone remodeling, resulting in decreased osteoblastic activity and increased osteoclastic activity, with subsequent increased release of calcium and phosphate from the skeleton and loss of bone mass. Serum PTH and 1,25(OH)$_2$D levels are usually suppressed, and urine calcium level is increased. This condition seems to be more common in states of increased bone turnover such as in Paget disease; it can also be seen in acute immobilization following head injuries, fractures, spinal cord injuries, and burns. Prolonged immobilization may result in decreased bone mineral density and possibly fractures. The hypercalcemia and hypercalciuria generally resolve with the onset of weight bearing.

SUMMARY

A thorough appreciation of the pathophysiology of hypercalcemia requires understanding of the normal physiology underlying calcium homeostasis. Conversely, examination of mechanisms underlying the development of clinical hypercalcemic states has led to expanded understanding of mechanisms defending the normal regulation of extracellular calcium. In concert, this has facilitated appropriate diagnosis of clinical conditions underlying a presentation of hypercalcemia, specific and appropriate therapy depending on the underlying pathophysiology, and insights into the likely prognosis of the clinical disorders. Continued advances in understanding the underlying mechanisms should continue to refine and advance our insights for the benefits of patients.

CLINICS CARE POINTS

- Sporadic PHPT is the most common cause of hypercalcemia and may be intermittently normocalcemic, and either symptomatic or asymptomatic.

- Identification of the underlying genetic defect in familial HPT can establish the correct prognosis and enhance appropriate diagnostic and therapeutic management.

- MAH, without or with skeletal metastases, is the most common cause of severe hypercalcemia and of hypercalcemia in hospitalized patients.

- Extrarenal production of calcitriol can occur in malignancies, and in infectious and noninfectious granulomatous diseases, and can cause hypercalcemia.

- Excess consumption of vitamin D either in precursor form (vitamin D and calcidiol) or in active form (alfacalcidol, calcitriol) can cause hypercalcemia.

ACKNOWLEDGMENTS

This work was supported by grants from the Canadian Institutes for Health Research (CIHR).

DISCLOSURE

The author has nothing to disclose.

REFERENCES

1. Vautour L, Goltzman D. Regulation of calcium homeostasis. In: Bilezikian JP, Bouillon R, Clemens T, et al, editors. Primer on the metabolic bone diseases and disorders of mineral metabolism. 9th edition. Hoboken (NJ): John Wiley & Sons; 2018. p. 163–72.
2. de Rouffignac C, Quamme GA. Renal magnesium handling and its hormonal control. Physiol Rev 1994;74(2):305–22.
3. Brenza HL, Kimmel-Jehan C, Jehan F, et al. Parathyroid hormone activation of the 25-hydroxyvitamin D3-1α-hydroxylase gene promoter. Proc Natl Acad Sci U S A 1998;95(4):1387–91.
4. Lieben L, Benn BS, Ajibade D, et al. Trpv6 mediates intestinal calcium absorption during calcium restriction and contributes to bone homeostasis. Bone 2010; 47(2):301–8.
5. Silverberg SJ, Shane E, de la Cruz L, et al. Skeletal disease in primary hyperparathyroidism. J Bone Miner Res 1989;4(3):283–91.
6. Lieben L, Verlinden L, Masuyama R, et al. Extra-intestinal calcium handling contributes to normal serum calcium levels when intestinal calcium absorption is suboptimal. Bone 2015;81:502–12.

7. Brown EM, Gamba G, Riccardi D, et al. Cloning and characterization of an extracellular Ca(2+)-sensing receptor from bovine parathyroid. Nature 1993; 366(6455):575–80.

8. Nesbit MA, Hannan FM, Howles SA, et al. Mutations affecting G protein subunit alpha11 in hypercalcemia and hypocalcemia. N Engl J Med 2013;368(26): 2476–86.

9. Bushinsky DA, Monk RD. Electrolyte quintet: calcium. Lancet 1998;352(9124): 306–11.

10. Riccardi D, Valenti G. Localization and function of the renal calcium-sensing receptor. Nature 2016;12:414–25.

11. Kolek OI, Hines ER, Jones MD, et al. 1alpha,25-Dihydroxyvitamin D3 upregulates FGF23 gene expression in bone: the final link in a renal-gastrointestinal-skeletal axis that controls phosphate transport. Am J Physiol Gastrointest Liver Physiol 2005;289:G1036–42.

12. Quinn SJ, Thomsen AR, Pang L, et al. Interactions between calcium and phosphorus in the regulation of the production of fibroblast growth factor 23 in vivo. Am J Physiol Endocrinol Metab 2013;304(3):E310–20.

13. Bilezikian JP, Cusano NE, Khan AA, et al. Primary hyperparathyroidism. Nat Rev Dis Primers 2016;2:16033.

14. Cetani F, Pardi E, Marcocci C. Parathyroid carcinoma. In: Brandi ML, editor. Parathyroid disorders. Focusing on Unmet Needs, vol. 51. Front Horm Res. Basel, Karger; 2019. p. 63–76.

15. Albright F, Reifenstein EC Jr. Parathyroid glands and metabolic bone disease. Baltimore, MD: Williams & Wilkins; 1948. p. 46–114.

16. Pawlowska M, Cusano NE. An overview of normocalcemic primary hyperparathyroidism. Curr Opin Endocrinol Diabetes Obes 2015;22(6):413–21.

17. Rejnmark L, Vestergaard P, Mosekilde L. Nephrolithiasis and renal calcifications in primary hyperparathyroidism. J Clin Endocrinol Metab 2011;96:2377–85.

18. Bilezikian JP. Primary Hyperparathyroidism. J Clin Endocrinol Metab 2018; 103(11):3993–4004.

19. Szalat A, Mazeh H, Freund HR. Lithium-associated hyperparathyroidism: report of four cases and review of the literature. Eur J Endocrinol 2009;160(2):317–23.

20. Griebeler ML, Kearns AE, Ryu E, et al. Thiazide-associated hypercalcemia: incidence and association with primary hyperparathyroidism over two decades. J Clin Endocrinol Metab 2016;101(3):1166–73.

21. Alon U, Lovell HB, Donaldson DL. Nephrocalcinosis, hyperparathyroidism and renal failure in familial hypophosphatemic rickets. Clin Pediatr 1992;21:180–3.

22. Goltzman D. Hypercalcemia. In: Feingold KR, Anawalt B, Boyce A, et al, editors. Endotext [Internet]. South Dartmouth (MA): MDText.com, Inc; 2019.

23. Marx SJ, Goltzman D. Evolution of our understanding of the hyperparathyroid syndromes: a historical perspective. J Bone Miner Res 2019;34(1):22–37.

24. Thakker RV. Multiple endocrine neoplasia type 1 (MEN1) and type 4 (MEN4). Mol Cell Endocrinol 2014;386(1–2):2–15.

25. Weinstein LS, Simonds WF. HRPT2, a marker of parathyroid cancer. N Engl J Med 2003;349(18):1691–2.

26. Guan B, Welch JM, Sapp JC, et al. GCM2-activating mutations in familial isolated hyperparathyroidism. Am J Hum Genet 2016;99(5):1034–44.

27. Zajickova K, Vrbikova J, Canaff L, et al. Identification and functional characterization of a novel mutation in the calcium-sensing receptor gene in familial hypocalciuric hypercalcemia: modulation of clinical severity by vitamin D status. J Clin Endocrinol Metab 2007;92(7):2616–23.

28. Zajíčková K, Dvořáková M, Moravcová J, et al. Familial hypocalciuric hypercalcemia in an index male: grey zones of the differential diagnosis from primary hyperparathyroidism in a 13-year clinical follow up. Physiol Res 2020;69(Suppl 2): S321–8.

29. Glaudo MLS, Quinkler M, Ulrich B, et al. Heterozygous inactivating CaSR mutations causing neonatal hyperparathyroidism: function, inheritance and phenotype. Eur J Endocrinol 2016;175(5):421–31.

30. Nesbit MA, Hannan FM, Howles SA, et al. Mutations in AP2S1 cause familial hypocalciuric hypercalcemia type 3. Nat Genet 2013;13(45):93–7.

31. Schipani E, Langman C, Hunzelman J, et al. A novel parathyroid hormone (PTH)/ PTH-related peptide receptor mutation in Jansen's metaphyseal chondrodysplasia. J Clin Endocrinol Metab 1999;84(9):3052–7.

32. Juppner H, Abou-Samra AB, Freeman MW, et al. G protein-linked receptor for parathyroid hormone and parathyroid hormone-related peptide. Science 1991; 254:1024–6.

33. Goltzman D, Hendy GN, Banville D. Parathyroid hormone-like peptide: Molecular characterization and biological properties. Trends Endocrinol Metab 1989;1: 39–44.

34. Morimoto T, Devora GA, Mibe M, et al. Parathyroid hormone-related protein and human myometrial cells: Action and regulation. Mol Cell Endocrinol 1997; 129:91–9.

35. Wysolmerski JJ, Mccaugherncarucci JF, Daifotis AG, et al. Overexpression of parathyroid hormone-related protein or parathyroid hormone in transgenic mice impairs branching morphogenesis during mammary gland development. Development 1995;121:3539–47.

36. Amizuka N, Warshawsky H, Henderson JE, et al. Parathyroid hormone-related peptide-depleted mice show abnormal epiphyseal cartilage development and altered endochondral bone formation. J Cell Biol 1994;126:1611–23.

37. Turner JJO. Hypercalcaemia - presentation management. Clin Med (Lond) 2017; 17:270–3.

38. Goltzman D. Nonparathyroid hypercalcemia. Front Horm Res 2019;51:77–90.

39. Henderson JE, Shustik C, Kremer R, et al. Circulating concentrations of parathyroid hormone-like peptide in malignancy and hyperparathyroidism. J Bone Miner Res 1990;5:105–13.

40. Ghaferi AA, Chojnacki KA, Long WD, et al. Pancreatic VIPomas: subject review and one institutional experience. J Gastrointest Surg 2008;12(2):382–93.

41. Kremer R, Shustik C, Tabak T, et al. Parathyroid-hormone-related peptide in hematologic malignancies. Am J Med 1996;100:406–11.

42. Mune T, Katakami H, Kato Y, et al. Production and secretion of parathyroid hormone-related protein in pheochromocytoma: participation of an alpha-adrenergic mechanism. J Clin Endocrinol Metab 1993;76(3):757–62.

43. Yasuda T, Banville D, Hendy GN, et al. Characterization of the human parathyroid hormone-like peptide gene. J Biol Chem 1989;264:7720–5.

44. Wysolmerski JJ. Parathyroid hormone-related protein: an update. J Clin Endocrinol Metab 2012;97:2947–56.

45. Fraher LJ, Hodsman AB, Jonas K, et al. A comparison of the in vivo biochemical responses to exogenous parathyroid hormone (1-34) [PTH 1-34] and PTH-related peptide (1-34) in man. J Clin Endocrinol Metab 1992;75:417–23.

46. Budayr AA, Nissenson RA, Klein RF, et al. Increased serum levels of parathyroid hormone-like protein in malignancy-associated hypercalcemia. Ann Intern Med 1989;111:807–12.

47. Mirrakhimov AE. Hypercalcemia of malignancy: an update on pathogenesis and management. North Am J Med Sci 2015;7:483–93.
48. Johnson RW, Nguyen MP, Padalecki SS, et al. TGF-beta promotion of Gli2-induced expression of parathyroid hormone-related protein, an important osteolytic factor in bone metastasis, is independent of canonical Hedgehog signaling. Cancer Res 2011;71:822–31.
49. Ikushima H, Miyazono K. TGFbeta signalling: a complex web in cancer progression. Nat Rev Cancer 2010;10:415–24.
50. Roodman GD. Pathogenesis of myeloma bone disease. J Cell Biochem 2010; 109:283–91.
51. Nielsen PK, Rasmussen AK, Feldt-Rasmussen U, et al. Ectopic production of intact parathyroid hormone by a squamous cell lung carcinoma in vivo and in vitro. J Clin Endocrinol Metab 1996;81:3793–6.
52. Holtz G, Johnson TR Jr, Schrock ME. Paraneoplastic hypercalcemia in ovarian tumors. Obstet Gynecol 1979;54:483–7.
53. VanHouten JN, Yu N, Rimm D, et al. Hypercalcemia of malignancy due to ectopic transactivation of the parathyroid hormone gene. J Clin Endocrinol Metab 2006; 91:580–3.
54. Shallis RM, Rome RS, Reagan JL. Mechanisms of hypercalcemia in non-hodgkin lymphoma and associated outcomes: a retrospective review. Clin Lymp Myel Leuke 2018;18:e123–9.
55. Hibi M, Hara F, Tomishige H, et al. 1,25-dihydroxyvitamin D-mediated hypercalcemia in ovarian dysgerminoma. Pediatr Hematol Oncol 2008;25:73–8.
56. Kallas M, Green F, Hewison M, et al. Rare causes of calcitriol-mediated hypercalcemia: a case report and literature review. J Clin Endocrinol Metab 2010;95: 3111–7.
57. Gwadera Ł, Białas AJ, Iwański MA, et al. Sarcoidosis and calcium homeostasis disturbances-Do we know where we stand? Chron Respir Dis 2019;16. 1479973119878713.
58. Deluca HF, Prahl JM, Plum LA. 1,25-Dihydroxyvitamin D is not responsible for toxicity caused by vitamin D or 25-hydroxyvitamin D. Arch Biochem Biophys 2011;505(2):226–30.
59. Schlingmann KP, Kaufmann M, Weber S, et al. Mutations in CYP24A1 and idiopathic infantile hypercalcemia. N Engl J Med 2011;365(5):410–21.
60. O'Keeffe DT, Tebben PJ, Kumar R, et al. A Clinical and biochemical phenotypes of adults with monoallelic and biallelic CYP24A1 mutations: evidence of gene dose effect Osteoporos. Int 2016;27:3121–5.
61. Rosen HN, Moses AC, Gundberg C, et al. Therapy with parenteral pamidronate prevents thyroid hormone-induced bone turnover in humans. J Clin Endocrinol Metab 1993;77:664–9.
62. Diamond T, Thornley S. Addisonian crisis and hypercalcaemia. Aust N Z J Med 1994;24:316.
63. Beall DP, Scofield RH. Milk-alkali syndrome associated with calcium carbonate consumption. Report of 7 patients with parathyroid hormone levels and an estimate of prevalence among patients hospitalized with hypercalcemia. Milk-alkali syndrome associated with calcium carbonate consumption. Medicine 1995;74: 89–96.
64. Ott SM, Maloney NA, Klein GL, et al. Aluminum is associated with low bone formation in patients receiving chronic parenteral nutrition. Ann Intern Med 1983; 96:910–4.

65. McPherson ML, Prince SR, Atamer ER, et al. Theophylline-induced hypercalcemia. Ann Intern Med 1986;105:52–4.
66. Barker ME, Blumsohn A. Is vitamin a consumption a risk factor for osteoporotic fracture? Proc Nutr Soc 2003;62:845–50.
67. Stewart AF, Adler M, Byers CM, et al. Calcium homeostasis in immobilization: An example of resorptive hypercalciuria. N Engl J Med 1982;306:1136–40.

Sporadic Primary Hyperparathyroidism

Stephanie J. Kim, MD, MPH[a],*, Dolores M. Shoback, MD[b]

KEYWORDS

- Primary hyperparathyroidism • Hypercalcemia • Parathyroid hormone
- Parathyroidectomy • Calcium-sensing receptor • Osteitis fibrosa cystica
- Calcimimetic • Nephrolithiasis

KEY POINTS

- Primary hyperparathyroidism is characterized by hypercalcemia and elevated or inappropriately normal parathyroid hormone levels, due to increased secretion of parathyroid hormone and expansion of parathyroid cell mass.
- Primary hyperparathyroidism has shifted from a symptomatic disease to an asymptomatic disease due to an increase in routine screening.
- Clinical manifestations of primary hyperparathyroidism when present can include skeletal, renal, cardiovascular, neuropsychiatric, gastrointestinal, and rheumatologic.
- Although parathyroidectomy remains the definitive treatment of primary hyperparathyroidism, pharmacologic options can be considered for patients who cannot undergo surgery.

INTRODUCTION

Primary hyperparathyroidism (PHPT) is due to an increased secretion of parathyroid hormone (PTH) by 1 or more parathyroid glands, characterized by hypercalcemia and elevated or inappropriately normal PTH levels. A majority of cases of PHPT present sporadically without other affected family members and without other endocrine gland involvement, and this form of PHPT is the focus of this article.

A majority of cases of PHPT are caused by a single parathyroid adenoma (80%), followed by 4-gland hyperplasia (10%–15%) and multiple adenomas (5%) and, rarely, atypical adenoma (2%–3%) and carcinoma (<1%).[1] Parathyroid carcinoma should be suspected when a patient presents with a palpable neck mass and significantly elevated calcium and PTH levels, as discussed in Filomena Cetani and colleagues' article, "Parathyroid Carcinoma and Ectopic Secretion of PTH," in this issue. Classic

[a] Division of Endocrinology and Metabolism, University of California, 400 Parnassus Avenue A549, San Francisco, CA 94143, USA; [b] Endocrine Research Unit - 111N, San Francisco Department of Veterans Affairs Medical Center, Division of Endocrinology and Metabolism, San Francisco VA Medical Center, University of California, 1700 Owens Street, 3rd floor Room 369, San Francisco, CA 94158, USA
* Corresponding author.
E-mail address: stephanie.kim@ucsf.edu

Endocrinol Metab Clin N Am 50 (2021) 609–628
https://doi.org/10.1016/j.ecl.2021.07.006
0889-8529/21/© 2021 Elsevier Inc. All rights reserved.

genetic forms of PHPT are discussed in Paul Newey's article, "Hereditary Primary Hyperparathyroidism," in this issue, although genetic abnormalities also been have described in sporadic parathyroid adenomas, as discussed later.

Long-term lithium therapy, external neck radiation, chronic low calcium intake, higher body weight, celiac disease (presumably from chronic malabsorption), hypertension, and furosemide intake all have been reported as risk factors for the development of sporadic PHPT.[2]

EPIDEMIOLOGY

PHPT occurs 3 times to 4 times more frequently in women than in men,[3] with female predominance in adult patients,[4] and is more common in postmenopausal versus premenopausal women.[1] PHPT commonly is diagnosed in the first decade after menopause, and the incidence of PHPT increases with age.[2] Although the incidence of PHPT varies worldwide, estimates vary from 0.4 to 82 cases per 100,000 person-years.[5–7] In North America, studies have reported the incidence of PHPT to be 21.6 per 100,000 person-years[6] and prevalence of 0.86%.[7] A contemporary study analyzed a large multiethnic series of more than 13,000 North American patients with PHPT and reported previously under-appreciated gender and racial differences in disease occurrence.[5] The incidence in women was on average 66 per 100,000 person-years (vs 25 per 100,000 person-years among men) with these differences more apparent with advanced age.[5] With regard to race, the incidence was higher in black individuals compared with whites, with lower incidences observed in Asian and Hispanic populations (**Table 1**).[5] The prevalence of PHPT also was noted to have tripled during the study period of 15 years (1995–2010), attributed to increased routine testing.[5]

Incidence and prevalence data for this disease in a given population depend on the extent of biochemical screening being done, because PHPT is seen more frequently and presents differently in countries that commonly utilize routine screening compared with those that do not. The advent of biochemical multichannel screening in the 1970s led to a shift from symptomatic to asymptomatic disease presentations in Western countries.[8] In less developed countries, however, routine screening for hypercalcemia typically is not performed. Therefore, symptomatic PHPT still is prevalent, because a diagnosis usually occurs when the patient presents with overt symptoms of hypercalcemia and/or PTH excess. For example, in India, a systematic review from 2011 reported that most patients with PHPT presented with bone disease (multiple fractures or brown tumors), renal disease, and psychiatric symptoms, whereas only 5.6% of patients with PHPT presented asymptomatically.[9] Additionally, due to the

Table 1
Primary hyperparathyroidism incidence by race and ethnic group in the United States

Race/Ethnicity	Incidence in Women (per 100,000)	Incidence in Men (per 100,000)
Black	92	46
White	81	29
Asian	52	28
Hispanic	52	28

Adapted from Yeh MW, Ituarte PH, Zhou HC, Nishimoto S, Liu IL, Harari A, Haigh PI, Adams AL. Incidence and prevalence of primary hyperparathyroidism in a racially mixed population. J Clin Endocrinol Metab. 2013 Mar;98(3):1122-9.

severity of their disease at diagnosis, these patients often present with large, palpable parathyroid glands, and hungry bone disease commonly is observed post-parathyroidectomy.[9]

More recent studies suggest a shift in numbers of patients with asymptomatic hypercalcemia in Asian countries, although a series from China indicates that most patients with PHPT still demonstrate classic symptoms.[10,11] Comparisons of patients with PHPT in Beijing and New York (1984–1999) showed that Chinese patients with PHPT have higher serum calcium and PTH and more skeletal lesions and kidney stones (97%) compared with their American counterparts (<20%).[10] Follow-up comparisons of patients in Shanghai and New York a decade later were reported in 2013. Although most of the patients with PHPT in the Beijing cohort (97%) were symptomatic, patients in Shanghai cohort (60%) trended toward asymptomatic disease due to biochemical screening. During the 10-year study period of patients in Shanghai, the percentage of asymptomatic patients rose from less than 20% to 40%. Chinese patients in that series, however, still had higher calcium and PTH and classical symptoms, including bone and renal manifestations, compared with patients in New York City.[11]

GENETIC ABNORMALITIES

Parathyroid adenomas primarily are monoclonal outgrowths derived from a single progenitor cell with an acquired growth advantage transmitted to its progeny.[12] Activation of proto-oncogenes and inactivation of tumor suppressor genes are involved in parathyroid tumorigenesis. Sporadic PHPT is associated with alterations of the *cyclin D1* and *MEN1* genes, located on chromosome 11; the loss of chromosome 11q is the most frequent genetic abnormality seen in parathyroid adenomas.[13]

Cyclin D1

Cyclin D1 (*CCND1*), an oncogene and regulator of the cell cycle located on chromosome 11q13, is involved in genesis of 5% to 8% of parathyroid adenomas.[13] Pericentromeric inversion of chromosome 11 places *cyclin D1* under the control of the PTH gene promoter sequence, resulting in the overexpression of *cyclin D1* mRNA and protein, which eventually leads to increased PTH production.[12,13] The overexpression of *cyclin D1* has been reported in up to 40% of parathyroid adenomas,[12,13] so it is hypothesized that mechanisms other than rearrangement, as described previously, also may be responsible for overexpression of the oncogene. Hypothesized mechanisms include impaired ubiquitin-mediated proteolytic degradation of *cyclin D1* and changes in *cyclin D1* phosphorylation sites (involved in the export of the protein from the nucleus to the cytoplasm, the site of ubiquitylation) and *cyclin D1b* (an alternatively spliced isoform of *cyclin D1*), which may contribute to tumorigenesis.[12]

MEN1

Another gene implicated in sporadic parathyroid adenomas is the tumor suppressor gene *MEN1* on chromosome 11q13 that encodes the protein menin.[13] The loss of functioning menin is responsible for the multiple endocrine neoplasia type 1 syndrome, discussed in Paul Newey's article, "Hereditary Primary Hyperparathyroidism," in this issue. Approximately 40% to 45% of sporadic parathyroid adenomas harbor *MEN1* gene mutations.[14] Sporadic parathyroid adenomas are associated most commonly with loss of heterozygosity (LOH) in the *MEN1* gene, seen in approximately 35% (range 26.2%–50.0%) of cases.[15] Because LOH can include other genes on chromosome 11q, however, the biallelic inactivation of *MEN1* may not be the only abnormality.[15]

Other genetic mechanisms involve in sporadic parathyroid adenomas that require further investigation include inactivation of cyclin-dependent kinase inhibitors, enhancers of zeste homolog 2, zinc finger X-linked (ZFX), components of the Wnt signaling pathway, and mutations in *GCM2* (transcription factor essential in parathyroid development) and in *CDC73* (gene responsible for the hyperparathyroidism–jaw tumor syndrome).[15]

CLINICAL PRESENTATION

Decades ago, PHPT was a chronic, symptomatic, and often devastating disorder with skeletal, renal, gastrointestinal, and psychological complications.[16] With enhanced screening and improved biochemical testing for PTH, now PHPT presents most often as asymptomatic hypercalcemia. When present, the signs and symptoms of PHPT generally manifest as those related to hypercalcemia, especially when the serum calcium level is elevated to greater than 12 mg/dL or if it rises rapidly, traditionally referred to as "stones, bones, abdominal groans and psychic moans." Typical symptoms of hypercalcemia include altered mental status, abdominal pain, constipation, nausea, vomiting, anorexia, fatigue, weakness, polyuria, and polydipsia. Clinical manifestations are outlined in **Table 2**.

Skeletal Manifestations

Although rare today, osteitis fibrosa cystica is the classic manifestation of PHPT and usually is seen in severe and prolonged PHPT. Osteitis fibrosa cystica refers to subperiosteal bone resorption on radiographic studies, especially of the phalanges (**Fig. 1**) as well as bone cysts and brown tumors that present as lytic lesions (**Fig. 2**) and a salt-and-pepper appearance of the skull. Clinically, patients present with bone pain, sometimes with pathologic fractures, and elevated alkaline phosphatase on laboratory evaluation, representing high bone turnover.

More commonly, osteoporosis is diagnosed by dual-energy x-ray absorptiometry (DXA) showing reduced bone mineral density (BMD) either for age and sex (by z score)

Table 2	
Manifestations of primary hyperparathyroidism by organ system	
Organ System	**Signs and Symptoms**
Skeletal	Osteitis fibrosa cystica, osteoporosis, osteosclerosis, fractures
Renal	Hypercalciuria, nephrolithiasis, nephrocalcinosis, and reduced renal function
Cardiovascular	Hypertension, conduction abnormalities and arrhythmias, diastolic dysfunction, atherosclerosis, vascular stiffness, left ventricular hypertrophy, calcification of the myocardium and heart valves
Neuropsychiatric/ cognitive/muscular	Fatigue, difficulty concentrating, poor memory, cognitive decline, anxiety, depression, personality changes and sleep disturbance, weakness
Gastrointestinal	Constipation, heartburn, nausea, and loss of appetite Not clearly established: acute pancreatitis, peptic ulcer disease, celiac disease
Rheumatologic	Chondrocalcinosis (pseudogout), gout

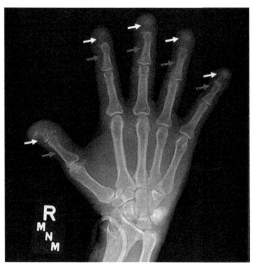

Fig. 1. Hand radiograph of a patient with a history of severe hyperparathyroidism showing multiple sites of subperiosteal bone resorption of radial aspect of the middle phalanges (*red arrows*) and tuftal resorption (*white arrows*).

or for sex-matched and ethnicity-matched young normal controls (by T score). Osteoporosis preferentially affects cortical bone in this disease classically at sites like the distal one-third radius rather than trabecular sites, such as the lumbar spine, because the catabolic effects of excessive PTH affect cortical sites preferentially, while sparing trabecular sites.[1] Therefore, an increased risk of peripheral fractures and decreased vertebral fracture risk would be expected, although not always observed.[17,18] High-

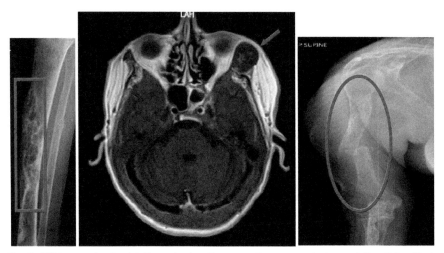

Fig. 2. Widespread mixed lytic and sclerotic expansile osseous lesions of the tibia, fibula ([*left*] *box*) and skull ([*middle*] *arrow*) and humerus, including a pathologic fracture ([*right*] *circle*) in a patient with severe PHPT left untreated for years.

resolution peripheral quantitative computed tomography (HRpQCT) and trabecular bone score (TBS) have provided insight into this inconsistency. HRpQCT measures volumetric bone density, bone geometry, skeletal microarchitecture, and bone strength in cortical and trabecular compartments. Both compartments are negatively affected in PHPT, with reduced volumetric densities, thinner cortices, and widely spaced and heterogeneously distributed trabeculae.[19] BMD increases following parathyroidectomy.[16,17]

PHPT is associated with elevated bone turnover markers, which are higher in patients with more active disease, even if they are asymptomatic.[19] Patients with asymptomatic PHPT present most often with bone turnover markers that are elevated or in the upper limit of the normal range.[20]

After parathyroidectomy, bone resorption markers fall precipitously, followed by a slower fall in bone formation markers.[21]

A recent meta-analysis of 12 studies found an increased risk of any fracture compared with controls[22] in patients with PHPT, with further analysis showing an increased risk at the forearm and spine. The risk of vertebral fractures was also increased if the analyses included studies with a healthy control group, patients with mild PHPT or postmenopausal women.[22] This increased risk of vertebral fractures in patients with PHPT has been demonstrated with fracture rates estimated to be 3-fold higher than the general population,[17] although the reported prevalence of vertebral fractures have varied widely, with some studies reporting less than 5%,[23] between 10% and 25%,[18,24] or greater than 35%.[25] Furthermore, there are inconsistent data looking at the trajectory of fracture risk after surgery. One study reported an increased risk for fractures during the first year following parathyroidectomy, which decreased to the same rate in the control population,[23,26] whereas other studies have observed decreased risk of fracture following surgery.[27]

Renal Manifestations

Renal involvement includes hypercalciuria, nephrolithiasis, nephrocalcinosis, and reduced renal function. In a series of patients with PHPT, symptomatic nephrolithiasis occurred in 10% to 20% of cases and was more common in men and patients with a younger onset of PHPT,[1,28] whereas nephrocalcinosis was less common. PTH increases the tubular reabsorption of calcium in the nephron, however, the renal excretion of calcium often is high in patients with PHPT.[28] This is because hypercalcemia leads to a proportional increase in filtered calcium in the glomerulus, leading to increased urinary calcium excretion. Therefore, hypercalciuria is thought to contribute to the pathophysiology of renal stone formation. Calcium oxalate stones are typical in patients with PHPT,[29] although slightly alkaline urine may be predispose to calcium phosphate stones.[29] Additionally, although patients who have nephrolithiasis are more likely to be hypercalciuric, less than one-third of hypercalciuric patients with PHPT develop renal stones.[29] Although there are limited data in this population, it is thought that the prevalence of asymptomatic nephrolithiasis is increased in patients with PHPT compared with the general population.[28]

Reduced renal function, defined as estimated glomerular filtration rate (eGFR) less than 60 mL/min, occurs in approximately 15% to 17% in patients with PHPT.[1] Traditional risk factors, such as age, hypertension, antihypertensive medication use, fasting glucose levels, and reduced 25-hydroxy (25-OH) vitamin D levels, were associated with renal dysfunction, rather than PHPT disease severity indices, including the history of nephrolithiasis.[30] Parathyroidectomy appears to have no effect on renal function,[31] although recent evidence suggests that surgical cure of PHPT prevents worsening of renal function in patients with PHPT and coexisting renal disease.[32]

Cardiovascular Manifestations

Cardiovascular manifestations, including hypertension, conduction abnormalities and arrhythmias, diastolic dysfunction, atherosclerosis, and vascular stiffness as well as structural anomalies, including left ventricular hypertrophy and calcification of the myocardium and heart valves,[33,34] are discussed in Marcella Walker and Shonni J. Silverberg's article, "Non-traditional Aspects of Sporadic Primary Hyperparathyroidism," in this issue.

Neuropsychiatric, Cognitive, and Muscular Manifestations

Symptoms include fatigue, difficulty concentrating, poor memory, cognitive decline, anxiety, depression, personality changes, and sleep disturbance in PHPT and are described in Marcella Walker and Shonni J. Silverberg's article, "Non-traditional Aspects of Sporadic Primary Hyperparathyroidism," in this issue.

Gastrointestinal Manifestations

Gastrointestinal manifestations in PHPT are nonspecific and thought to be due to atony of the smooth muscle.[35] Most common symptoms are constipation, heartburn, nausea and loss of appetite, reported in 1 study as 33%, 30%, 24% and 15% of cases, respectively,[36] and are discussed in Marcella Walker and Shonni J. Silverberg's article, "Non-traditional Aspects of Sporadic Primary Hyperparathyroidism," in this issue.

Rheumatologic Manifestations

Uncommon manifestations of PHPT include chondrocalcinosis (pseudogout) and gout,[37] discussed in Marcella Walker and Shonni J. Silverberg's article, "Non-traditional Aspects of Sporadic Primary Hyperparathyroidism," in this issue.

Normocalcemic hyperparathyroidism is characterized by consistently normal albumin adjusted serum calcium or ionized calcium. Additionally, criteria for diagnosis includes thorough elimination of secondary causes of hyperparathyroidism, including vitamin D deficiency, decreased creatinine clearance, medications associated with elevated PTH like hydrochlorothiazide and lithium, hypercalciuria, and calcium malabsorption.[38]

DIAGNOSIS

Diagnosis of PHPT should rely on the laboratory evaluation summarized in **Table 3**. Hypercalcemia should be established by 1 or more plasma measurements, with concomitant intact PTH measurements. Ionized calcium measurements, if done reliably, can substitute for plasma total calcium levels. The plasma total calcium concentration is corrected for albumin with the following formula:

Corrected calcium = $[0.8 \times (4.0 \text{ g/dL} - \text{patient's albumin})]$ + serum calcium level

Screening for familial hypocalciuric hypercalcemia (FHH) always should be considered in patients with longstanding, asymptomatic, and usually mild hypercalcemia. The urinary calcium and creatinine (24-h sample) always should be measured along with simultaneous plasma calcium and creatinine, and the calcium-to-creatinine clearance ratio should be calculated with the formula:

Calcium-to-creatinine clearance ratio = (24-hour urine calcium $\times$ plasma creatinine) $\div$ (plasma calcium $\times$ 24-h urine creatinine)

Calcium-to-creatinine clearance ratios of less than 0.01, coupled with a family history of hypercalcemia and/or prior unsuccessful parathyroid surgery, support the diagnosis of possible FHH, and further testing should be strongly considered as

Table 3	
Recommended workup for primary hyperparathyroidism	
Laboratory evaluation	Blood levels of PTH, calcium, phosphorus, alkaline phosphatase activity, creatinine (with eGFR), and 25-OH vitamin D; 24-h urine calcium and creatinine
	Stone risk profile (if urinary calcium >400 mg/d)
Imaging	DXA (lumbar spine, hip, distal-third radius)
	Vertebral spine assessment (radiograph, CT, vertebral fracture assessment by DXA)
	Abdominal imaging (radiograph, ultrasonography, CT scan)
Optional	HRpQCT, TBS by DXA, bone turnover markers, DNA testing if genetic basis for PHPT is suspected

Adapted from Bilezikian JP, Brandi ML, Eastell R, Silverberg SJ, Udelsman R, Marcocci C, et al. Guidelines for the Management of Asymptomatic Primary Hyperparathyroidism: Summary Statement from the Fourth International Workshop. J Clin Endocrinol Metab. 2014 Oct 1;99(10):3561–9; with permission.

described in Paul Newey's article, "Hereditary Primary Hyperparathyroidism," in this issue.

Imaging to evaluate for end-organ involvement includes DXA to assess BMD, including the distal-third radius, and vertebral imaging, given vertebral involvement in asymptomatic PHPT. Abdominal imaging also should be obtained to rule out asymptomatic nephrolithiasis and/or nephrocalcinosis.

TREATMENT
Surgical Management

Definitive treatment of PHPT is parathyroidectomy. According to the Fourth International Workshop on for the Management of Asymptomatic Primary Hyperparathyroidism, parathyroidectomy is indicated and/or may be strongly considered if 1 or more criteria are met: age less than 50 years, persistent hypercalcemia greater than 1 mg/dL above the upper limit of normal, presence of osteoporosis or fragility fracture, nephrolithiasis, hypercalciuria, risk factors for stones, and reduced kidney function (**Table 4**).

Additionally, the American Association of Endocrine Surgeons recommends parathyroidectomy for patients with neurocognitive and/or neuropsychiatric symptoms attributable to PHPT. Their guidelines also recommend considering offering surgery to patients with cardiovascular disease (other than hypertension), muscle weakness, impaired functional capacity, and abnormal sleep patterns as well as gastroesophageal reflux and fibromyalgia symptoms.[39]

Localization

Preoperative parathyroid localization is helpful in the successful management of PHPT, especially for the use of the minimally invasive approach, which is very popular. With positive localization studies and an experienced surgeon, cure rates are in the range of 95% or better.[40] The advantages and disadvantages, as well as the reported sensitivity and positive predictive value, of each imaging modality varies (**Table 5**).

Although the choice of imaging modality varies by the medical team and institution, ultrasound and sestamibi imaging are the most commonly employed first-line modalities, although recently, 4-dimensional CT (4-D) computed tomography (CT) has become more popular.[41] Ultrasound (**Fig. 3**) is the least costly and it is widely

Table 4	
Indications for parathyroidectomy	
Age	<50 Years Old
Serum calcium	>1 mg/dL above upper limit of normal
Skeletal involvement	T-score < −2.5 (lumbar spine, total hip or distal-third radius) Vertebral fracture (radiograph, CT, vertebral fracture assessment by DXA, MRI)
Renal involvement	Nephrolithiasis or nephrocalcinosis on abdominal imaging Hypercalciuria (>400 mg/d) + risk for renal stones on stone risk profile Creatinine clearance <60 mL/min
Additional recommendations from the American Association of Endocrine Surgeons: Neurocognitive and/or neuropsychiatric symptoms, cardiovascular disease (other than hypertension), muscle weakness, impaired functional capacity, abnormal sleep patterns gastroesophageal reflux and fibromyalgia symptoms	

Data from Refs.[39,49]

available. The success of ultrasound is dependent on operator experience, and the technique is limited in visualizing multiglandular disease and enlarged glands outside the neck. The radioisotope used most commonly in parathyroid scintigraphy is technetium Tc 99m sestamibi. Sestamibi imaging (**Fig. 4**) depends on the uptake and retention of radiotracer in mitochondria-rich cells like parathyroid chief cells. Various sestamibi protocols are used including dual phase, Iodine 131 subtraction, single-photon emission CT (SPECT), and SPECT-CT imaging. SPECT provides 3-dimensional imaging for better visualization of posterior low-lying superior adenomas, not well seen on ultrasound, and can localize glands in ectopic locations like the mediastinum.[39] Combining ultrasound and sestamibi improves the sensitivity and localization accuracy.[39] A 4-D–CT (**Fig. 5**) provides detailed anatomic and functional data; however, there with increased radiation exposure, and costs than ultrasound. Under ideal conditions, a radiologist, experienced in analyzing the results, does the interpretation. Magnetic resonance imaging (MRI) and venous sampling are not recommended routinely.[39] Fluorine 18 (^{18}F)-fluorocholine PET/CT or PET/MRI (**Fig. 6**) is a modality currently being studied, with promising results.[42–44] Choline is part of the phospholipid layer in the cell membrane. It is hypothesized that hyperfunctioning parathyroid cells increase the phospholipid/calcium-dependent protein kinase activity thus leading to increased choline uptake.[44] Therefore, radiolabeled choline tracer (such as ^{18}F-fluorocholine) can improve detection of abnormal parathyroid glands. The technique can positively localize adenomas with high accuracy and provide detailed anatomic information in settings where conventional imaging results are inconclusive.[44]

The 2 approaches for surgical treatment of PHPT are the minimally invasive parathyroidectomy (MIP) and the bilateral neck exploration, with the former favored for the high cure and low complication rates in for patients with a single parathyroid adenoma.[45] Intraoperative PTH monitoring is key, especially in patients who may have multiglandular disease (with nonlocalizing imaging studies) as well as when a focused or MIP is done. Immediately after surgical excision of a single adenoma, intraoperative PTH should decrease by at least 50% and should decrease to the normal range within 15 minutes to 30 minutes postoperatively.[3] Cure rates in the hands of experienced surgeons exceed 95%.[41] Although rare, surgical complications include recurrent laryngeal nerve injury, hypoparathyroidism due to unintended removal of or damage to

Table 5
Imaging for parathyroid localization

Imaging Modality	Advantages	Disadvantages	Sensitivity (%)[64,a]	Positive Predictive Value (%)[64,a]
Ultrasound	• Assesses concomitant thyroid disease • No ionizing radiation or contrast • Low cost • Widely available • Ease of use	• Operator dependent • False positive from thyroid or lymph node pathology • Poor visualization in obese patients, multiglandular disease, posterior low-lying superior or inferior glands	76.1	93.2
Technetium Tc 99m-labeled sestamibi	• Assesses function of parathyroid tissue • Low ionizing radiation • Visualizes deep cervical, ectopic glands	• Cannot assess thyroid disease • False-positive results if thyroid or lymph node pathology • Poor visualization in patients with multiglandular disease • Higher costs	78.9	90.7
4-D-CT	• Detailed anatomic and functional data (including ectopic gland localization) • Visualizes normal parathyroid glands • Useful for localization in reoperations	• Increased radiation exposure • High cost • Not widely available • Specially trained radiologist to interpret results • Requires contrast administration	89.4	93.5
18F-fluorocholine PET/CT or PET/MRI	• Higher uptake in parathyroid than thyroid tissue • Localizes multiglandular disease and ectopic glands • Shorter study time	• Higher costs • Not widely available • Not Food and Drug Administration approved for this indication	90–94[38,39]	97–100[20,21]

[a] Note: specificity and negative predictive values were not calculated as the inclusion criteria included biochemical confirmation of PHPT.

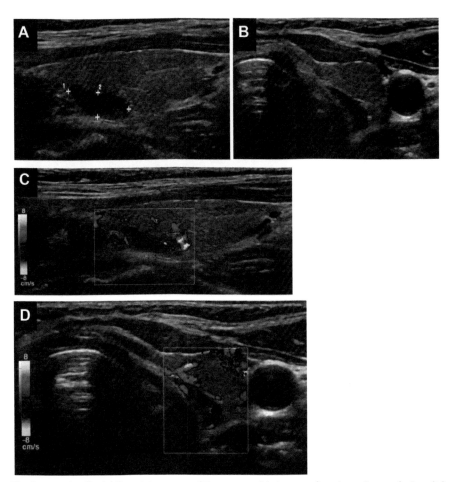

Fig. 3. Longitudinal (*A*) and transverse (*B*) sonographic images showing a hypoechoic solid structure (delineated by electronic calipers) deep to the left thyroid lobe, consistent with a parathyroid adenoma in a patient with PHPT. Color Doppler ultrasound is used to show vascularity within the lesion (longitudinal [*C*] and transverse [*D*]).

parathyroid glands, bleeding, and infection. In addition, recurrent or persistent hyperparathyroidism can be seen in approximately 2% to 5% of patients.[46]

Medical Management

Asymptomatic patients with PHPT, who do not meet surgical criteria, and patients who decline parathyroidectomy or are deemed to be poor surgical candidates can be managed medically with conservative follow-up. An observational study over a 10-year period showed that the biochemistries of patients with PHPT who did not undergo parathyroidectomy often remained stable for many years.[31] Although when looked at after 15 years, the BMD of those medically followed patients showed declines at cortical sites after a decade with progression of disease in nearly 40% of patients.[47]

Recommendations for surveillance include annual plasma calcium and plasma creatinine and eGFR; monitoring for end-organ damage with DXA scanning every 1

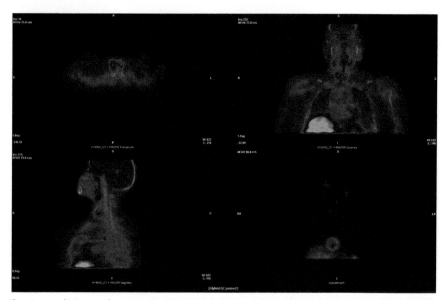

Fig. 4. Localizing technetium Tc 99m sestamibi parathyroid imaging study. Delayed tomographic images showed delayed persistent uptake in the inferior right thyroid region, consistent with a single parathyroid adenoma.

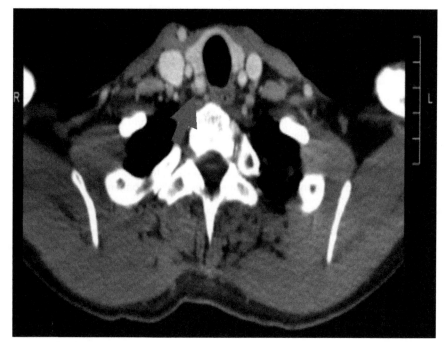

Fig. 5. Right upper parathyroid adenoma (*arrow*) identified in the arterial phase of the 4-D–CT in a patient with PHPT.

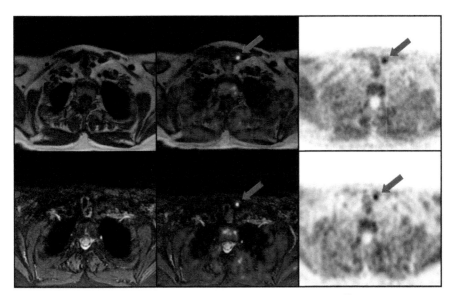

Fig. 6. Left inferior parathyroid adenoma (*red arrows*) identified on ^{18}F-fluorocholine PET/ MRI ([*left upper* and *lower panels*] MRI, [*middle upper* and *lower panels*] fused PET/MRI, [*right upper* and *lower panels*] ^{18}F-fluorocholine PET) in a patient with PHPT.

years to 2 years and vertebral fracture assessment; and abdominal imaging to evaluate nephrolithiasis, all as clinically indicated (**Table 6**). Although there is no curative medical therapy for PHPT, any pharmacologic intervention should address bone disease, hypercalcemia, and hypercalciuria as appropriate for the individual patient.

Calcium and Vitamin D Intake

Restricting dietary calcium is not recommended, because doing so can stimulate parathyroid tissue and increase PTH levels.[48,49] Studies of patients with PHPT support the idea that those with mild PHPT and mild hypercalcemia should consume diets that are not calcium restricted. Should the patient with PHPT have low bone mass or osteoporosis, then modest calcium supplementation can be considered, in the range of 500 mg per day, with careful monitoring of plasma calcium values in such individuals.[50] In a small study of patients with mild PHPT, calcium supplementation (500 mg daily) was given if the baseline calcium intake was less than 450 mg daily, whereas those whose baseline calcium intake exceeded 450 mg daily did not receive supplementation. Patients who received calcium supplementation exhibited a significant decrease in PTH as well as a significant increase in femoral neck BMD, as well as nonsignificant increases in serum calcium and urinary calcium excretion.[50]

A large proportion of patients with mild PHPT have reduced serum 25-OH vitamin D levels. In many cases, those levels are deemed insufficient for the maintenance of optimal skeletal health, especially in postmenopausal women. Restoring those levels of 25-OH vitamin D to what is considered sufficient based on country-wide standards can be challenging. Additionally, there are few systematic studies supporting a regimen that safely accomplishes this goal. In a randomized trial, patients with PHPT were randomized to treatment with 2800 international units (IU) of vitamin D_3 daily (N = 20) or placebo (N = 20), and their biochemical and densitometric parameters were compared.[51] Reductions in serum PTH were observed with vitamin D

Table 6
Surveillance of medically managed primary hyperparathyroidism

Test	Frequency
Laboratory	
Serum calcium	Annual
Serum creatinine and eGFR	Annual
Skeletal involvement	
DXA (lumbar spine, total hip or distal-third radius)	Every 1–2 y
Vertebral fracture (radiograph, CT, vertebral fracture assessment by DXA, MRI)	As clinically indicated
Renal involvement	
Abdominal imaging (radiograph, ultrasonography, CT scan)	As clinically indicated

Adapted from Bilezikian JP, Brandi ML, Eastell R, Silverberg SJ, Udelsman R, Marcocci C, et al. Guidelines for the Management of Asymptomatic Primary Hyperparathyroidism: Summary Statement from the Fourth International Workshop. J Clin Endocrinol Metab. 2014 Oct 1;99(10):3561–9; with permission.

repletion by 17% and BMD rose by 2.5% in the lumbar spine in those individuals over 6 months, compared with placebo-treated patients.[51] Hypercalcemia and hypercalciuria did not differ between groups, and vitamin D supplementation overall was well-tolerated. Despite this study, older reports of worsening hypercalcemia and hypercalciuria exist; thus, it remains prudent to monitor closely serum and urinary calcium with vitamin D repletion in patients with PHPT.[48] Recommended dosages for vitamin D repletion are 600 IU to 1000 IU of cholecalciferol daily in patients with low serum 25-OH vitamin D to achieve a goal serum 25-OH vitamin D level to greater than or equal to 50 nmol/L (20 ng/mL) at a minimum, or greater than or equal to 75 nmol/L (30 ng/mL).[48,52] Adequate hydration also should be encouraged.

Osteoporosis

Estrogen therapy in patients with PHPT may decrease bone resorption and improve BMD in postmenopausal women[53] and may be considered in women with menopausal symptoms without contraindications to estrogen.[48]

There are limited data on the selective estrogen response modulator raloxifene from an 8-week study in postmenopausal women (N = 18) with asymptomatic PHPT.[54] Serum calcium significantly decreased, as did bone turnover markers, whereas serum PTH; 1,25-OH vitamin D; total alkaline phosphatase; and urinary calcium excretion remained unchanged.[54]

Alendronate has been studied more widely in patients with PHPT and osteoporosis, with limited data on other bisphosphonates. Alendronate treatment increases BMD significantly at the lumbar spine and the hip after 1 year or 2 years, although not at the distal radius.[55–58] Changes in serum total and ionized calcium, PTH, and urine calcium excretion were not observed, and bone turnover markers were suppressed and remained below baseline.[58] There are no data regarding fracture rate reduction or fracture risk, however, because these studies were under-powered for such endpoints.

A small study of denosumab in postmenopausal women with PHPT or osteoporosis showed that after 2 years, there were significantly greater increases in BMD at the spine, total hip, and femoral neck in women with PHPT compared with those seen in women with osteoporosis.[59] Additionally, serum and urinary calcium and serum

PTH levels were higher in patients with PHPT. Although these results are promising, further studies evaluating the role of denosumab in the medical management of PHPT are warranted.

Cinacalcet

Cinacalcet is a calcimimetic that binds to the calcium-sensing receptor and increases its sensitivity to the ambient calcium concentration, thereby enhancing the inhibition of PTH secretion. Approved indications for its use in the United States in PHPT include treatment of hypercalcemia in patients with parathyroid cancer and in patients with PHPT indicated for surgery but unable to undergo it. In Europe, cinacalcet is approved for patients with PHPT who meet surgical criteria on the basis of serum calcium levels although cannot undergo parathyroidectomy.[60,61]

Several studies support the use of cinacalcet in patients with PHPT who are not surgical candidates. A large meta-analysis of 28 studies of patients with PHPT treated with cinacalcet reported that the higher the baseline serum calcium level, the greater the calcium reduction with cinacalcet.[62] A phase 3, multicenter, randomized trial of 67 patients who met surgical criteria for parathyroidectomy but were unable or unwilling to undergo parathyroidectomy showed that cinacalcet normalized calcium levels by 28 weeks.[61] Additionally, a similar reduction in serum calcium over 16 weeks was observed in a study of patients with intractable PHPT (defined as a serum calcium >12.5 mg/dL and did not respond to parathyroid surgery or for whom surgery was contraindicated).[63]

In a 1-year study of cinacalcet in patients with mild to moderate PHPT, serum calcium normalized, plasma PTH levels declined, bone turnover markers increased, and BMD remained stable.[64] Cinacalcet also increased serum phosphate levels and reduced fasting and 24-hour urinary calcium excretion. Patients were followed for an additional 4.5 years, and normocalcemia was maintained across the spectrum of serum calcium concentrations, plasma PTH levels were reduced, and alkaline phosphatase activity levels increased, although no significant changes in BMD were demonstrated.[65] Cinacalcet generally was well tolerated; reported side effects included arthralgia, myalgias, diarrhea, upper respiratory symptoms, and nausea. Cinacalcet has not been shown to decrease the risk of developing nephrolithiasis, but patients with renal stones and/or at high risk of recurrent stones are often not included in these trials, because surgery often is performed expeditiously. The effects of cinacalcet therapy on bone turnover markers are not consistent across studies; however, the data are limited.

Cinacalcet also may be useful in the management of moderate to significant hypercalcemia in the perioperative period. A small study of 23 patients with hypercalcemia (serum [Ca] >12.5 mg/dL) awaiting parathyroidectomy showed that cinacalcet rapidly reduced serum [Ca] to 11.3 mg/dL or lower with minimal side effects.[66]

Combination therapy with cinacalcet and a bisphosphonate like alendronate may be considered in patients with significant hypercalcemia and low BMD.[67] Combining the 2 agents has been shown to maintain and/or increase BMD while lowering serum calcium, whereas cinacalcet alone in the comparison group in this study showed similarly controlled serum calcium and PTH levels but no change in BMD.[67] To date, randomized controlled trials with that study design have not been conducted.

Cinacalcet and denosumab have been studied in a randomized placebo-controlled trial in PHPT. Patients were randomized to receive denosumab (N = 16), denosumab and cinacalcet (N = 15), or placebo (N = 15).[68] Larger increases in BMD were observed in those receiving denosumab, regardless of whether or not they received cinacalcet.

SUMMARY

PHPT is a common cause of hypercalcemia, especially in postmenopausal women. Although previously a symptomatic disorder with skeletal, renal, gastrointestinal, and psychological complications, it now is a largely asymptomatic disease in countries where routine screening and biochemical testing are done. Surgery is the definitive treatment, with cure rates exceeding 95% with an experienced surgeon and accurate preoperative localization. For those patients who are unable to undergo parathyroidectomy, medical management with close biochemical and BMD monitoring is a possible option.

CLINICS CARE POINTS

- PHPT is a common cause of hypercalcemia, especially in postmenopausal women. It is characterized by elevated or inappropriately normal PTH levels, due to an increased secretion of PTH.

- Sporadic PHPT is associated with genetic alterations of the *cyclin D1* and *MEN1* genes, located on chromosome 11.

- Although routine screening and biochemical testing have led to PHPT presenting asymptomatically at the present time, appropriate screening for end-organ complications is recommended.

- Parathyroidectomy is the definitive treatment of PHPT, with high cure rates given an experienced surgeon and preoperative localization. For patients who cannot undergo surgery, close monitoring and pharmacologic approaches, including cinacalcet, can be considered.

ACKNOWLEDGMENTS

The authors appreciate Vickie Feldstein, MD; Miguel Pampaloni, MD; Quan-Yang Duh, MD; and Insoo Suh, MD, for sharing of images and insights.

DISCLOSURE

The authors have nothing to disclose.

REFERENCES

1. Walker MD, Silverberg SJ. Primary hyperparathyroidism. Nat Rev Endocrinol 2018;14(2):115–25.
2. Walker MD, Bilezikian JP. Primary hyperparathyroidism: recent advances. Curr Opin Rheumatol 2018;30(4):427–39.
3. Bilezikian JP. Primary hyperparathyroidism. J Clin Endocrinol Metab 2018; 103(11):3993–4004.
4. Miller BS, Dimick J, Wainess R, et al. Age- and sex-related incidence of surgically treated primary hyperparathyroidism. World J Surg 2008;32(5):795–9.
5. Yeh MW, Ituarte PHG, Zhou HC, et al. Incidence and prevalence of primary hyperparathyroidism in a racially mixed population. J Clin Endocrinol Metab 2013; 98(3):1122–9.
6. Wermers RA, Khosla S, Atkinson EJ, et al. Incidence of primary hyperparathyroidism in Rochester, Minnesota, 1993-2001: an update on the changing epidemiology of the disease. J Bone Miner Res 2006;21(1):171–7.

7. Press DM, Siperstein AE, Berber E, et al. The prevalence of undiagnosed and unrecognized primary hyperparathyroidism: a population-based analysis from the electronic medical record. Surgery 2013;154(6):1232–7 [discussion: 1237–8].

8. Silverberg SJ, Walker MD, Bilezikian JP. Asymptomatic primary hyperparathyroidism. J Clin Densitom 2013;16(1):14–21.

9. Pradeep PV, Jayashree B, Mishra A, et al. Systematic review of primary hyperparathyroidism in India: the past, present, and the future trends. Int J Endocrinol 2011;2011:921814.

10. Bilezikian JP, Meng X, Shi Y, et al. Primary hyperparathyroidism in women: a tale of two cities–New York and Beijing. Int J Fertil Womens Med 2000;45(2):158–65.

11. Liu J, Cusano NE, Silva BC, et al. Primary hyperparathyroidism: a tale of two cities revisited — New York and Shanghai. Bone Res 2013;1(1):162–9.

12. Arnold A, Shattuck TM, Mallya SM, et al. Molecular pathogenesis of primary hyperparathyroidism. J Bone Miner Res 2002;17(Suppl 2):N30–6.

13. DeLellis RA. Parathyroid tumors and related disorders. Mod Pathol 2011;24(2):S78–93.

14. Mizamtsidi M, Nastos C, Mastorakos G, et al. Diagnosis, management, histology and genetics of sporadic primary hyperparathyroidism: old knowledge with new tricks. Endocr Connect 2018;7(2):R56–68.

15. Brewer K, Costa-Guda J, Arnold A. Molecular genetic insights into sporadic primary hyperparathyroidism. Endo Rel Canc 2019;26(2):R53–72.

16. Cope O. The study of hyperparathyroidism at the Massachusetts General Hospital. N Engl J Med 1966;274(21):1174–82.

17. Khosla S, Melton LJ, Wermers RA, et al. Primary hyperparathyroidism and the risk of fracture: a population-based study. J Bone Min Res 1999;14(10):1700–7.

18. Vignali E, Viccica G, Diacinti D, et al. Morphometric vertebral fractures in postmenopausal women with primary hyperparathyroidism. J Clin Endocrinol Metab 2009;94(7):2306–12.

19. Bandeira F, Cusano NE, Silva BC, et al. Bone disease in primary hyperparathyroidism. Arq Bras Endocrinol Metabol 2014;58(5):553–61.

20. Silverberg SJ, Gartenberg F, Jacobs TP, et al. Longitudinal measurements of bone density and biochemical indices in untreated primary hyperparathyroidism. J Clin Endocrinol Metab 1995;80(3):723–8.

21. Christiansen P, Steiniche T, Brixen K, et al. Primary hyperparathyroidism: short-term changes in bone remodeling and bone mineral density following parathyroidectomy. Bone 1999;25(2):237–44.

22. Ejlsmark-Svensson H, Rolighed L, Harsløf T, et al. Risk of fractures in primary hyperparathyroidism: a systematic review and meta-analysis. Osteoporos Int 2021;32:1053–60. Available at: https://doi.org/10.1007/s00198-021-05822-9. Accessed March 21, 2021.

23. Vestergaard P, Mosekilde L. Fractures in patients with primary hyperparathyroidism: nationwide follow-up study of 1201 patients. World J Surg 2003;27(3):343–9.

24. Ejlsmark-Svensson H, Bislev LS, Lajlev S, et al. Prevalence and Risk of Vertebral Fractures in Primary Hyperparathyroidism: A Nested Case-Control Study. J Bone Miner Res 2018;33(9):1657–64.

25. Cipriani C, Biamonte F, Costa AG, et al. Prevalence of kidney stones and vertebral fractures in primary hyperparathyroidism using imaging technology. J Clin Endocrinol Metab 2015;100(4):1309–15.

26. Vestergaard P, Mosekilde L. Cohort study on effects of parathyroid surgery on multiple outcomes in primary hyperparathyroidism. BMJ 2003;327(7414):530–4.

27. VanderWalde LH, Liu I-LA, O'Connell TX, et al. The effect of parathyroidectomy on bone fracture risk in patients with primary hyperparathyroidism. Arch Surg 2006; 141(9):885–9 [discussion: 889–91].

28. Rejnmark L, Vestergaard P, Mosekilde L. Nephrolithiasis and renal calcifications in primary hyperparathyroidism. J Clin Endocrinol Metab 2011;96(8):2377–85.

29. Lila AR, Sarathi V, Jagtap V, et al. Renal manifestations of primary hyperparathyroidism. Indian J Endocrinol Metab 2012;16(2):258–62.

30. Walker MD, Nickolas T, Kepley A, et al. Predictors of renal function in primary hyperparathyroidism. J Clin Endocrinol Metab 2014;99(5):1885–92.

31. Silverberg SJ, Shane E, Jacobs TP, et al. A 10-year prospective study of primary hyperparathyroidism with or without parathyroid surgery. N Engl J Med 1999; 341(17):1249–55.

32. Tassone F, Guarnieri A, Castellano E, et al. Parathyroidectomy halts the deterioration of renal function in primary hyperparathyroidism. J Clin Endocrinol Metab 2015;100(8):3069–73.

33. Walker MD, Rubin M, Silverberg SJ. Non-traditional manifestations of primary hyperparathyroidism. J Clin Densitom 2013;16(1):40–7.

34. Walker MD, Silverberg SJ. Cardiovascular aspects of primary hyperparathyroidism. J Endocrinol Invest 2008;31(10):925–31.

35. Abboud B, Daher R, Boujaoude J. Digestive manifestations of parathyroid disorders. World J Gastroenterol 2011;17(36):4063–6.

36. Chan AK, Duh QY, Katz MH, et al. Clinical manifestations of primary hyperparathyroidism before and after parathyroidectomy. A case-control study. Ann Surg 1995;222(3):402–14.

37. Silva BC, Cusano NE, Bilezikian JP. Primary hyperparathyroidism. Best Pract Res Clin Endocrinol Metab 2018;32(5):593–607.

38. Cusano NE, Silverberg SJ, Bilezikian JP. Normocalcemic Primary Hyperparathyroidism. J Clin Densitom 2013;16(1):33–9.

39. Wilhelm SM, Wang TS, Ruan DT, et al. The American Association of Endocrine Surgeons Guidelines for Definitive Management of Primary Hyperparathyroidism. JAMA Surg 2016;151(10):959–68.

40. Singh Ospina NM, Rodriguez-Gutierrez R, Maraka S, et al. Outcomes of parathyroidectomy in patients with primary hyperparathyroidism: a systematic review and meta-analysis. World J Surg 2016;40(10):2359–77.

41. Kuzminski SJ, Sosa JA, Hoang JK. Update in parathyroid imaging. Magn Reson Imaging Clin N Am 2018;26(1):151–66.

42. Kim S-J, Lee S-W, Jeong SY, et al. Diagnostic performance of F-18 Fluorocholine PET/CT for parathyroid localization in hyperparathyroidism: a systematic review and meta-analysis. Horm Canc 2018;9(6):440–7.

43. Uslu-Beşli L, Sonmezoglu K, Teksoz S, et al. Performance of F-18 Fluorocholine PET/CT for detection of hyperfunctioning parathyroid tissue in patients with elevated parathyroid hormone levels and negative or discrepant results in conventional imaging. Korean J Radiol 2020;21(2):236–47.

44. Kluijfhout WP, Pasternak JD, Gosnell JE, et al. 18F Fluorocholine PET/MR imaging in patients with primary hyperparathyroidism and inconclusive conventional imaging: a prospective pilot study. Radiology 2017;284(2):460–7.

45. Ruda JM, Hollenbeak CS, Stack BC. A systematic review of the diagnosis and treatment of primary hyperparathyroidism from 1995 to 2003. Otolaryngol Head Neck Surg 2005;132(3):359–72.

46. Mazotas IG, Yen TWF, Doffek K, et al. Persistent/recurrent primary hyperparathyroidism: does the number of abnormal glands play a role? J Surg Res 2020;246: 335–41.
47. Rubin MR, Bilezikian JP, McMahon DJ, et al. The natural history of primary hyperparathyroidism with or without parathyroid surgery after 15 years. J Clin Endocrinol Metab 2008;93(9):3462–70.
48. Marcocci C, Bollerslev J, Khan AA, et al. Medical management of primary hyperparathyroidism: proceedings of the fourth International Workshop on the Management of Asymptomatic Primary Hyperparathyroidism. J Clin Endocrinol Metab 2014;99(10):3607–18.
49. Bilezikian JP, Brandi ML, Eastell R, et al. Guidelines for the Management of Asymptomatic Primary Hyperparathyroidism: Summary Statement from the Fourth International Workshop. J Clin Endocrinol Metab 2014;99(10):3561–9.
50. Jorde R, Szumlas K, Haug E, et al. The effects of calcium supplementation to patients with primary hyperparathyroidism and a low calcium intake. Eur J Nutr 2002;41(6):258–63.
51. Rolighed L, Rejnmark L, Sikjaer T, et al. Vitamin D treatment in primary hyperparathyroidism: a randomized placebo controlled trial. J Clin Endocrinol Metab 2014; 99(3):1072–80.
52. Cetani F, Saponaro F, Marcocci C. Non-surgical management of primary hyperparathyroidism. Best Pract Res Clin Endocrinol Metab 2018;32(6):821–35.
53. Grey AB, Stapleton JP, Evans MC, et al. Effect of hormone replacement therapy on bone mineral density in postmenopausal women with mild primary hyperparathyroidism. A randomized, controlled trial. Ann Intern Med 1996;125(5):360–8.
54. Rubin MR, Lee KH, McMahon DJ, et al. Raloxifene lowers serum calcium and markers of bone turnover in postmenopausal women with primary hyperparathyroidism. J Clin Endocrinol Metab 2003;88(3):1174–8.
55. Rossini M, Gatti D, Isaia G, et al. Effects of oral alendronate in elderly patients with osteoporosis and mild primary hyperparathyroidism. J Bone Miner Res 2001;16(1):113–9.
56. Parker CR, Blackwell PJ, Fairbairn KJ, et al. Alendronate in the treatment of primary hyperparathyroid-related osteoporosis: a 2-year study. J Clin Endocrinol Metab 2002;87(10):4482–9.
57. Chow CC, Chan WB, Li JKY, et al. Oral alendronate increases bone mineral density in postmenopausal women with primary hyperparathyroidism. J Clin Endocrinol Metab 2003;88(2):581–7.
58. Khan AA, Bilezikian JP, Kung AWC, et al. Alendronate in primary hyperparathyroidism: a double-blind, randomized, placebo-controlled trial. J Clin Endocrinol Metab 2004;89(7):3319–25.
59. Eller-Vainicher C, Palmieri S, Cairoli E, et al. Protective effect of denosumab on bone in older women with primary hyperparathyroidism. J Am Geriatr Soc 2018;66(3):518–24.
60. Rothe HM, Liangos O, Biggar P, et al. Cinacalcet treatment of primary hyperparathyroidism. Int J Endocrinol 2011;2011.
61. Khan A, Bilezikian J, Bone H, et al. Cinacalcet normalizes serum calcium in a double-blind randomized, placebo-controlled study in patients with primary hyperparathyroidism with contraindications to surgery. Eur J Endocrinol 2015; 172(5):527–35.
62. Ng CH, Chin YH, Tan MHQ, et al. Cinacalcet and primary hyperparathyroidism: systematic review and meta regression. Endocr Connect 2020;9(7):724–35.

63. Marcocci C, Chanson P, Shoback D, et al. Cinacalcet reduces serum calcium concentrations in patients with intractable primary hyperparathyroidism. J Clin Endocrinol Metab 2009;94(8):2766–72.

64. Peacock M, Bilezikian JP, Klassen PS, et al. Cinacalcet hydrochloride maintains long-term normocalcemia in patients with primary hyperparathyroidism. J Clin Endocrinol Metab 2005;90(1):135–41.

65. Peacock M, Bolognese MA, Borofsky M, et al. Cinacalcet treatment of primary hyperparathyroidism: biochemical and bone densitometric outcomes in a five-year study. J Clin Endocrinol Metab 2009;94(12):4860–7.

66. Misiorowski W, Zgliczyński W. Cinacalcet as symptomatic treatment of hypercalcaemia in primary hyperparathyroidism prior to surgery. Endokrynol Pol 2017; 68(3):306–10.

67. Faggiano A, Di Somma C, Ramundo V, et al. Cinacalcet hydrochloride in combination with alendronate normalizes hypercalcemia and improves bone mineral density in patients with primary hyperparathyroidism. Endocrine 2011;39(3): 283–7.

68. Leere JS, Karmisholt J, Robaczyk M, et al. Denosumab and cinacalcet for primary hyperparathyroidism (DENOCINA): a randomised, double-blind, placebo-controlled, phase 3 trial. Lancet Diabetes Endocrinol 2020;8(5):407–17.

Nontraditional Aspects of Sporadic Primary Hyperparathyroidism

Marcella Walker, MD, MS[a], Shonni J. Silverberg, MD[b],*

KEYWORDS

- Cardiovascular • Mortality • Quality of life • Cognition
- Nontraditional manifestations • Primary hyperparathyroidism
- Cardiovascular effects • Neuropsychological effects

KEY POINTS

- Cardiovascular disease, such as hypertension, left ventricular hypertrophy, and increased vascular stiffness, has inconsistently been associated with the modern form of primary hyperparathyroidism.
- Similarly, neuropsychological symptoms, including but not limited to fatigue, anxiety, depression, and altered cognition, have been reported variably.
- The reversibility of such symptoms after parathyroidectomy has not been shown clearly.

INTRODUCTION

Nontraditional aspects of primary hyperparathyroidism (PHPT) refer to the condition's clinical manifestations in organ systems other than the skeletal and kidney. These include its cardiovascular (CV), neuropsychological, gastrointestinal, and rheumatic effects. Despite the term "nontraditional" manifestations, classical PHPT, as described in the early part of the twentieth century, was clearly a multisystemic disorder.[1] It was not only characterized by nephrolithiasis and severe parathyroid bone disease, but also cardiac, neurologic, gastrointestinal, and rheumatic features.[1] The presentation of PHPT has evolved over the last century and today most patients are "asymptomatic," that is, lacking overt symptoms of hypercalcemia or the classical renal, skeletal, and neuromuscular features.[2–4] Whether subtle neuropsychological symptoms as well as CV disease are part of the clinical picture of modern PHPT remains controversial.[5,6] Gastrointestinal and rheumatic sequelae, although rarely studied today, do not seem to be a part of the clinical spectrum of modern PHPT. None of

[a] Division of Endocrinology, Department of Medicine, Columbia University Irving Medical Center, New York, NY 10032, USA; [b] Division of Endocrinology, Department of Medicine, Columbia University, Columbia University Irving Medical Center, New York, NY 10032, USA
* Corresponding author.
E-mail address: Sjs5@columbia.edu

Endocrinol Metab Clin N Am 50 (2021) 629–647
https://doi.org/10.1016/j.ecl.2021.07.007
0889-8529/21/© 2021 Elsevier Inc. All rights reserved.

endo.theclinics.com

the nontraditional manifestations are considered sole indications for recommending parathyroidectomy (PTX) by most experts owing to inconsistent findings with regard to improvement after surgery.[5] This article reviews the nonclassical features of PHPT and reviews recent advances in the literature. We also allude to several nontraditional presentations of PHPT, that is, presentations that are neither classical nor asymptomatic, including acute PHPT, parathyroid cancer, and PHPT in pregnancy, which are covered in greater detail elsewhere in this volume.

CARDIOVASCULAR DISEASE

Definitive conclusions regarding the association between present-day PHPT and CV disease remain uncertain owing to varied results between studies. One explanation for the inconsistencies is the evolution of the clinical profile of PHPT over time, which has led to great variability between cohorts with regard to the biochemical severity of their underlying disease. Some studies suggest that cohorts with the most marked hypercalcemia and hyperparathyroidism have the most CV involvement.[7] Because it is hypothesized that serum calcium and parathyroid hormone (PTH) themselves mediate the CV effects, variability between studies in extent of elevation of serum calcium and PTH could yield inconsistencies.[8] For example, hypercalcemia can increase blood pressure (BP) and cause vasoconstriction and has been associated with a short QT interval, as well as calcification of the myocardium, heart valves, and coronary arteries.[9–11] PTH has been shown to have vascular effects and to potentially act as a hypertrophic factor on myocardial muscle cells, thereby inducing left ventricular hypertrophy.[12–14] Recent studies, however, have included mostly those with relatively mild disease (which has been inconsistently defined in various studies but is often used to refer to those with a serum calcium or a study average serum calcium of <1 mg/dL above the upper limit of normal); these studies, however, have also yielded conflicting results, making it unclear whether this explanation fully accounts for the discrepancies. Modern studies have focused mostly on subclinical CV disease, including hypertension, CV risk factors, valve calcification, left ventricular hypertrophy, cardiac function, and vascular function and stiffness, whereas fewer have investigated coronary artery disease and mortality.

Cardiovascular Mortality

There is evidence to suggest CV mortality is increased in severe classical PHPT, but this finding tends to contrast with data in those with milder disease.[7,15–19] A study from Mayo Clinic may provide insight into these inconsistencies. In mildly hypercalcemic individuals, the overall mortality and CV mortality were decreased, but in those whose serum calcium was in the highest quartile, CV mortality was increased.[7] The concept that the more common asymptomatic form of PHPT is not associated with increased mortality is supported by data from studies in which more recently enrolled subjects had better survival than those who were enrolled earlier and presumably had more active disease.[20]

Hypertension

Hypertension has been reported to be more frequent in those with asymptomatic PHPT than in those without PHPT in a number of studies. A recent study that included 37,922 inpatients with PHPT who were identified as having PHPT by *International Classification of Diseases* coding, indicated that the risk for hypertension was increased by 30% compared with those without PHPT.[21] The mechanism of this association is unknown, and the condition does not clearly remit after cure of the hyperparathyroid state.[22] Some investigators have suggested that the association is due to surveillance bias. Other studies suggest relationships with PTH or other factors. BP increased across PTH tertiles in a recent study.[23] The aldosterone–renin ratio was related to BP and depended on the PTH level in another study of 136 patients with mild PHPT.[24] Observational studies often indicate that the BP improves after PTX.[25] A larger recent retrospective analysis (n = 2380) showed self-selection to PTX decreased BP and antihypertensive use compared with observation.[26] In contrast, 2 randomized clinical trials, the 10-year Scandinavian Investigation of PHPT (SIPH) trial (n = 119) and a smaller, shorter Danish randomized controlled trial (n = 79) as well as other randomized controlled trials (**Table 1**), however, found no benefit of PTX in mild PHPT, suggesting that the relationship is either not causal or is irreversible.[27,28]

Cardiac Risk Factors

Data regarding the associations between PHPT and the metabolic syndrome are conflicting. A meta-analysis indicated higher indices of insulin resistance, but not body mass index, in those with PHPT compared with controls.[29] The SIPH randomized controlled trial, however, found no benefit of PTX on glucose or indices of insulin resistance, fat mass, or cholesterol at 5 years after randomization in patients with asymptomatic PHPT.[30] In contrast, the Danish randomized controlled trial reported that PTX decreased cholesterol in patients with mild PHPT, but this effect was only investigated until 3 months after PTX, raising the possibility that this is a short-term benefit. The latter study did not investigate insulin resistance.[27]

Coronary Artery Disease, Atherosclerosis, and Cardiovascular Events

Data on atherosclerosis are conflicting. Some data suggest that when coronary artery disease is present in PHPT, it is most likely due to traditional risk factors rather than the disease itself.[22,31] A recent study showed higher coronary artery calcification scores were present in a cohort that included those with both mild and classical PHPT (n = 130) compared with controls, but the presence of coronary artery calcification was related to cardiac risk factors, not PTH or serum calcium.[32] In another study that included patients with mild PHPT, there was no association between PHPT and coronary artery calcification.[33] Data on CV events are limited, and prospective studies have reported inconsistent improvement in such events related to atherosclerosis after PTX. A 21-year population-based study found no differences in myocardial infarction, stroke, or death in men with PHPT versus controls.[34] In contrast, a retrospective study indicated atherosclerotic CV events were decreased in those self-selecting to PTX.[35] The SIPH randomized controlled trial showed no difference in CV events at 5 years after randomization to PTX or observation, but events were rare and the study lacked the statistical power for this end point (see **Table 1**).[36]

Atherosclerosis in other parts of the vasculature has also been recently investigated. A recent study suggested that those with moderately severe PHPT (n = 140) had a higher prevalence of abdominal aortic calcifications that were more severe compared with controls without PHPT.[37] The PTH level was significantly associated with calcification severity.[37] The average carotid intima-media thickness, a subclinical marker of atherosclerosis, was higher in patients with mild PHPT compared with controls, but not reversible after PTX.[38] In contrast, a case-control study (n = 204) indicated no association between carotid or femoral plaque or intima-media thickness[23] and biochemically mild PHPT in a cohort that was composed of patients with both symptomatic and asymptomatic disease. Changes in atherosclerosis after PTX are also inconsistent.[39,40]

Table 1
Randomized controlled trials of PTX versus observation on CV outcomes

Study	Study Duration	Serum Calcium	Symptomatic/ Asymptomatic	N	BP	Diastolic Function	LVMI	PWV	CV Vents	Arrhythmia/ Conduction/ VPBs
Almqvist et al,[45] 2002	2 y	10.5 mg/dL	Symptomatic and asymptomatic	50	Not reported	No benefit	**Benefit at 2 y**	Not reported	Not reported	Not reported
Ambrogini et al,[55] 2007	1 y	10.2 mg/dL	Asymptomatic	50	Not reported	No benefit	No benefit	Not reported	Not reported	Not reported
Ejlsmark-Svensson et al,[27] 2019	3 mo	Ionized ca 1.41 mmol/L	Symptomatic and asymptomatic	79	No benefit	Not reported	Not reported	No Benefit	Not reported	Not reported
SIPH Trial Godang et al,[30] 2018; Lundstam et al,[36] 2015 Persson et al,[54] 2011	2–5 y	Albumin adjusted calcium 2.63 mmol/L or 10.5 mg/dL-10.8	Asymptomatic	119 49	No Benefit	No benefit	"Borderline effect"	Not reported	No Benefit	reported
Pepe et al,[79] 2013	6 mo	10.8 mg/dL	Symptomatic and asymptomatic	24	No benefit	No benefit	Not reported No effect on IVS or PWT	Not reported	Not reported	**Benefit**
Pepe et al,[80] 2018	6 mo	Ionized calcium 1.4 mmol/L or 10.9 mg/dL	Symptomatic and asymptomatic	26 pts|/26 controls	Not reported	Reported	Not reported	Not reported	Not reported	**Benefit**

Abbreviations: IVS, interventricular septum thickness; LVMI, left ventricular mass index; PWT, posterior wall thickness; PWV, pulse wave velocity.

Valve Calcification

Valve calcification is present in severe PHPT.[41] Data from those with milder disease are limited. In 1 study, there was no difference in the frequency of valve calcification in those with mild PHPT compared with non-PHPT controls.[42] However, valve calcification, when present, has been shown to be more extensive (ie, there was greater calcification area) in those with mild PHPT versus controls.[38,42] The association may be mediated by PTH, because the PTH level was associated with the valve calcification area, but it is not reversible with PTX.[38]

Cardiac Structure and Function

Left ventricular hypertrophy has been associated with PHPT in many, but not all, studies.[22] A 2015 meta-analysis indicated that PTX is associated with a decrease in left ventricular mass and that higher levels of PTH preoperatively predicted greater regression of left ventricular hypertrophy after surgery. However, this effect tended to be present only in observational studies and not randomized controlled trials (see **Table 1**). Calcium and PTH levels were higher, however, in observational studies than randomized controlled trials, making it difficult to dissociate disease severity from study design.[14] A second meta-analysis (with fewer studies) found that PTX did not improve left ventricular mass.[43]

Diastolic dysfunction has been shown in a number of PHPT studies, although the attribution of causality to PHPT is difficult, because many investigations did not control for BP.[44–50] Two recent studies in mild PHPT in which relevant CV risk factors were excluded or accounted for showed no increase in diastolic function in PHPT.[51,52] In contrast, a third study, which did not adjust for CV risk factors, found evidence of diastolic dysfunction.[53] Diastolic dysfunction was also reported in a study in which patients had higher average calcium levels (10.9 mg/dL vs 10.5 mg/dL in the other 2 studies), which might impair cardiac relaxation to a greater extent.[48] Data on improvement with PTX are also conflicting but, as shown in **Table 1**, randomized controlled trials did not reveal a benefit of PTX on diastolic function.[45,54,55] Although most studies have not indicated that systolic cardiac function is affected in PHPT, a small study suggests that left ventricular asynchrony may be present.[56] A recent meta-analysis showed no change in the left ventricular ejection fraction after PTX.[43]

Endothelial Function

Vascular endothelial dysfunction has been reported to be both normal and abnormal in those with severe or symptomatic PHPT using differing methodologies.[57–60] In those with more moderate hypercalcemia, 1 study showed flow-mediated dilation was impaired and negatively correlated with calcium levels.[61] Studies in those with mild disease have been inconsistent.[62–65] One US study (n = 45) in mild symptomatic and asymptomatic PHPT (mean serum calcium of 10.6 mg/dL) found no evidence of abnormal flow-mediated dilation and no change after PTX.[63] Two other studies indicated lower flow-mediated dilation in patients with PHPT versus controls and improvement after PTX.[64,65] Calcium and PTH were associated with flow-mediated dilation in both studies, but both studies were also characterized by very high mean levels of PTH, which may limit the applicability of these results to many of today's patients with PHPT.

Vascular Stiffness

Several, but not all, studies indicate increased vascular stiffness in various parts of the vasculature in patients with mild PHPT.[39,66–71] In 1 study, PHPT was a stronger predictor of increased aortic stiffness than many traditional CV risk factors, and stiffness was associated with the extent of PTH elevation.[69] Aortic pulse wave velocity, augmentation index and retinal vessel narrowing were worse in PHPT (n = 30) versus controls in a recent study, but only retinal findings were independent of hypertension and correlated with PTH.[72] Several observational studies indicate aortic stiffness improves after PTX, but this may be due to changes in BP postoperatively.[39,66,67] Carotid stiffness has also been shown to be increased in some studies, but not others.[51,70] In 1 study, higher PTH levels predicted greater stiffness, independent of age and renal function, but stiffness did not improve after PTX.[38,51] Recently, a randomized controlled trial has addressed the issue of reversibility of aortic stiffness in PHPT. A Danish randomized controlled trial found no benefit of PTX on vascular function overall, but in a subgroup analysis in those with the highest calcium, pulse wave velocity improved 3 months after PTX, suggesting a possible benefit in those with the most severe disease.[27]

Cardiac Arrhythmias

Although several case reports of arrhythmia appeared in the 1970s and 1980s,[73,74] relatively few studies since have investigated cardiac arrhythmias and conduction disturbances systematically in PHPT. In 1992, Rosenqvist and colleagues[75] studied 20 patients with PHPT and found no increase in the prevalence of cardiac arrhythmias, but did find that the QT interval increased after PTX. The short QT interval in PHPT has been confirmed by multiple other reports.[76–78] More recent studies looked for arrhythmia. In a cohort that included patients with both symptomatic and asymptomatic PHPT, PTX reduced ventricular premature beats during exercise testing and restored normal exercise-induced QT interval adaptations.[79] A small randomized controlled trial that included symptomatic and asymptomatic patients meeting criteria for PTX (n = 26) showed PHPT (mean calcium of 10.9 mg/dL) was associated with a higher prevalence of premature beats and a shorter QT interval. PTX improved these indices versus observation, but only 13 patients were randomized to surgery.[80] Such findings, although suggestive, would benefit from confirmation.

NEUROLOGIC, PSYCHOLOGICAL, AND COGNITIVE FEATURES

Descriptions of classical PHPT indicate neurologic and psychological features.[1] The biochemical hallmarks of PHPT have the potential to affect the nervous system. Calcium has a key role in regulating the release of neurotransmitters at synapses, and hypercalcemia could interfere with that process. In contrast, the long-known vascular effects of PTH could also affect cognition and mood by altering cerebrovascular function.[12] Whether PHPT is causally associated with such symptoms today, however, is controversial.

Neuromuscular Disease

Classic PHPT was previously associated with a distinct neuromuscular syndrome characterized by type II muscle cell atrophy.[81] The syndrome, originally described in 1949, was characterized by easy fatigability, symmetric proximal muscle weakness, and muscle atrophy. Both the clinical and electromyographic features of this disorder were reversible after PTX.[82] In the milder, less symptomatic form of the disease that is, common today, this disorder is rarely seen. Several studies have recently readdressed this issue by assessing more subtle effects on physical function. In asymptomatic PHPT, 1 study suggested reduced knee extension and flexion muscle strength, as well as postural stability compared with controls.[83] Another study showed abnormal muscle strength and performance of the upper and lower limbs in both hypercalcemic and normocalcemic patients with PHPT.[84] Data on the reversibility of such symptoms after PTX are not yet available.

Psychological Symptoms and Quality of Life

Classical PHPT, as described in the early twentieth century, had clear psychological features.[1] Whether psychiatric symptoms and reduced quality of life (QOL) are present in PHPT as it is seen today remains a source of controversy. A retrospective analysis of patients with more severe disease showed a 23% incidence of psychiatric symptomatology (n = 441).[85] However, even those with disease commonly considered "asymptomatic" because of the absence of renal stones or overt bone disease often report depression, anxiety, fatigue, decreased QOL, sleep disturbances, and cognitive dysfunction.[55,86–108] Whether neuropsychological symptoms are specifically attributable to PHPT and reversible after PTX is controversial, and results from both observational studies and randomized trials have been conflicting.[55,95,98,99,109]

As shown in **Table 2**, 3 short-term (1–2 year) randomized controlled trials have investigated the reversibility of decreased QOL and psychiatric symptoms.[55,98,99] Despite being of similar design and using similar assessment tools, all 3 randomized controlled trials came to different conclusions; 1 randomized controlled trial suggested PTX prevents worsening of QOL and improves psychiatric symptoms,[99] another randomized controlled trial indicated no benefit, and the third randomized controlled trial demonstrated improvement in QOL.[55,98] Pretorius and colleagues[110] recently described the 10-year end of study SIPH results on these outcomes (see **Table 2**). This randomized controlled trial of PTX versus observation in patients with mild PHPT addresses the long-term effect of intervention on QOL and psychological indices. After PTX, there was no consistent, global improvement in QOL detected, but also no deterioration in QOL in those who did not undergo surgery. Both the surgical and observation groups had improved psychological function over the decade with no treatment effect. Thus, most data do not indicate a clear benefit of surgery.

Cognition

Observational studies and 1 small randomized controlled trial have investigated cognition.[90,95,100–105,109,111] Although many, but not all, suggest memory to be affected and improvement in memory or other cognitive domains after PTX, the lack of longitudinal surgical or nonsurgical controls in many studies makes attribution of improvement to cure of PHPT difficult.[90,95,100,102–105,111–114] Improvement in noncontrolled studies may be due to learning or placebo effects of surgery.[115] The results of studies in which longitudinal surgical control groups are compared with those undergoing PTX are inconsistent.[90,100,103,113,116] Recent work has turned to the potential mechanisms that contribute to cognitive dysfunction in PHPT. One recent study investigated whether cerebrovascular dysfunction (ie, vascular stiffness) might underlie cognitive changes in patients with PHPT. Although PTH correlated with cerebrovascular function as measured by transcranial Doppler, there was no consistent association between cerebrovascular function and cognitive performance[117] or improvement after PTX.

Functional MRI, a noninvasive tool that maps brain function based on changes in blood flow, was recently used to assess whether cerebral neuronal activation is altered by PHPT.[118] In this study, PHPT was associated with differences in task-related neural activation patterns on MRI, but no difference in cognitive performance. This finding may indicate neuronal compensation in PHPT to maintain the

Table 2
Randomized controlled trials of QOL and psychiatric symptoms

Study	Duration	Serum Calcium	Symptomatic/ Asymptomatic	N	Psychiatric Symptoms	QOL (SF-36)
Talpos et al,[99] 2000; Rao et al,[145] 2004	2 y	10.4 mg/dL	Asymptomatic	53	Benefit on anxiety and phobia	Benefit social and emotional role function
Ambrogini et al,[55] 2007	1 y	10.2 mg/dL	Asymptomatic	50	No benefit	Benefit on bodily pain; general health; vitality; mental health
SIPH						
Bollerslev et al,[98] 2007	2 y	10.8 mg/dL	Asymptomatic	191	No benefit	No benefit
Pretoriuset al,[110] 2021	10 y	10.6	Asymptomatic	129 at 10 y	No benefit	Benefit on vitality only, uncertain clinical significance

same cognitive function, but there was no clear improvement in neural activation after PTX.[118] At present, most experts do not recognize cognitive or psychiatric symptoms as a sole indication for PTX. Reasons for this include the failure to clearly demonstrate reversibility in randomized controlled trials, the inability to predict which patients might improve, and the lack of a clear mechanism to explain such findings.[5]

OTHER SYSTEMIC INVOLVEMENT

Many organ systems were affected by the hyperparathyroid state in the past. Anemia, band keratopathy, and loose teeth are no longer seen in PHPT. Gout and pseudogout are observed very infrequently, and their etiologic relationship to PHPT is not clear. The gastrointestinal system is rarely affected except in multiple endocrine neoplasia type 1 that includes gastrinoma as a part of the syndrome.

Rheumatological Disease

Classical PHPT was rarely associated with hyperuricemia, gout, and calcium pyrophosphate crystal deposition disease.[119–121] Pseudogout, a complication of calcium pyrophosphate crystal deposition disease in which calcium pyrophosphate crystal deposition causes synovitis, has been reported after the surgical cure of PHPT,[122] although the mechanism of this association is unclear.[122] Overt rheumatologic manifestations are mainly a historical phenomenon and not part of the clinical spectrum of modern disease.[123]

Gastrointestinal Manifestations

Classic PHPT was associated with peptic ulcer disease. There is no clear causal association between the modern phenotype of sporadic PHPT and peptic ulcer disease. In multiple endocrine neoplasia type 1 syndrome, about 40% of patients have clinically apparent gastrinomas (Zollinger–Ellison syndrome).[124] Gastrinoma is more severe in those with coexisting PHPT, and Zollinger–Ellison syndrome improves with surgical treatment of PHPT.[124] However, medical therapy is very effective and thus PTX is not necessarily recommended in those with gastrinoma.

Gastrointestinal symptoms related to severe hypercalcemia such as abdominal pain, nausea, vomiting, and constipation are virtually never observed in the United States today given the mild degree of hypercalcemia. In contrast, in the developing world, a minority present with gastrointestinal symptoms.[125] Pancreatitis is virtually never observed as a complication of modern PHPT given its usual mild degree of hypercalcemia.[8] Recent work indicates that patients with celiac disease are at increased risk for developing PHPT.[126] It is unclear whether this association is causal.

Cancer

There are inconsistent data regarding whether cancer is more common in patients with PHPT. Several studies report an increased risk of cancer and cancer deaths.[19,127,128] Some data suggest the risk persists even after PTX.[129] Several types of cancer have been associated with PHPT, including gastrointestinal and genitourinary malignancies and multiple myeloma, as well as breast and thyroid cancers, among others. A US study, however, suggested risk of cancer death was decreased, rather than increased, in patients with PHPT.[7] It is important to consider that the associations observed between PHPT and cancer in some investigations might not be causal, but secondary to confounding or surveillance bias.

UNUSUAL PRESENTATIONS

PHPT is typically asymptomatic today, although a minority of patients have symptomatic nephrolithiasis or fractures. Hypercalcemia is usually mild and the disease most often presents in women after menopause. Unusual presentations include parathyroid cancer (covered in Filomena Cetani and colleagues' article, "Parathyroid Carcinoma and Ectopic Secretion of PTH," in this issue), acute primary hyperparathyroidism, both of which are characterized by marked hypercalcemia, and presenting during pregnancy (covered in Karel Dandurand and colleagues' article, "Hypercalcemia in Pregnancy," in this issue).

Acute Primary Hyperparathyroidism

Acute PHPT, also known as parathyroid crisis, parathyroid poisoning, parathyroid intoxication, and parathyroid storm, describes an episode of life-threatening hypercalcemia of sudden onset in a patient with PHPT. Clinical manifestations of acute PHPT are mainly related to the severe hypercalcemia. Nephrocalcinosis, nephrolithiasis, and radiologic evidence of subperiosteal bone resorption may be present. Laboratory evaluation is remarkable for very high serum calcium levels and PTH levels that may be 20 times normal.[130] Thus, acute PHPT resembles parathyroid carcinoma, biochemically. In about 25% of patients, there is a history of antecedent, persistent mild hypercalcemia. The risk of developing acute PHPT in mild asymptomatic PHPT is very low and acute hyperparathyroidism remains a rare phenomenon. Intercurrent medical illness with immobilization may precipitate acute PHPT. Early diagnosis, with aggressive medical therapy followed by surgical cure, is recommended. Acute PHPT may be mistaken for hypercalcemia of malignancy in those without a prior known history of hypercalcemia. The PTH level, however, usually quickly elucidates the diagnosis.

Parathyroid Cancer

Parathyroid carcinoma, which represents less than 1% of cases of PHPT, is indolent, but life threatening and often incurable.[131] The clinical profile of parathyroid cancer is distinct from that of benign PHPT in several notable ways.[132] First, parathyroid carcinoma is typically characterized by marked hypercalcemia. The elevations are greater than those seen with benign PHPT. Similarly, PTH levels tend to be far higher compared with those with benign adenomas or hyperplasia. In those with carcinoma, there is no female predominance. Ultimately, the main morbidity of parathyroid carcinoma is typically due to hypercalcemia itself. However, because the hyperparathyroid disease is much more severe, the classic targets of PTH excess are affected in most cases. Nephrolithiasis or nephrocalcinosis is seen in up to 60% of patients, and overt radiologic evidence of skeletal involvement is seen in 35% to 90% of patients.[132,133]

A palpable neck mass, unusual in benign PHPT, has been reported in 30% to 76% of patients with parathyroid carcinoma.[134] On pathology, malignant glands are large, sometimes exceeding 12 g. Glands are often adherent to adjacent structures, but the disease tends to spread slowly in the neck.[134] A late finding is metastatic disease. The most common sites are lung (40%), liver (10%), and lymph nodes (30%). Parathyroid carcinoma may be part of a hereditary syndromes, particularly hyperparathyroidism-jaw tumor syndrome.[135–139] Parathyroid carcinoma has also been reported in familial isolated hyperparathyroidism[136,140] and multiple endocrine neoplasia type 1.[141–143] Thus, a family history may be present, which is unusual in those with benign disease.

Primary Hyperparathyroidism in Pregnancy

PHPT in pregnancy is primarily of concern related to its potential effects on the fetus and neonate. Potential complications of PHPT in pregnancy include spontaneous abortion, low birth weight, supravalvular aortic stenosis, and neonatal tetany. The latter results from fetal parathyroid gland suppression by high levels of maternal calcium, which readily crosses the placenta during pregnancy. These infants, acclimated to hypercalcemia in utero, have functional, reversible hypoparathyroidism after birth, and can develop hypocalcemia and tetany in the first few days of life. Although infrequent, neonatologists should be made aware of this possibility before delivery. Today, an individualized approach to the management of the pregnant patient with mild PHPT is advised. A recent retrospective study suggested that the modern form of PHPT does not increase the risk of abortion, low birth weight, or a low Apgar score.[144] Thus, many of those with mild disease can be followed safely, without surgery. However, PTX during the second trimester remains the conventional recommendation for this condition.

SUMMARY

Today, PHPT typically presents with mild hypercalcemia in otherwise asymptomatic patients. In a minority of patients, symptomatic nephrolithiasis or fractures may be present. Unusual presentations include acute hyperparathyroidism, parathyroid cancer, and detection during pregnancy. Neuropsychological symptoms such as altered mood and cognition are commonly reported by patients with the modern form of PHPT and variably demonstrated in studies. Overt CV disease does not seem to be part of mild PHPT. Subclinical CV disease has been detected, although causality remains controversial. The majority of evidence does not support reversibility of neuropsychiatric or CV manifestations after PTX and therefore neither is considered a sole indication for recommending surgery. An individualized approach to PHPT that takes into account particular patient concerns, preferences, and risk factors as well as the availability of an experienced surgeon has, however, always been recommended when considering surgery or observation. This approach is advisable in patients with nonclassical manifestations as well, but it is important to set appropriate evidence-based expectations regarding the lack of robust data to indicate improvement of such manifestations after PTX.

CLINICS CARE POINTS

- Data regarding the nontraditional manifestations of PHPT continue to evolve.
- Currently, clinical evaluation for nontraditional features of PHPT including CV, neuropsychological, gastrointestinal disease, is not recommended.
- Nonclassical manifestations are not considered a sole indication for PTX, but it is important to take into account patient-specific and physician factors in this decision.

DISCLOSURE

The authors have nothing to disclose.

REFERENCES

1. Albright F, Aub J, Bauer W. Hyperparathyroidism: common and polymorphic condition as illustrated by seventeen proven cases in one clinic. JAMA 1934; 102:1276.

2. Walker MD, Silverberg SJ. Primary hyperparathyroidism. Nat Rev Endocrinol 2018;14(2):115–25.

3. Cope O. The study of hyperparathyroidism at the Massachusetts General Hospital. N Engl J Med 1966;274(21):1174–82.

4. Silverberg SJ, et al. A 10-year prospective study of primary hyperparathyroidism with or without parathyroid surgery. N Engl J Med 1999;341(17):1249–55.

5. Bilezikian JP, et al. Guidelines for the management of asymptomatic primary hyperparathyroidism: summary statement from the Fourth International Workshop. J Clin Endocrinol Metab 2014;99(10):3561–9.

6. Silverberg SJ, et al. Current issues in the presentation of asymptomatic primary hyperparathyroidism: proceedings of the Fourth International Workshop. J Clin Endocrinol Metab 2014;99(10):3580–94.

7. Wermers RA, et al. Survival after the diagnosis of hyperparathyroidism: a population-based study. Am J Med 1998;104(2):115–22.

8. Silverberg SJ. Non-classical target organs in primary hyperparathyroidism. J Bone Miner Res 2002;17(Suppl 2):N117–25.

9. Ellison DH, et al. Effects of calcium infusion on blood pressure in hypertensive and normotensive humans. Hypertension 1986;8(6):497–505.

10. Ahmed R, Hashiba K. Reliability of QT intervals as indicators of clinical hypercalcemia. Clin Cardiol 1988;11(6):395–400.

11. Roberts WC, Waller BF. Effect of chronic hypercalcemia on the heart. An analysis of 18 necropsy patients. Am J Med 1981;71(3):371–84.

12. Collip JB, Clark EP. Further studies on the physiological action of a parathyroid hormone. J Biol Chem 1925;64:485–507.

13. Schluter KD, Piper HM. Cardiovascular actions of parathyroid hormone and parathyroid hormone-related peptide. Cardiovasc Res 1998;37(1):34–41.

14. McMahon DJ, et al. Effect of parathyroidectomy upon left ventricular mass in primary hyperparathyroidism: a meta-analysis. J Clin Endocrinol Metab 2015; 100(12):4399–407.

15. Hedback G, et al. Premature death in patients operated on for primary hyperparathyroidism. World J Surg 1990;14(6):829–35 [discussion: 836].

16. Hedback G, Oden A, Tisell LE. The influence of surgery on the risk of death in patients with primary hyperparathyroidism. World J Surg 1991;15(3):399–405 [discussion: 406–7].

17. Hedback G, Oden A. Increased risk of death from primary hyperparathyroidism–an update. Eur J Clin Invest 1998;28(4):271–6.

18. Palmer M, et al. Mortality after surgery for primary hyperparathyroidism: a follow-up of 441 patients operated on from 1956 to 1979. Surgery 1987;102(1):1–7.

19. Yu N, et al. Increased mortality and morbidity in mild primary hyperparathyroid patients. The Parathyroid Epidemiology and Audit Research Study (PEARS). Clin Endocrinol (Oxf) 2010;73(1):30–4.

20. Nilsson IL, et al. Clinical presentation of primary hyperparathyroidism in Europe–nationwide cohort analysis on mortality from nonmalignant causes. J Bone Miner Res 2002;17(Suppl 2):N68–74.

21. Kalla A, et al. Primary hyperparathyroidism predicts hypertension: results from the National Inpatient Sample. Int J Cardiol 2017;227:335–7.

22. Walker MD, Silverberg SJ. Cardiovascular aspects of primary hyperparathyroidism. J Endocrinol Invest 2008;31(10):925–31.

23. Stamatelopoulos K, et al. Hemodynamic markers and subclinical atherosclerosis in postmenopausal women with primary hyperparathyroidism. J Clin Endocrinol Metab 2014;99(8):2704–11.

24. Verheyen N, et al. Parathyroid hormone, aldosterone-to-renin ratio and fibroblast growth factor-23 as determinants of nocturnal blood pressure in primary hyperparathyroidism: the eplerenone in primary hyperparathyroidism trial. J Hypertens 2016;34(9):1778–86.

25. Storvall S, et al. Surgery significantly improves neurocognition, sleep, and blood pressure in primary hyperparathyroidism: a 3-year prospective follow-up study. Horm Metab Res 2017;49(10):772–7.

26. Graff-Baker AN, et al. Parathyroidectomy for patients with primary hyperparathyroidism and associations with hypertension. JAMA Surg 2019;155(1):32–9.

27. Ejlsmark-Svensson H, Rolighed L, Rejnmark L. Effect of parathyroidectomy on cardiovascular risk factors in primary hyperparathyroidism: a randomized clinical trial. J Clin Endocrinol Metab 2019;104(8):3223–32.

28. Bollerslev J, et al. Effect of surgery on cardiovascular risk factors in mild primary hyperparathyroidism. J Clin Endocrinol Metab 2009;94(7):2255–61.

29. Sun Q, et al. Glucose metabolic disorder in primary hyperparathyroidism: a systematic review and meta-analysis. Int J Clin Exp Med 2019;12(9):11964–73.

30. Godang K, et al. The effect of surgery on fat mass, lipid and glucose metabolism in mild primary hyperparathyroidism. Endocr Connect 2018;7(8):941–8.

31. Vestergaard P, et al. Cardiovascular events before and after surgery for primary hyperparathyroidism. World J Surg 2003;27(2):216–22.

32. Koubaity O, et al. Coronary artery disease is more severe in patients with primary hyperparathyroidism. Surgery 2020;167(1):149–54.

33. Streeten EA, et al. Coronary artery calcification in patients with primary hyperparathyroidism in comparison with control subjects from the multi-ethnic study of atherosclerosis. Endocr Pract 2008;14(2):155–61.

34. Kontogeorgos G, et al. Hyperparathyroidism in men - morbidity and mortality during 21 years' follow-up. Scand J Clin Lab Invest 2020;80(1):6–13.

35. Nana M, et al. Primary hyperparathyroidism: comparing cardiovascular morbidity and mortality in patients treated with parathyroidectomy versus conservative management. J Endocrinol Metab 2019;9(4):95–107.

36. Lundstam K, et al. Effects of parathyroidectomy versus observation on the development of vertebral fractures in mild primary hyperparathyroidism. J Clin Endocrinol Metab 2015;100(4):1359–67.

37. Pepe J, et al. High prevalence of abdominal aortic calcification in patients with primary hyperparathyroidism as evaluated by Kauppila score. Eur J Endocrinol 2016;175(2):95–100.

38. Walker MD, et al. Effect of parathyroidectomy on subclinical cardiovascular disease in mild primary hyperparathyroidism. Eur J Endocrinol 2012;167(2):277–85.

39. Cansu GB, et al. Parathyroidectomy in asymptomatic primary hyperparathyroidism reduces carotid intima-media thickness and arterial stiffness. Clin Endocrinol (Oxf) 2016;84(1):39–47.

40. Dural C, et al. A pilot study investigating the effect of parathyroidectomy on arterial stiffness and coronary artery calcification in patients with primary hyperparathyroidism. Surgery 2016;159(1):218–24.

41. Stefenelli T, et al. Primary hyperparathyroidism: incidence of cardiac abnormalities and partial reversibility after successful parathyroidectomy. Am J Med 1993;95(2):197–202.

42. Iwata S, et al. Aortic valve calcification in mild primary hyperparathyroidism. J Clin Endocrinol Metab 2011;97(1):132–7.

43. Best CAE, et al. Echocardiogram changes following parathyroidectomy for primary hyperparathyroidism: a systematic review and meta-analysis. Medicine (Baltimore) 2017;96(43):e7255.
44. Baykan M, et al. Assessment of left ventricular diastolic function and the Tei index by tissue Doppler imaging in patients with primary hyperparathyroidism. Clin Endocrinol (Oxf) 2007;66(4):483–8.
45. Almqvist EG, et al. Cardiac dysfunction in mild primary hyperparathyroidism assessed by radionuclide angiography and echocardiography before and after parathyroidectomy. Surgery 2002;132(6):1126–32 [discussion: 1132].
46. Dalberg K, et al. Cardiac function in primary hyperparathyroidism before and after operation. An echocardiographic study. Eur J Surg 1996;162(3):171–6.
47. Nuzzo V, et al. Increased intima-media thickness of the carotid artery wall, normal blood pressure profile and normal left ventricular mass in subjects with primary hyperparathyroidism. Eur J Endocrinol 2002;147(4):453–9.
48. Ozdemir D, et al. Evaluation of left ventricle functions by tissue Doppler, strain, and strain rate echocardiography in patients with primary hyperparathyroidism. Endocrine 2014;47(2):609–17.
49. Yilmazer MM, et al. Improvement in cardiac structure and functions early after transcatheter closure of secundum atrial septal defect in children and adolescents. Turk J Pediatr 2013;55(4):401–10.
50. Aktas Yilmaz B, et al. Cardiac structure and functions in patients with asymptomatic primary hyperparathyroidism. J Endocrinol Invest 2013;36(10):848–52.
51. Walker MD, et al. Carotid vascular abnormalities in primary hyperparathyroidism. J Clin Endocrinol Metab 2009;94(10):3849–56.
52. Farahnak P, et al. Cardiac function in mild primary hyperparathyroidism and the outcome after parathyroidectomy. Eur J Endocrinol 2010;163(3):461–7.
53. Luigi P, et al. Arterial hypertension, metabolic syndrome and subclinical cardiovascular organ damage in patients with asymptomatic primary hyperparathyroidism before and after parathyroidectomy: preliminary results. Int J Endocrinol 2012;2012:408295.
54. Persson A, et al. Effect of surgery on cardiac structure and function in mild primary hyperparathyroidism. Clin Endocrinol (Oxf) 2011;74(2):174–80.
55. Ambrogini E, et al. Surgery or surveillance for mild asymptomatic primary hyperparathyroidism: a prospective, randomized clinical trial. J Clin Endocrinol Metab 2007;92(8):3114–21.
56. Kiris A, et al. The assessment of left ventricular systolic asynchrony in patients with primary hyperparathyroidism. Echocardiography 2011;28(9):955–60.
57. Nilsson IL, et al. Endothelial vasodilatory dysfunction in primary hyperparathyroidism is reversed after parathyroidectomy. Surgery 1999;126(6):1049–55.
58. Neunteufl T, et al. Impairment of endothelium-independent vasodilation in patients with hypercalcemia. Cardiovasc Res 1998;40(2):396–401.
59. Kosch M, et al. Impaired flow-mediated vasodilation of the brachial artery in patients with primary hyperparathyroidism improves after parathyroidectomy. Cardiovasc Res 2000;47(4):813–8.
60. Agarwal G, et al. Cardiovascular dysfunction in symptomatic primary hyperparathyroidism and its reversal after curative parathyroidectomy: results of a prospective case control study. Surgery 2013;154(6):1394–403 [discussion: 1403–4].
61. Baykan M, et al. Impairment of flow mediated vasodilatation of brachial artery in patients with primary hyperparathyroidism. Int J Cardiovasc Imaging 2007; 23(3):323–8.

62. Virdis A, et al. The sulfaphenazole-sensitive pathway acts as a compensatory mechanism for impaired nitric oxide availability in patients with primary hyperparathyroidism. Effect of surgical treatment. J Clin Endocrinol Metab 2010; 95(2):920–7.
63. Carrelli AL, et al. Endothelial function in mild primary hyperparathyroidism. Clin Endocrinol (Oxf) 2013;78(2):204–9.
64. Ekmekci A, et al. Endothelial function and endothelial nitric oxide synthase intron 4a/b polymorphism in primary hyperparathyroidism. J Endocrinol Invest 2009; 32(7):611–6.
65. Tuna MM, et al. Impaired endothelial function in patients with mild primary hyperparathyroidism improves after parathyroidectomy. Clin Endocrinol (Oxf) 2015;83(6):951–6.
66. Rosa J, et al. Pulse wave velocity in primary hyperparathyroidism and effect of surgical therapy. Hypertens Res 2011;34(3):296–300.
67. Schillaci G, et al. Large-artery stiffness: a reversible marker of cardiovascular risk in primary hyperparathyroidism. Atherosclerosis 2011;218(1):96–101.
68. Smith JC, et al. Augmentation of central arterial pressure in mild primary hyperparathyroidism. J Clin Endocrinol Metab 2000;85(10):3515–9.
69. Rubin MR, et al. Arterial stiffness in mild primary hyperparathyroidism. J Clin Endocrinol Metab 2005;90(6):3326–30.
70. Barletta G, et al. Cardiovascular effects of parathyroid hormone: a study in healthy subjects and normotensive patients with mild primary hyperparathyroidism. J Clin Endocrinol Metab 2000;85(5):1815–21.
71. Tordjman KM, et al. Cardiovascular risk factors and arterial rigidity are similar in asymptomatic normocalcemic and hypercalcemic primary hyperparathyroidism. Eur J Endocrinol 2010;162(5):925–33.
72. Pepe J, et al. Retinal micro-vascular and aortic macro-vascular changes in postmenopausal women with primary hyperparathyroidism. Sci Rep 2018;8(1): 16521.
73. Dubois F, et al. [Primary hyperparathyroidism disclosed by heart arrhythmia]. Arch Mal Coeur Vaiss 1989;82(12):2071–4.
74. Baumgartl P. [Changes in the ECG caused by electrolyte changes in primary hyperparathyroidism]. Z Kardiol 1975;64(4):359–62.
75. Rosenqvist M, et al. Cardiac conduction in patients with hypercalcaemia due to primary hyperparathyroidism. Clin Endocrinol (Oxf) 1992;37(1):29–33.
76. Curione M, et al. Increased risk of cardiac death in primary hyperparathyroidism: what is a role of electrical instability? Int J Cardiol 2007;121(2):200–2.
77. Vazquez-Diaz O, et al. Reversible changes of electrocardiographic abnormalities after parathyroidectomy in patients with primary hyperparathyroidism. Cardiol J 2009;16(3):241–5.
78. Pepe J, et al. Arrhythmias in primary hyperparathyroidism evaluated by exercise test. Eur J Clin Invest 2013;43(2):208–14.
79. Pepe J, et al. Parathyroidectomy eliminates arrhythmic risk in primary hyperparathyroidism, as evaluated by exercise test. Eur J Endocrinol 2013;169(2): 255–61.
80. Pepe J, et al. Reduction of arrhythmias in primary hyperparathyroidism, by parathyroidectomy, evaluated with 24-h ECG monitoring. Eur J Endocrinol 2018; 179(2):117–24.
81. Vicale CT. Diagnostic features of muscular syndrome resulting from hyperparathyroidism, osteomalacia owing to renal tubular acidosis and perhaps related disorders of calcium metabolism. Trans Am Neurol Assoc 1949;74:143–7.

82. Rollinson RD, Gilligan BS. Primary hyperparathyroidism presenting as a proximal myopathy. Aust N Z J Med 1977;7(4):420–1.

83. Rolighed L, et al. Muscle function is impaired in patients with "asymptomatic" primary hyperparathyroidism. World J Surg 2014;38(3):549–57.

84. Voss L, et al. Impaired physical function and evaluation of quality of life in normocalcemic and hypercalcemic primary hyperparathyroidism. Bone 2020;141:115583.

85. Joborn C, et al. Psychiatric morbidity in primary hyperparathyroidism. World J Surg 1988;12(4):476–81.

86. Liu JY PB, Mlaver E, Patel SG, et al. Neuropsychologic changes in primary hyperparathyroidism after parathyroidectomy from a dual-institution prospective study. Surgery 2021;169(1):114–9.

87. Kearns AE, Espiritu R, Vickers Douglass K, et al. Clinical characteristics and depression score response after parathyroidectomy in primary hyperparathyroidism. Clin Endocrinol (Oxf) 2019;91(3):464–70.

88. Shah-Becker S, Derr J, Oberman BS, et al. Early neurocognitive improvements following parathyroidectomy for primary hyperparathyroidism. Laryngoscope 2018;128(3):775–80.

89. Liu JY, Saunders N, Chen A, et al. Neuropsychological changes in primary hyperparathyroidism after parathyroidectomy. Am Surg 2016;82(9):839–45.

90. Lourida I, et al. Parathyroid hormone, cognitive function and dementia: a systematic review. PLoS ONE [Electronic Resource] 2015;10(5):e0127574.

91. Weber T, Eberle J, Messelhäuser U, et al. Parathyroidectomy, elevated depression scores, and suicidal ideation in patients with primary hyperparathyroidism: results of a prospective multicenter study. JAMA Surg 2013;148(2):109–15.

92. Trombetti A CE, Henzen C, Gold G, et al. Clinical presentation and management of patients with primary hyperparathyroidism of the Swiss Primary Hyperparathyroidism Cohort: a focus on neuro-behavioral and cognitive symptoms. J Endocrinol Invest 2016;39(5):567–76.

93. Yılmaz BA, et al. Neuropsychological changes and health-related quality of life in patients with asymptomatic primary hyperparathyroidism. Asemptomatik primer hiperparatiroidizmi olan hastalarda nöropsiklojik değişiklikler ve yaşam kalitesi 2017;21(1):9–14.

94. Webb SM, et al. Validation of PHPQoL, a disease-specific quality-of-life questionnaire for patients with primary hyperparathyroidism. J Clin Endocrinol Metab 2016;101(4):1571–8.

95. Walker MD, et al. Neuropsychological features in primary hyperparathyroidism: a prospective study. J Clin Endocrinol Metab 2009;94(6):1951–8.

96. Sheldon DG, et al. Surgical treatment of hyperparathyroidism improves health-related quality of life. Arch Surg 2002;137(9):1022–6 [discussion: 1026–8].

97. Amstrup AK, Rejnmark L, Mosekilde L. Patients with surgically cured primary hyperparathyroidism have a reduced quality of life compared with population-based healthy sex-, age-, and season-matched controls. Eur J Endocrinol 2011;165(5):753–60.

98. Bollerslev J, et al. Medical observation, compared with parathyroidectomy, for asymptomatic primary hyperparathyroidism: a prospective, randomized trial. J Clin Endocrinol Metab 2007;92(5):1687–92.

99. Talpos GB, et al. Randomized trial of parathyroidectomy in mild asymptomatic primary hyperparathyroidism: patient description and effects on the SF-36 health survey. Surgery 2000;128(6):1013–20 [discussion: 1020–1].

100. Roman SA, et al. Parathyroidectomy improves neurocognitive deficits in patients with primary hyperparathyroidism. Surgery 2005;138(6):1121–8 [discussion: 1128–9].

101. Benge JF, et al. Cognitive and affective sequelae of primary hyperparathyroidism and early response to parathyroidectomy. J Int Neuropsychol Soc 2009; 15(6):1002–11.

102. Perrier ND, et al. Prospective, randomized, controlled trial of parathyroidectomy versus observation in patients with "asymptomatic" primary hyperparathyroidism. Surgery 2009;146(6):1116–22.

103. Chiang CY, et al. A controlled, prospective study of neuropsychological outcomes post parathyroidectomy in primary hyperparathyroid patients. Clin Endocrinol (Oxf) 2005;62(1):99–104.

104. Numann PJ, Torppa AJ, Blumetti AE. Neuropsychologic deficits associated with primary hyperparathyroidism. Surgery 1984;96(6):1119–23.

105. Babinska D, et al. Evaluation of selected cognitive functions before and after surgery for primary hyperparathyroidism. Langenbecks Arch Surg 2012; 397(5):825–31.

106. Veras A, et al. Lower quality of life in longstanding mild primary hyperparathyroidism. Arq Bras Endocrinol Metab 2013;57(2):139–43.

107. Webb SM, et al. Development of a new tool for assessing health-related quality of life in patients with primary hyperparathyroidism. Health Qual Life Outcomes 2013;11:97.

108. Ryhänen EM, et al. Health-related quality of life is impaired in primary hyperparathyroidism and significantly improves after surgery: a prospective study using the 15D instrument. Endocr Connect 2015;4(3):179–86.

109. Walker MD, Silverberg SJ. Parathyroidectomy in asymptomatic primary hyperparathyroidism: improves "bones" but not "psychic moans. J Clin Endocrinol Metab 2007;92(5):1613–5.

110. Pretorius M, et al. Effects of parathyroidectomy on quality of life: 10 years: data from a prospective randomized controlled trial on primary hyperparathyroidism (the SIPH-study). J Bone Miner Res 2021;36(1):3–11.

111. Prager G, et al. Parathyroidectomy improves concentration and retentiveness in patients with primary hyperparathyroidism. Surgery 2002;132(6):930–5 [discussion: 935–6].

112. Cogan MG, et al. Central nervous system manifestations of hyperparathyroidism. Am J Med 1978;65(6):963–70.

113. Goyal A, et al. Neuropsychiatric manifestations in patients of primary hyperparathyroidism and outcome following surgery. Indian J Med Sci 2001;55(12): 677–86.

114. Mittendorf EA, et al. Improvement of sleep disturbance and neurocognitive function after parathyroidectomy in patients with primary hyperparathyroidism. Endocr Pract 2007;13(4):338–44.

115. Wartolowska K, et al. Use of placebo controls in the evaluation of surgery: systematic review. BMJ 2014;348:g3253.

116. Dotzenrath CM, et al. Neuropsychiatric and cognitive changes after surgery for primary hyperparathyroidism. World J Surg 2006;30(5):680–5.

117. Liu M, et al. Cognition and cerebrovascular function in primary hyperparathyroidism before and after parathyroidectomy. J Endocrinol Invest 2020;43(3): 369–79.

118. Gazes Y, et al. Functional magnetic resonance imaging in primary hyperparathyroidism. Eur J Endocrinol 2020;183(1):21–30.

119. Broulik PD, Stepan JJ, Pacovsky V. Primary hyperparathyroidism and hyperuri-caemia are associated but not correlated with indicators of bone turnover. Clin Chim Acta 1987;170(2–3):195–200.

120. Rynes RI, Merzig EG. Calcium pyrophosphate crystal deposition disease and hyperparathyroidism: a controlled, prospective study. J Rheumatol 1978;5(4): 460–8.

121. Alexander GM, et al. Pyrophosphate arthropathy: a study of metabolic associa-tions and laboratory data. Ann Rheum Dis 1982;41(4):377–81.

122. Bilezikian JP, et al. Pseudogout after parathyroidectomy. Lancet 1973;1(7801): 445–6.

123. Rubin MR, Silverberg SJ. Rheumatic manifestations of primary hyperparathy-roidism and parathyroid hormone therapy. Curr Rheumatol Rep 2002;4(2): 179–85.

124. Brandi ML, et al. Guidelines for diagnosis and therapy of MEN type 1 and type 2. J Clin Endocrinol Metab 2001;86(12):5658–71.

125. Yadav SK, et al. Primary hyperparathyroidism in developing world: a systematic review on the changing clinical profile of the disease. Arch Endocrinol Metab 2020;64(2):105–10.

126. Ludvigsson JF, et al. Primary hyperparathyroidism and celiac disease: a population-based cohort study. J Clin Endocrinol Metab 2012;97(3):897–904.

127. Pickard AL, et al. Hyperparathyroidism and subsequent cancer risk in Denmark. Cancer 2002;95(8):1611–7.

128. Michels KB, et al. Hyperparathyroidism and subsequent incidence of breast cancer. Int J Cancer 2004;110(3):449–51.

129. Palmer M, et al. Increased risk of malignant diseases after surgery for primary hyperparathyroidism. A nationwide cohort study. Am J Epidemiol 1988;127(5): 1031–40.

130. Bayat-Mokhtari F, et al. Parathyroid storm. Arch Intern Med 1980;140(8):1092–5.

131. Bilezikian JP, et al. Hyperparathyroidism. Lancet 2018;391(10116):168–78.

132. Marcocci C, et al. Parathyroid carcinoma. J Bone Miner Res 2008;23(12): 1869–80.

133. Shane E. Clinical review 122: parathyroid carcinoma. J Clin Endocrinol Metab 2001;86(2):485–93.

134. LiVolsi V. Morphology of the parathyroid glands. In: Becker KL, editor. Principles and practice of endocrinology and metabolism. Lippincott Williams and Wilkins: Philadelphia.

135. Streeten EA, et al. Studies in a kindred with parathyroid carcinoma. J Clin Endo-crinol Metab 1992;75(2):362–6.

136. Wassif WS, et al. Familial isolated hyperparathyroidism: a distinct genetic entity with an increased risk of parathyroid cancer. J Clin Endocrinol Metab 1993; 77(6):1485–9.

137. Yoshimoto K, et al. Familial isolated primary hyperparathyroidism with parathy-roid carcinomas: clinical and molecular features. Clin Endocrinol (Oxf) 1998; 48(1):67–72.

138. Marx SJ, Simonds WF, Agarwal SK, et al. Hyperparathyroidism in hereditary syn-dromes: special expressions and special managements. J Bone Mineral Res 2002;17:N37–43.

139. Chen JD, et al. Hyperparathyroidism-jaw tumour syndrome. J Intern Med 2003; 253(6):634–42.

140. Simonds WF, et al. Familial isolated hyperparathyroidism: clinical and genetic characteristics of 36 kindreds. Medicine (Baltimore) 2002;81(1):1–26.

141. Dionisi S, et al. Concurrent parathyroid adenomas and carcinoma in the setting of multiple endocrine neoplasia type 1: presentation as hypercalcemic crisis. Mayo Clin Proc 2002;77(8):866–9.
142. Agha A, et al. Parathyroid carcinoma in multiple endocrine neoplasia type 1 (MEN1) syndrome: two case reports of an unrecognised entity. J Endocrinol Invest 2007;30(2):145–9.
143. Haven CJ, et al. Identification of MEN1 and HRPT2 somatic mutations in paraffin-embedded (sporadic) parathyroid carcinomas. Clin Endocrinol (Oxf) 2007;67(3):370–6.
144. Abood A, Vestergaard P. Pregnancy outcomes in women with primary hyperparathyroidism. Eur J Endocrinol 2014;171(1):69–76.
145. Rao DS, et al. Randomized controlled clinical trial of surgery versus no surgery in patients with mild asymptomatic primary hyperparathyroidism. J Clin Endocrinol Metab 2004;89(11):5415–22.

Tertiary and Postrenal Transplantation Hyperparathyroidism

Carlo Alfieri, MD[a,b], Deborah Mattinzoli[c],
Piergiorgio Messa, MD[a,b,*]

KEYWORDS

- Kidney transplantation • Hyperparathirodism • Calcium • Bone disease

KEY POINTS

- Patients who have undergone kidney transplantation are a distinctive population, characterized by the persistence of some metabolic anomalies present during end-stage renal disease.
- Posttransplant hyperparathyroidism, especially in the tertiary form, is responsible for several posttransplant complications, such as vascular calcifications and bone disorders, and finally the extreme cardiovascular risk present in this cohort of patients.
- The treatment of posttransplant hyperparathyroidism might be sometimes difficult, but fortunately, different therapeutic options can be used.
- Medical therapy should be also focused to ameliorate bone mineral density and possibly reduce fracture risk. Parathyroidectomy should be reserved for those patients who have undergone KTx in whom a THP is present and cannot be managed with drug therapy.

INTRODUCTION

Kidney transplantation (KTx) is considered the best therapy for end-stage renal disease (ESRD). Nevertheless, patients who have undergone KTx (KTxps) are a distinctive population, characterized by the persistence of some metabolic anomalies present during ESRD.

Mineral metabolism (MM) parameters are frequently altered after KTx, also in the presence of complete renal function recovery. These anomalies, involving calcium (Ca), phosphorus (P), vitamin D, and parathormone (PTH), are frequently responsible for post-KTx mineral and bone disorders and impact significantly in long term patients and KTx outcomes.[1]

[a] Department of Nephrology, Dialysis and Renal Transplantation, Fondazione IRCCS Ca' Granda Ospedale Policlinico, Via Commenda 15, Milan 20122, Italy; [b] Department of Clinical Sciences and Community Health, University of Milan, Via Festa del Perdono, 7, Milan 20122, Italy; [c] Renal Research Laboratory Fondazione IRCCS Ca' Granda Ospedale Policlinico, Via Pace 9, Milan 20122, Italy
* Corresponding author. Department of Nephrology, Dialysis and Renal Transplantation, Fondazione IRCCS Ca' Granda Ospedale Policlinico, Via Commenda 15, Milan 20122, Italy.
E-mail addresses: piergiorgio.messa@unimi.it; piergiorgio.messa@policlinico.mi.it

Endocrinol Metab Clin N Am 50 (2021) 649–662
https://doi.org/10.1016/j.ecl.2021.08.004
0889-8529/21/© 2021 Elsevier Inc. All rights reserved.

During ESRD, a condition of hyperparathyroidism (hyper-PTH) is frequent and can be characterized by the increase of PTH related to uremic factors and reduction of Ca and vitamin D and hyperphosphatemia, namely, secondary hyperparathyroidism (SHP). In the presence for a long time of hyper-PTH, especially if not well controlled during the pre-KTx time, an evolution toward an uncontrolled form, namely, tertiary hyperparathyroidism (THP) is possible. THP is determined by an abnormal secretion of PTH from the parathyroid glands and by the complete loss of Ca control in the modulation of parathyroid activity. Biochemically THP is characterized by the presence of abnormally high levels of PTH associated, differently to SHP, to hypercalcemia (hyper-Ca).[2]

Post-KTx hyper-PTH and especially THP are considered important causal factors responsible for several post-KTx complications, such as vascular calcifications and bone disorders and finally the extreme cardiovascular risk present in this cohort of patients.[3]

In this article, the prevalence and epidemiologic and clinical impact of post-KTx hyper-PTH are presented. In addition, the principal biochemical and instrumental investigations and the therapeutic options for these conditions are reported.

PREVALENCE AND CASUAL FACTORS OF PARATHORMONE ANOMALIES AFTER KIDNEY TRANSPLANTATION

Considering the important impact of hyper-PTH, several studies tried to detect the prevalence of this metabolic disarrangement in KTxps. An initial decrease in the PTH levels is usually found within the first 12 months posttransplant.[4] Of note, in up to 50% of cases, also in the presence of a well-functional KTx, a persistent increase of PTH levels can be present.[5] These data reported in the literature have also been mostly confirmed in our experience. As reported in **Fig. 1**, in fact, in our experience, the prevalence of high levels of PTH, considering the level of glomerular filtration rate, in a cohort of 600 KTxps at 24 months after KTx is around 48%.

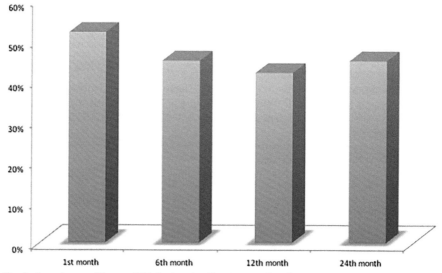

Fig. 1. Prevalence of hyper-PTH during the first 24 months after KTx in a cohort of 600 KTxps followed in our department.

Several factors, including dialysis vintage, older age, and presence of severe pre-KTx hyper-PTH, influence the development of THP post-KTx, present in almost 20% KTxps.[6]

Post-KTx THP is frequently observed in patients with chronic SHP treated usually for several years by dialysis. At the basis of THP, there is a hypertrophied parathyroid gland enlargement (**Fig. 2**). In this condition, a continuous overtime secretion of PTH, autonomous of Ca levels with minimal response to therapeutic agents, is present and establishes the development of hyper-Ca.

Physiologically, parathyroid cells are strongly sensible to Ca modifications through a membrane receptor, the calcium-sensing receptor (CaSR). CaSR controls PTH release and synthesis.[7,8] An important modulating effect on PTH release has been described for vitamin D, fibroblast growth factor 23 (FGF-23), and αKlotho. In the presence of chronic kidney disease (CKD) and ESRD, a reduction of CaSR expression on parathyroid cells and a modification of the set point for the Ca-controlled PTH release determine the augmented secretion of PTH and the final development of SHP.[9] In the initial phases of SHP, experimental studies have reported that after an increase of calcium and vitamin D levels and with the use of calcimimetics, an increase in CaSR density is present. Moreover, in these conditions an increase in the expression of CYP27B1, the enzyme responsible for the synthesis of calcitriol, was evidenced. These observations can imply a possible compensatory autocrine/paracrine mechanism in the attempt of reducing PTH production.[10] In possible agreement with this concept, in an extreme condition as THP, the expressions of CYP27B1, CaSR, and vitamin D receptors are generally reduced.[11–13]

The presence of high levels of PTH in the KTx setting, associated with the recovery of the target organs to the PTH calcemic effect (including obviously a functioning kidney) is the principal, but not the unique, mechanism explaining the occurrence of hyper-Ca after KTx.[14] According to our data, reported in **Fig. 3**, a condition of hyper-Ca, defined as Ca levels greater than 10.4 mg/dL, is present in almost 25% of KTxps during the first year of KTx.

In addition to the recovery of PTH receptor sensitivity to PTH, certainly the increased availability of calcitriol, in the presence of a normal tubular function, can play a role in the development of hyper-Ca after KTx.

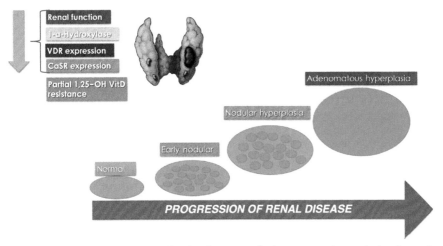

Fig. 2. At the basis of THP there is the development of adenomatous hyperplasia of parathyroid glands, responsible for an uncontrolled secretion of PTH. VDR, vitamin D receptor.

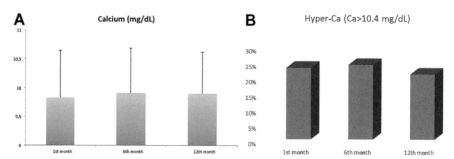

Fig. 3. Calcium levels (*A*) and prevalence of Hyper-Ca (*B*) during the first year of transplantation after KTx in a cohort of 600 KTxps followed in our department.

Hyper-Ca is frequently associated with hyperphosphatemia. However, it is important to remember that hypo-Pi is relatively frequent in KTx and can be related to the use of some medications (eg, immunosuppressive drugs) that can increase urinary phosphorus wasting.

CLINICAL IMPACT OF PARATHORMONE DISORDERS IN PATIENTS WHO HAVE UNDERGONE KIDNEY TRANSPLANTATION

Bone disease associated with disarrangement of Ca, P, and PTH is almost invariably present in CKD. Chronically increased PTH levels are responsible for an increased bone turnover, strictly determined by an overactivation of osteoclasts associated with a reduction of mineral bone content and an altered structural bone quality.[15,16] The principal clinical manifestations of this process are bone pain, muscular-skeletal structural disarrangements, fractures, and, especially when high levels of PTH are present, as in THP, the development of severe bone osteoclast and fibroblast proliferative process, namely, brown tumors.[17] Of note, in KTxps there is a demonstration of a pronounced reduction of bone density during the first year of KTx, which can be evidenced by biochemical and instrumental evaluations. This explains the fact that those patients present a strong risk of novel fractures during the early period after KTx.[18]

The persistence of high levels of PTH after KTx per se, accompanied by the associated changes of other MM components (increased Pi, Ca, alkaline phosphatase [ALP], FGF-23, or decreased vitamin D, Klotho) or by other metabolic changes, frequently promoted by immunosuppressive therapy (dyslipidemia, impaired insulin sensitivity, or secretion), might determine the development of cardiovascular pathologic events.[19–22]

Making this picture certainly more complicated it is important to remember that elevated levels of PTH, especially in the initial phases, can influence the recovery from anemia by PTH-related resistance to erythropoietin.[23] A correlation has also been demonstrated with immunologic dysfunction and glucose and lipid metabolic changes. All these effects are frequently reversed or of a reduced entity after the control of hyper-PTH (**Fig. 4**).[24–26]

BIOCHEMICAL AND INSTRUMENTAL EVALUATION OF PARATHORMONE DISORDERS IN PATIENTS WHO HAVE UNDERGONE KIDNEY TRANSPLANTATION
Biochemical Evaluation of Hyperparathyroidism in Patients Who Have Undergone Kidney Transplantation

Generally, as in ESRD, in KTxps also the finding of a condition of hyper-PTH, should be associated with the investigation of the clinical history of the patients and all the main parameters of MM.

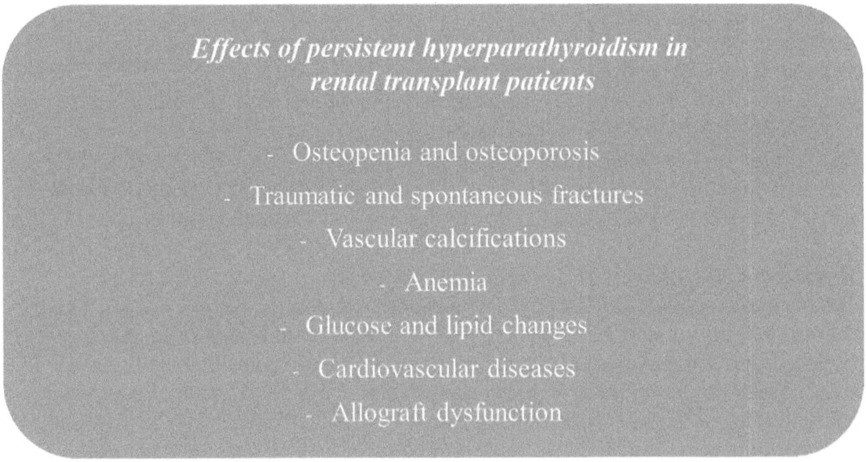

Effects of persistent hyperparathyroidism in renal transplant patients

- Osteopenia and osteoporosis
- Traumatic and spontaneous fractures
- Vascular calcifications
- Anemia
- Glucose and lipid changes
- Cardiovascular diseases
- Allograft dysfunction

Fig. 4. Principal effects of persistent hyperparathyroidism in patients who have undergone renal transplantation.

Some difficulties can be present in the evaluation of PTH. As well recognized, circulating PTH is a complex of the intact PTH molecule (84 amino acids). In this context, the existence of a group of different PTH fragments with some possible biological activity that are differently cleared by the kidneys according to glomerular filtration rate was demonstrated.[27,28] Actually, the clinically use of measuring PTH fragments is still a matter of debate.

Another important point is that at the moment there is no uniformity regarding the best assay and way to measure PTH levels, with several differences among the nephrological centers.[29]

A correct evaluation of Ca levels and the anamnesis of the patient can permit an assessment of discrimination among primary hyperparathyroidism (PHP), SHP, and THP. In the presence of a normal renal function, all the forms of hyper-PTH can be associated with low-normal serum phosphate levels, due to the phosphaturic effects of PTH.

As PTH, Ca levels measurement can present some peculiarities.

Even if ionized Ca is the metabolic form of Ca, in clinical practice usually total Ca level is measured. This fact assumes, incorrectly, an acceptable correlation between total and ionized calcium levels. For example, the frequent finding of reduced albumin levels, due to malnutrition or inflammation syndrome, might determine some improper findings in total Ca levels. For this reason, the use of specific correcting formulas is recommended even if they do not consider interfering factors such as pH and accumulation of inorganic and organic anions that might influence total Ca levels.[30–32]

In KTxps, a possible influence in the development of high levels of Ca can be attributed to the use of some immunosuppressive drugs. Some evidence of increased bone resorption mediated by calcineurin inhibitors, in particular cyclosporine, is present; this might promote the development of hyper-Ca.[33] On the other hand, it was reported that KTxps on rapamycin therapy would be more prone to develop persistent SHP, frequently with high levels of Ca.[34]

Steroids have been related to several effects that can potentially affect calcium metabolism (anti-vitamin D effect, calciuretic activity, induction of osteoblast apoptosis, etc.). Most of these effects are, however, expected to induce more hypocalcemia rather than hyper-Ca.[35] According to our opinion, a direct measurement of ionized serum calcium might be the preferable way to obtain a precise evaluation of Ca status, especially in the characterization of PTH anomalies.

In the presence of hyper-PTH, and normal renal function, low levels of phosphate are frequently found and are related to the inhibitory effect of PTH on Na-phosphate cotransporters in the renal tubules. In addition, in KTxps a tubular effect of FGF-23, particularly high up to the sixth month of KTx and the influence of some immunosuppressant drugs that specifically act to reduce the tubular reabsorption of P are also present.

The assessment of vitamin D and ALP levels deserves some clarifications.

The evaluation of both native (25-OH-VitD) and active form (1,25-OH-VitD) of vitamin D is important. Increased availability of 1,25-OH-VitD contributes to the development of hyper-Ca in KTxps by the induction of renal 1-α-OH-ase activity in the presence of a normal tubular function and of PTH concentrations higher than those expected for the renal function level.[36] This mechanism may be partially masked by the low levels of calcitriol precursors (25-OH-VitD), a condition that is very frequent in KTxps especially in the early phases of KTx (**Figs. 5** and **6**).[37] So, it is important to study the 2 forms of vitamin D before starting supplementation.

Especially in the past, ALP was considered a marker of bone turnover in renal disease. Taking into account all the possible limits of this marker, a strict association of high values of ALP with the risk for bone fractures and mortality in patients with CKD has been reported.[38]

The clinical utility of assessing the serum or plasma levels of newer bone biomarkers (FGF-23, αKlotho, sclerostin, OPG, periostin, etc) is still debatable. In our opinion, their dosage can have a rationale only in clinical research or in specific clinical conditions.[39]

Instrumental Evaluation of Parathormone Anomalies in Patients Who Have Undergone Kidney Transplantation

Morphologic and functional evaluation of parathyroid glands

Both morphologic and functional approaches are present to evaluate the characteristics of hyperplastic parathyroid glands. In particular, the study of their volume has certainly great importance, especially in the function of following surgical evaluation or for monitoring of medical therapy. High-resolution sonography with color Doppler,

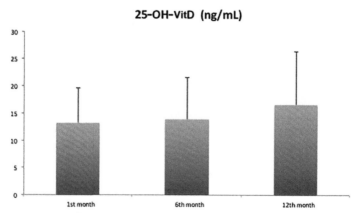

Fig. 5. Native vitamin D levels during the first 12 months after KTx in a cohort of 600 KTxps followed in our department.

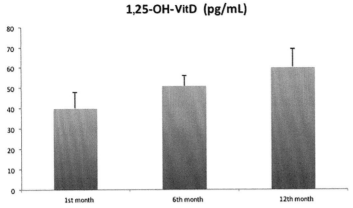

Fig. 6. Active vitamin D levels during the first 12 months after KTx in a cohort of 600 KTxps followed in our department.

99mTc-MIBI scintigraphy, computed tomography (CT), MRI, PET, and single-photon emission computed tomography can be valid methods of evaluation, especially if performed by expert staff.[40]

Radiological evaluations

Basal radiographic examination of multiple sites such as hands, skull, pelvis, and spine can give some important information about the bone status and identify subclinical spontaneous fractures. In addition, some information about vascular calcifications, especially aortic, might be found.[41,42]

In KTxps much information can be obtained by the evaluation of bone mass and bone mineral density (BMD), well obtained with dual-energy x-ray absorptiometry (DXA) whose results indicate alterations in bone mass (osteopenia/osteoporosis) and are also reliable predictors of the future fracture events.[43]

Advanced techniques of imaging will add in the future some important elements, diagnostic and prognostic, in the evaluation of mineral and bone disorders in the general population and in KTxps. Quantitative CT (QCT) and high-resolution peripheral QCT (HR-pQCT) are useful in obtaining diagnostic results representative of those obtained with histologic diagnosis and so can significantly increase the predictivity of the risk of fracture.[44] Interesting in this area are the micro-CT and micro-MRI; their resolution is higher than that of HR-pQCT.[45] Unfortunately, at present, the availability of these techniques is limited to few highly specialized centers and they have been used almost exclusively in experimental studies.

Bone biopsy

Histomorphometric analysis obtained with a bone biopsy is the gold standard for the diagnosis of bone disease in CKD and KTxps and is an important tool for assessing the effects of therapy. This study gives information about variations in bone turnover, mineralization rate, and bone volume. Bone biopsy is performed after 2 brief courses of tetracycline administration, separated 10 to 12 days from each other. Unfortunately, because of its invasiveness, bone biopsy frequently is not well accepted by the patients and is rarely performed, and it is analyzed by only few centers because it requires specific technical training and specialized personnel for preparation, reading, and interpretation. For these reasons, a bone biopsy is performed rarely, for specific indications, and only in specialized centers.[46–49]

THERAPEUTIC MANAGEMENT

In the management of PTH alteration in KTxps, strong importance is represented by the condition in which patients arrive at the KTx. In consideration of this, good pre-KTx management is mandatory and can minimize post-KTx hyper-PTH and the related MM anomalies in the first period after KTx.

After KTx, unfortunately, there are no large randomized controlled trials to guide treatment decisions and there is little consensus about the correct monitoring and management of PTH disorders.

The recent Kidney Disease Improving Global Outcomes (KDIGO) guidelines suggest, unfortunately with a low grade of evidence, just to test with particular regard for the first year post-KTx, Ca, P, PTH, ALP, and 25-OH-VitD levels in intervals, according to the stage of renal function.[50]

This lack of clear guidelines determines the fact that the management of the post-KTx PTH disarrangements and the related mineral bone abnormalities varies between transplant centers.

Fortunately, some drugs are useful in treating mineral and bone alterations after KTx.

Vitamin D and Analogues

In consideration of the role of kidneys in the synthesis of calcitriol, the active vitamin D metabolite, in the presence of CKD, the use of the active form of vitamin D has certainly strong importance in SHP control. In the presence of SHP in a functioning KTx, the dosage of native vitamin D is needed. Recent insights have demonstrated some essential roles of native and active vitamin D, assigning also to native vitamin D some pleiotropic effects, both in patients with CKD and in KTxps. This important point was reviewed recently by our group.[51,52]

Some studies have demonstrated that the use of vitamin D metabolites is associated with a reduction in immediate bone loss by decreasing the effect of glucocorticoid on intestinal absorption or by suppressing PTH secretion.[53,54] This is an important point, also in consideration of the strong prevalence of hypovitaminosis D at the moment and during the early KTx time. However, the presence of autonomous parathyroid adenomas with decreased calcitriol, FGF-23, or CaSR expression makes it difficult to achieve a successful outcome, and many cases of post-KTx persistent HPT become refractory to treatment with calcium and vitamin D analogues assuming the semblance of THP.

In the management of PTH alterations during KTx, we suggest using 25-OH-VitD supplementation, when indicated, as the primary choice. Native vitamin D supplementation does not exclude the use of the active form of vitamin D. So, in agreement with what the guidelines support, the 2 forms should be considered not in contrast but potentially together in the treatment of SHP and, probably, in bone health. More trials in the future might provide information about the lack of classical effectiveness of 25-OH-VitD supplementation in patients with CKD in clinical practice.

Calcimimetics

Although cinacalcet has a proven efficacy in the control of SHP in patients undergoing dialysis and in KTx recipients, its use resulted in a relatively high rate of gastrointestinal discomfort and relatively low compliance of patients to its use.

The possibility to use oral calcimimetics in KTxps has radically reduced the recurrence of parathyroidectomy (PTX) both before and after KTx.

Cinacalcet allosterically activates the CaSR resulting in an inhibition of PTH secretion and a consequent reduction in serum calcium levels.[55,56]

Some data have demonstrated that cinacalcet is effective in reducing PTH levels in KTxps. In addition, the drug had a good safe for the graft, both in the short and in long term.[57,58]

In a randomized placebo-controlled 52-week trial including 114 hyper-Ca KTxps with persistent post-KTx hyper-PTH, normalization in Ca levels and a significant reduction of PTH were observed after the initiation of cinacalcet. These results were significantly different compared with the placebo group. On the other hand, compared with the placebo group, no improvement in BMD at the femoral neck, lumbar spine, or distal one-third radius was found.[59]

In clinical practice, as in patients with CKD, nephrologists should take advantage of the combined use of all the therapies available. Certainly, when possible and necessary, vitamin D supplementations should be prescribed, whereas calcimimetics should be used as the starting drugs in those cases characterized by high calcium levels and severe forms of hyper-PTH. After the reduction of Ca levels an association between low doses of vitamin D and calcimimetics can be indicated.[60]

Antiresorptive Agents Related to Osteopenia and Osteoporosis Posttransplant

The presence of a persistent hyper-PTH after KTx is frequently associated with bone disease and osteopenia/osteoporosis. These alterations are particularly important during the first 6 months of KTx. Many immunosuppressive drugs, like steroids and tacrolimus, have been associated with a worsening of bone density. To ameliorate bone status some drugs are available. Before their use, however, a deep evaluation of all the principal MM parameters is important.

Bisphosphonates are agents able to induce osteoclastic apoptosis, through a reduction of osteoclastic activity; this results in a reduction of bone resorption. Even though several studies have demonstrated a good efficacy for this class of drugs in preserving BMD in the early time after KTx, there is a high concern about their use in KTxps, mostly related to their potential nephrotoxicity and the limited data on their efficacy in preventing novel fractures.[61,62]

Recently, denosumab, a fully humanized monoclonal antibody to receptor activator of nuclear factor-κB ligand (RANKL) that blocks its binding to RANK resulting in an inhibition of the development and activity of osteoclast has been released. Data obtained in the general population have demonstrated that denosumab can be used as an optimal alternative to bisphosphonate in preventing osteoporosis and bone fractures. Unfortunately, data concerning its role in KTx are still limited. In a recent paper published by our group, BMD variations, the development of novel spontaneous vertebral fractures, the modifications of the renal function and MM parameters, and the safety of 1-year denosumab therapy was evaluated. According to our experience, denosumab had good bone efficacy and general safety in KTxps also.[63]

Little evidence concerning the use of teriparatide, a recombinant human parathyroid hormone 1 to 34, in KTxps is present.[64]

Parathyroidectomy

In the cases of severe THP, the indication of PTX, either before or after KTx, was strong in the past. An important question to face is the indication to pre-KTx parathyroidectomy. At the moment, thanks to the availability of specific treatments, PTX is reserved only for specific conditions such as strong diseases characterized by several fractures or long-term medical failure.[65]

Compared with cinacalcet therapy, the surgical procedure of subtotal parathyroidectomy seems to guarantee a higher prevalence of normocalcemia and PTH normalization, with substantial benefits on BMD.[66] In any case, it is recommended to well evaluate the indication to surgical approach, in consideration also of the patient preference and the patient surgical and postsurgical risk.[67] According to our opinion, a strong indication of pre-KTx PTX can be represented by the presence of a severe hyper-PTH not controlled by medical therapy, or in case of intolerance to oral calcimimetics.[68]

SUMMARY

PTH anomalies in KTxps and related bone disorders are important clinical problems that require an early diagnosis and management.

The treatment of these disorders might be sometimes difficult, but fortunately, different therapeutic options can be used. Medical therapy should be focused also on ameliorating BMD and possibly reduce the fracture risk. Parathyroidectomy should be reserved for those KTxps in whom a THP is present and cannot be managed with drug therapy.

The expectation for the future is to have even more specific data concerning mineral and bone disorders in KTxps, to increase the evidence and the specificity of international guidelines, and make the management of these anomalies more uniform worldwide.

CLINICS CARE POINTS

- When you study a patient for a future transplantation be careful to evaluate MM parameters, and to characterize deeply his hyper-PTH.
- In the evaluation of hyper-PTH after KTx look for its impact both on bone health and on systemic health, for example, anemia and cardiovascular risk.
- When you monitor calcium levels, look also for ionized calcium.
- Before starting the supplementation of vitamin D in hyper-PTH look for 2 forms of vitamin D.
- In consideration of the strong BMD reduction during the first year of KTx look for DXA both at the beginning and after 1 year of transplantation.
- In clinical practice, take advantage of the combined use of all the therapies available.
- A strong indication of pretransplantation parathyroidectomy can be represented by the presence of a severe hyper-PTH not controlled by medical therapy, or in case of intolerance to oral calcimimetics.

DISCLOSURE

The authors do not have disclosure related to this manuscript to declare.

REFERENCES

1. Egbuna OI, Taylor JG, Bushinsky DA, et al. Elevated calcium phosphate product after renal transplantation is a risk factor for graft failure. Clin Transplant 2007;21: 558–66.
2. Evenepoel P, Claes K, Kuypers D, et al. Natural history of parathyroid function and calcium metabolism after kidney transplantation: a single-centre study. Nephrol Dial Transplant 2004;19(5):1281–7.

3. Pihlstrøm H, Dahle DO, Mjøen G, et al. Increased risk of all-cause mortality and renal graft loss in stable renal transplant recipients with hyperparathyroidism. Transplantation 2015;99(2):351–9.
4. Reinhardt W, Bartelworth H, Jockenhovel F, et al. Sequential changes of biochemical bone parameters after kidney transplantation. Nephrol Dial Transplant 1998; 13(2):436–42.
5. Muirhead N, Zaltman JS, Gill JS, et al. Hypercalcemia in renal transplant patients: prevalence and management in Canadian transplant practice. Clin Transplant 2014;28(2):161–5.
6. Sutton W, Chen X, Patel P, et al. Prevalence and risk factors for tertiary hyperparathyroidism in kidney transplant recipients. Surgery 2021. https://doi.org/10.1016/j.surg.2021.03.067.
7. Morrison NA, Qi JC, Tokita A, et al. Prediction of bone density from vitamin D receptor alleles. Nature 1994;367(6460):284–7.
8. Brown EM. Extracellular Ca2+ sensing, regulation of parathyroid cell function, and role of Ca2+ and other ions as extracellular (first) messenger. Physiol Rev 1991;71:371–411.
9. Messa P, Sindici C, Cannella G, et al. Persistent secondary hyperparathyroidism after renal transplantation. Kidney Int 1998;54(5):1704–13.
10. Ritter C, Miller B, Coyne DW, et al. Paricalcitol and cinacalcet have disparate actions on parathyroid oxyphil cell content in patients with chronic kidney disease. Kidney Int 2017;92(5):1217–22.
11. Ritter CS, Haughey BH, Miller B, et al. Differential gene expression by oxyphil and chief cells of human parathyroid glands. J Clin Endocrinol Metab 2012;97(8): E1499–505.
12. Brown AJ, Dusso A, Lòpez – Hilker S, et al. 1,25-(OH)2D receptors are decreased in parathyroid glands from chronically uremic dogs. Kidney Int 1989;35:19–23.
13. Kumata C, Mizobuchi M, Ogata H, et al. Involvement of Alpha – Klotho and fibroblast growth factor receptor in the development of secondary hyperparathyroidism. Am J Nephrol 2010;31:230–8.
14. Messa P, Cafforio C, Alfieri C. Clinical impact of hypercalcemia in kidney transplant. Int J Nephrol 2011;2011:906832.
15. Wei K, Yin Z, Xie Y. Roles of the kidney in the formation, remodeling and repair of bone. J Nephrol 2016;29(3):349–57.
16. Zheng CM, Zheng JQ, Wu CC, et al. Bone loss in chronic kidney disease: quantity or quality? Bone 2016;87:57–70.
17. Selvi F, Cakarer S, Tanakol R, et al. Brown tumour of the maxilla and mandible: a rare complication of tertiary hyperparathyroidism. Dentomaxillofac Radiol 2009; 38(1):53–8.
18. Brandenburg VM, Politt D, Ketteler M, et al. Early rapid loss followed by long-term consolidation characterizes the development of lumbar bone mineral density after kidney transplantation. Transplantation 2004;77:1566–71.
19. Messa P. Skeletal fractures in patients on renal replacement therapy: how large still is the knowledge gap? Nephrol Dial Transplant 2016;31(10):1554–6.
20. Block G, Port FK. Calcium phosphate metabolism and cardiovascular disease in patients with chronic kidney disease. Semin Dial 2003;16:140–7.
21. Moe SM, Drüeke T, Lameire N, et al. Chronic kidney disease-mineral-bone disorder: a new paradigm. Adv Chronic Kidney Dis 2007;14(1):3–12.
22. Kestenbaum B, Katz R, de Boer I, et al. Vitamin D, parathyroid hormone, and cardiovascular events among older adults. J Am Coll Cardiol 2011;58(14):1433–41.

23. Zingraff J, Drüeke T, Marie P, et al. Anemia and secondary hyperparathyroidism. Arch Intern Med 1978;138(11):1650–2.

24. Tanaka M, Yoshida K, Fukuma S, et al. Effects of secondary hyperparathyroidism treatment on improvement in anemia: results from the MBD-5D Study. PLoS One 2016;11(10):e0164865.

25. Lim AK, Kansal A, Kanellis J. Factors associated with anaemia in kidney transplant recipients in the first year after transplantation: a cross-sectional study. BMC Nephrol 2018;19:252.

26. Hörl WH. The clinical consequences of secondary hyperparathyroidism: focus on clinical outcomes. Nephrol Dial Transplant 2004;19(Suppl 5):V2–8.

27. Herberth J, Fahrleitner-Pammer A, Obermayer-Pietsch B, et al. Changes in total parathyroid hormone (PTH), PTH-(1-84) and large C-PTH fragments in different stages of chronic kidney disease. Clin Nephrol 2006;65(5):328–34.

28. D'Amour P. Acute and chronic regulation of circulating PTH: significance in health and in disease. Clin Biochem 2012;45(12):964–9.

29. Souberbielle JC, Roth H, Fouque DP. Parathyroid hormone measurement in CKD. Kidney Int 2010;77(2):93–100.

30. Payne RB, Little AJ, Williams RB, et al. Interpretation of serum calcium in patients with abnormal serum proteins. Br Med J 1973;4(5893):643–6.

31. Gauci C, Moranne O, Fouqueray B, et al, NephroTest Study Group. Pitfalls of measuring total blood calcium in patients with CKD. J Am Soc Nephrol 2008;19(8):1592–8.

32. Sakaguchi Y, Hamano T, Kubota K. Anion gap as a determinant of ionized fraction of divalent cations in hemodialysis patients. Clin J Am Soc Nephrol 2018;13(2):274–81.

33. Westeel FP, Mazouz H, Ezaitouni F, et al. Cyclosporine bone remodeling effect prevents steroid osteopenia after kidney transplantation. Kidney Int 2000;58(4):1788–96.

34. Wu MS, Hung CC, Chang CT. Renal calcium handling after rapamycin conversion in chronic allograft dysfunction. Transpl Int 2006;19(2):140–5.

35. Julian BA, Laskow DA, Dubovsky J, et al. Rapid loss of vertebral mineral density after renal transplantation. N Engl J Med 1991;325(8):544–50.

36. Saha HH, Salmela KT, Ahonen PJ, et al. Sequential changes in vitamin D and calcium metabolism after successful renal transplantation. Scand J Urol Nephrol 1994;28(1):21–7.

37. Stavroulopoulos A, Cassidy MJ, Porter CJ, et al. Vitamin D status in renal transplant recipients. Am J Transplant 2007;7(11):2546–52.

38. Maruyama Y, Taniguchi M, Kazama JJ, et al. A higher serum alkaline phosphatase is associated with the incidence of hip fracture and mortality among patients receiving hemodialysis in Japan. Nephrol Dial Transplant 2014;29(8):1532–8.

39. Tan SJ, Cai MM. Is there a role for newer biomarkers in chronic kidney disease-mineral and bone disorder management? Nephrology (Carlton) 2017;22(Suppl 2):14–8.

40. Fuster D, Torregrosa JV, Setoain X, et al. Localising imaging in secondary hyperparathyroidism. Minerva Endocrinol 2008;33(3):203–12.

41. Alexander AJ, Jahangir D, Lazarus M, et al. Imaging in chronic kidney disease-metabolic bone disease. Semin Dial 2017;30(4):361–8.

42. Meneghini M, Regalia A, Alfieri C, et al. Calcium and osteoprotegerin levels predict the progression of the abdominal aortic calcifications after kidney transplantation. Transplantation 2013;96(1):42–8.

43. West SL, Lok CE, Langsetmo L, et al. Bone mineral density predicts fractures in chronic kidney disease. J Bone Miner Res 2015;30(5):913–9.
44. Cejka D, Patsch JM, Weber M, et al. Bone microarchitecture in hemodialysis patients assessed by HR-pQCT. Clin J Am Soc Nephrol 2011;6(9):2264–71.
45. Hopper TA, Wehrli FW, Saha PK, et al. Quantitative microcomputed tomography assessment of intratrabecular, intertrabecular, and cortical bone architecture in a rat model of severe renal osteodystrophy. J Comput Assist Tomogr 2007;31(2): 320–8.
46. Malluche HH, Mawad H, Monier-Faugere MC. Effects of treatment of renal osteodystrophy on bone histology. Clin J Am Soc Nephrol 2008;3(Suppl 3):S157–63.
47. Hernandez JD, Wesseling K, Pereira R, et al. Technical approach to iliac crest biopsy. Clin J Am Soc Nephrol 2008;3(Suppl 3):S164–9.
48. Gal-Moscovici A, Sprague SM. Role of bone biopsy in stages 3 to 4 chronic kidney disease. Clin J Am Soc Nephrol 2008;3(Suppl 3):S170–4.
49. Jorgetti V. Review article: bone biopsy in chronic kidney disease: patient level end point or just another test? Nephrology (Carlton) 2009;14(4):404–7.
50. Ketteler M, Block GA, Evenepoel P, et al. Executive summary of the 2017 KDIGO chronic kidney disease-mineral and bone disorder (CKD-MBD) guideline update: what's changed and why it matters. Kidney Int 2017;92(1):26–36.
51. Alfieri C, Ruzhytska O, Vettoretti S, et al. Native hypovitaminosis D in CKD patients: from experimental evidence to clinical practice. Nutrients 2019;11(8):1918.
52. Messa P, Regalia A, Alfieri CM. Nutritional Vitamin D in renal transplant patients: speculations and reality. Nutrients 2017;9(6):550.
53. Hahn TJ, Halstead LR, Baran DT. Efects of short term glucocorticoid administration on intestinal calcium absorption and circulating vitamin D metabolite concentrations in man. J Clin Endocrinol Metab 1981;52(1):111–5.
54. Lieben L, Carmeliet G, Masuyama R. Calcemic actions of vitamin D: effects on the intestine, kidney and bone. Best Pract Res Clin Endocrinol Metab 2011; 25(4):561–72.
55. Rodriguez M, Nemeth E, Martin D. The calcium-sensing receptor: a key factor in the pathogenesis of secondary hyperparathyroidism. Am J Physiol Renal Physiol 2005;288(2):F253–64.
56. Messa P, Alfieri C, Brezzi B. Cinacalcet: pharmacological and clinical aspects. Expert Opin Drug Metab Toxicol 2008;4(12):1551–60.
57. Leonard N, Brown JH. Persistent and symptomatic post-transplant hyperparathyroidism: a dramatic response to cinacalcet. Nephrol Dial Transplant 2006;21(6): 1736.
58. Serra AL, Savoca R, Huber AR, et al. Effective control of persistent hyperparathyroidism with cinacalcet in renal allograft recipients. Nephrol Dial Transplant 2007; 22(2):577–83.
59. Evenepoel P, Cooper K, Holdaas H, et al. A randomized study evaluating cinacalcet to treat hypercalcemia in renal transplant recipients with persistent hyperparathyroidism. Am J Transplant 2014;14(11):2545–55.
60. Messa P, Alfieri CM. Secondary and tertiary hyperparathyroidism. Front Horm Res 2019;51:91–108.
61. Abediazar S, Nakhjavani MR. Effect of alendronate on early bone loss of renal transplant recipients. Transplant Proc 2011;43(2):565–7.
62. Conley E, Muth B, Samaniego M, et al. Bisphosphonates and bone fractures in long-term kidney transplant recipients. Transplantation 2008;86:231–7.

63. Alfieri C, Binda V, Malvica S, et al. Bone effect and safety of one-year denosumab therapy in a cohort of renal transplanted patients: an observational monocentric study. J Clin Med 2021;10(9):1989.
64. Wilson LM, Rebholz CM, Jirru E, et al. Benefits and harms of osteoporosis medications in patients with chronic kidney disease: a systematic review and meta-analysis. Ann Intern Med 2017;166(9):649–58.
65. Lorenz K, Bartsch DK, Sancho JJ, et al. Surgical management of secondary hyperparathyroidism in chronic kidney disease– a consensus report of the European Society of Endocrine Surgeons. Langenbecks Arch Surg 2015;400:907–27.
66. Cruzado JM, Moreno P, Torregrosa JV, et al. A Randomized study comparing parathyroidectomy with cinacalcet for treating hypercalcemia in kidney allograft recipients with hyperparathyroidism. J Am Soc Nephrol 2016;27:2487–94.
67. Fukagawa M, Drueke TB. Parathyroidectomy or calcimimetic to treat hypercalcemia after kidney transplantation? J Am Soc Nephrol 2016;27:2221–4.
68. Messa P, Regalia A, Alfieri CM, et al. Current indications to parathyroidectomy in CKD patients before and after renal transplantation. J Nephrol 2013;26(6): 1025–32.

Hereditary Primary Hyperparathyroidism

Paul J. Newey, MBChB (Hons), DPhil, FRCP*

KEYWORDS

- Genetic testing • Primary hyperparathyroidism
- Familial hypocalciuric hypercalcemia (FHH) • Multiple endocrine neoplasia (MEN)
- Familial isolated hyperparathyroidism (FIHP)
- Hyperparathyroidism–jaw tumor syndrome (HPT-JT)

KEY POINTS

- Hereditary forms of primary hyperparathyroidism (PHPT) account for up to 10% of cases of PHPT and include several multiple tumor syndromes or the occurrence of PHPT as an isolated endocrinopathy.
- Multiple tumor syndromes associated with hereditary PHPT include multiple endocrine neoplasia (MEN) type 1 (MEN1), MEN type 2A, MEN type 4, and the hyperparathyroidism–jaw tumor (HPT-JT) syndrome, each inherited in an autosomal dominant manner.
- Familial isolated hyperparathyroidism (FIHP) describes the familial occurrence of PHPT without the additional manifestations associated with hereditary PHPT syndromes. In a majority of FIHP kindreds, the genetic basis of the disorder is undefined, although 15% to 20% of families harbor activating mutations in the *GCM2* gene.
- Kindreds manifesting apparent FIHP, but harboring pathogenic variants in *MEN1* or *CDC73* genes, should usually be diagnosed and managed in accordance with the associated PHPT syndrome (ie, MEN1 and HPT-JT, respectively).
- It is important to distinguish PHPT from FHH, which has a similar biochemical phenotype to PHPT but is characterized by hypocalciuria. Three forms of FHH are recognized, resulting from pathogenic variants in *CASR* (FHH1), *GNA11* (FHH2), and *AP2S1* (FHH3).
- Genetic testing should be offered to patients in whom hereditary PHPT or FHH is suspected to improve clinical management and to identify other family members who may be at risk of disease.

INTRODUCTION

Although a majority of patients presenting with primary hyperparathyroidism (PHPT) have a nonfamilial (ie, sporadic) etiology, up to 10% of cases occur as part of a hereditary disorder, either as part of a multiple neoplasia syndrome or as an isolated

Division of Molecular and Clinical Medicine, Ninewells Hospital and Medical School, Jacqui Wood Cancer Centre, James Arrott Drive, Dundee, Scotland DD1 9SY, UK
* Corresponding author.
E-mail address: p.newey@dundee.ac.uk

Endocrinol Metab Clin N Am 50 (2021) 663–681
https://doi.org/10.1016/j.ecl.2021.08.003
0889-8529/21/© 2021 Elsevier Inc. All rights reserved.

endo.theclinics.com

endocrinopathy (**Table 1**).[1–8] Although identifying those with hereditary forms of PHPT may be challenging in a busy clinic, establishing a genetic diagnosis may have several benefits for the patient and wider family. These include ensuring the most appropriate management of the PHPT (eg, determining the optimal surgical approach), facilitating the identification of any associated comorbidities, and allowing clinical evaluation and/ or cascade testing of family members. Although several features in the clinical evaluation may indicate a higher likelihood of a hereditary form of PHPT, it is important to consider the possibility of such a diagnosis in all PHPT patients. Germline genetic testing forms an important part of the clinical assessment of those in whom a hereditary PHPT disorder is suspected but requires judicious use to avoid potential diagnostic confusion and patient harms.[9]

In this review, each of the major forms of hereditary PHPT is reviewed, focusing on the parathyroid phenotype and briefly reviewing the molecular/genetic basis of the respective disorder. The hereditary forms of PHPT covered include multiple endocrine neoplasia (MEN) type 1 (MEN1),[3,10,11] MEN type 2A (MEN2A),[8,12] MEN type 4 (MEN4),[13] hyperparathyroidism–jaw tumor (HPT-JT) syndrome,[2,14,15] and familial isolated hyperparathyroidism (FIHP) (see **Table 1**).[5,16] A recently described disorder described as possible MEN type 5, due to germline *MAX* mutations, is not included because a clear association with PHPT has not been established.[17] Given the overlapping clinical and biochemical features with PHPT (and the potential for diagnostic confusion), each of the familial hypocalciuric hypercalcemic (FHH) disorders (ie, FHH1, FHH2, and FHH3) is reviewed,[18,19] as is neonatal severe hyperparathyroidism (NSHPT).[1,19–22] Finally, a suggested clinical and genetic testing workflow is provided.

CLINICAL EVALUATION: IDENTIFICATION OF PATIENTS WITH HEREDITARY PRIMARY HYPERPARATHYROIDISM
History and Examination

The possibility of a hereditary disorder should be considered in all PHPT patients, and a failure to do so may lead to delays in establishing a correct diagnosis, suboptimal or inappropriate patient management, and a missed opportunity to identify other family members who may be at risk of disease. Although the clinical features in those with hereditary PHPT do not typically differ from those of sporadic PHPT, several features may alert a clinician to the possibility of a genetic disorder. For example, although sporadic PHPT most commonly affects those greater than 50 years old, with a 3:1 female predominance, hereditary forms of PHPT frequently have a younger age of onset, with equal sex distribution (ie, due to autosomal patterns of inheritance). For children presenting with PHPT, the likelihood of a hereditary disorder approaches 50%; whereas, approximately 10% of adults with PHPT less than 40 years old may have a hereditary cause.[1,23,24]

During the initial evaluation of the patient, the presence (or history) of clinical manifestations associated with each of the respective hereditary syndromes should be established. Although PHPT most frequently is the presenting features of MEN1 and HPT-JT, in some instances it follows a preceding tumor (eg, prolactinoma or insulinoma in MEN1). Likewise, in young patients presenting with PHPT, the clinical assessment should establish whether there are features of synchronous MEN-associated tumors. Similarly, a careful examination of the patient might provide diagnostic clues; for example, cutaneous manifestations, such as facial angiofibroma or lipomas, might indicate underlying MEN1,[3] whereas more overt findings, such as a concurrent neck mass or hypertension, may indicate MEN2A (ie, from medullary thyroid carcinoma [MTC] or phaeochromocytoma, respectively).[8] In addition, there should be a high clinical

Table 1
Syndromic and nonsyndromic conditions associated with primary hyperparathyroidism

Disorder	Gene	Chromosomal Position	Inheritance	Variant Type	Notes on Disease-Associated Variants/Primary Hyperparathyroidism Phenotype
Syndromic forms of hereditary PHPT					
MEN1	*MEN1*	11q13.1	AD	ms, LOF, del[b]	Pathogenic *MEN1* variants occur throughout the coding region, with no clear genotype-phenotype correlation. MEN1-associated variants result in reduced/loss of function.
MEN2A	*RET*	10q11.21	AD	ms	A majority of MEN2A-associated *RET* affect cysteine residues in the ECD. Additional variants occur in ICD. Strong genotype-phenotype correlation
MEN4	*CDKN1B*	12p13.1	AD	ms, LOF	Limited number of kindred reported to date, no known genotype-phenotype correlation
HPT-JT syndrome	*CDC73*	1q31.2	AD	ms, LOF, del[b]	No clear genotype-phenotype correlation (possible increased risk of PC in those with high-impact *CDC73* mutations)
Nonsyndromic forms of hereditary PHPT, including FHH					
FIHP	*GCM2*	6p24.2	AD	ms,	FIHP associated with *GCM2* variants occur predominantly in C-terminal conserved inhibitory domain but likely are associated with reduced disease penetrance.
	(*MEN1*[a])	11q13.1	AD	ms, LOF	FIHP kindreds with pathogenic *MEN1* variant should be classified as MEN1.
	(*CDC73*[a])	1q31.2	AD	ms, LOF	FIHP kindreds with pathogenic *CDC73* variant should be classified as HPT-JT.
	(*CASR*[a])	3q13.33-q21.1	AD	ms, LOF	It is unclear whether kindreds reported to have FIHP due to *CASR* mutations represent a distinct entity from FHH1.

(continued on next page)

Table 1
(continued)

Disorder	Gene	Chromosomal Position	Inheritance	Variant Type	Notes on Disease-Associated Variants/Primary Hyperparathyroidism Phenotype
FHH1	CASR	3q13.3-q21.1	AD	ms, LOF	A majority of FHH1-associated CASR variants are missense (80%), of which the majority are reported in the ECD with remainder in TM domain.
FHH2	GNA11	19p13.3	AD	ms, (if-del)	Only a small number of FHH2 associated GNA11 variants are reported to date, comprising missense variants and an in-frame deletion reported to reduce protein function.
FHH3	AP2S1	19q13.32	AD	ms (Arg15)	FHH3 results from amino acid substitutions of Arg15 residue. Patients typically manifest a higher calcium than FHH1/2 and may display additional clinical features.
NSHPT	CASR	3q13.33-q21.1	AR	ms, LOF	Associated with homozygous/compound heterozygous CASR variants. Presents in neonatal period with features related to severe hypercalcemia
NHPT	CASR	3q13.33-q21.1	AD	ms, LOF	Associated with heterozygous CASR mutation; neonatal hypercalcemia typically is less severe than NSHPT and may improve over time with nonsurgical management.

LOF variants include nonsense mutations (ie, resulting from a single-nucleotide variant introducing a premature stop codon), small insertions, or deletions (indels), resulting most frequently in a frameshift in the coding sequence and early introduction of a stop codon, and those affected canonical splice sites resulting in aberrant transcript processing.

Abbreviations: aCGH, array comparative genomic hybridization; AD, autosomal dominant; AR, autosomal recessive; comp, het, compound, heterozygous; del, deletion (indicating large-scale whole or partial gene deletion); ECD, extracellular domain; FISH, fluorescence in situ hybridization; hom, homozygous; ICD, intracellular domain; if-del, in-frame deletion; LOF, loss-of-function; MLPA, multiplex ligation-dependent probe amplification; ms, missense; TM, transmembrane domain.

[a] Although kindreds with FIHP have been identified to harbor MEN1, CDC73, and CASR mutations, these likely represent incomplete/atypical expression of the associated syndromic PHPT/FHH disorder. Typically, those harboring pathogenic/likely pathogenic variants in MEN1 and CDC73 genes should be classified as having MEN1 and HPT-JT, respectively. Although a small number of individuals/kindreds with inactivating CASR mutations have been reported to have features more typical of PHPT (ie, hypercalcemia, hypercalciuria, and parathyroid adenoma/hyperplasia), most have a biochemical phenotype more typical of FHH, which is not improved with surgery.

[b] Several monogenic disorders may result from partial or whole gene deletions, which may not be detected by single-gene or gene-panel testing. In this setting, alternate methods may be required, including MLPA, aCGH, or FISH. Some next-generation sequencing platforms, including those used in gene-panel testing, also may detect these large-scale deletions.

suspicion of a genetic diagnosis in those with recurrent or persistent biochemical features of PHPT following previous parathyroid surgery (ie, raising the possibility of FHH or other hereditary hyperparathyroid syndrome).

Family History

Elucidating a patient's family history is paramount in identifying a potential hereditary disorder and should evaluate the presence of family members with a history of PHPT or other MEN or HPT-JT–associated tumors. A positive family history has been reported to be the strongest predictor of a genetic cause in those undergoing genetic testing for PHPT and/or FHH.[25,26] There are several reasons, however, that may limit the availability of such information. For example, a patient may be unaware of their relatives' medical history due to information not being shared between family members or geographic and/or social separation of the kindred.[9] In addition, affected family members may be asymptomatic and remain undiagnosed, whereas certain disorders (eg, HPT-JT due to CDC73 variants and FIHP due to GCM2 variants) are not fully penetrant, such that some affected family members (ie, those harboring the disease-associated variant) may remain disease-free.[16,27,28] Although a majority of familial PHPT disorders have an autosomal dominant mode of inheritance, in some instances, neither parent is affected. For example, a proportion of MEN1, CDC73, and RET pathogenic variants occur de novo (ie, appearing for the first time in the affected individual), whereas in rare instances there may be germline mosaicism, in which the disease-associated mutation occurs in a proportion of 1 parent's gametes, such that apparently unaffected parents may give rise to multiple affected offspring. Recent studies report both germline and somatic mosaicism in kindreds with MEN1.[29,30] In contrast, a history of parental consanguinity may be evident in those with autosomal recessive disorders (for example, NSPHT due to a homozygous calcium-sensing receptor [CASR] mutation).

Biochemical, Radiologic, and Pathologic Evaluations

During the diagnostic work-up, biochemical and radiologic features may help establish a potential genetic diagnosis. For example, the presence of long-standing mild hypercalcemia associated with inappropriately normal or elevated serum PTH and low 24-hour urinary calcium and/or reduced calcium:creatinine clearance ratio (eg, <0.01) may suggest FHH.[1,19,22] Reviewing historic medical records for evidence of a prior normal albumin-corrected calcium may help clarify whether the hypercalcemia is acquired (ie, in keeping in PHPT). The presence of multigland parathyroid involvement on preoperative imaging or at the time of surgery (multigland hyperplasia or adenomas) should raise the possibility of a hereditary disorder, whereas the presence of parathyroid carcinoma (PC) or atypical parathyroid adenoma(s) may suggest HPT-JT.[7]

HEREDITARY CAUSES OF PRIMARY HYPERPARATHYROIDISM
Multiple Endocrine Neoplasia Type 1

Definition/epidemiology

MEN1 is an autosomal dominant disorder characterized by the presence of parathyroid, pituitary, and pancreatic endocrine tumors, although additional tumors, including thymic and bronchial carcinoids and adrenal cortical tumors, also are observed.[3,10,31] MEN1 has an estimated population prevalence of approximately 1 in 30,000 and results from heterozygous germline inactivating mutation of the MEN1 gene. A clinical diagnosis of MEN1 is made in a patient presenting with at least 2 of the 3 main clinical features, whereas a genetic diagnosis of MEN1 describes an individual harboring a known pathogenic MEN1 variant who may not yet manifest any clinical manifestations.[3] Although PHPT in MEN1 almost always is benign, its early age of onset and almost universal occurrence may result in significant morbidity.[3]

Primary hyperparathyroidism clinical features and management. PHPT occurs with almost complete penetrance (>95%) in MEN1 patients, with equal sex distribution (male = female) and is the first manifestation of disease in 75% to 90% of patients.[3] Typically, PHPT presents in early adulthood with a mean age of onset of approximately 20 years, whereas greater than 90% of patients manifest PHPT by age 50 years. PHPT in MEN1 is unusual before 10 years of age, although asymptomatic and symptomatic cases have been reported as early as 4 years and 8 years of age, respectively.[32] Often the biochemical features of PHPT are mild and patients are asymptomatic, although clinical presentations with symptomatic hypercalcemia or end organ involvement are reported (eg, nephrolithiasis). Synchronous or asynchronous involvement of all 4 parathyroid glands typically is observed, whereas the histologic appearances most commonly reveal chief cell hyperplasia, although there is marked variation.[7] Severe hypercalcemia is rare in MEN1, whereas PC has been reported only occasionally.[3]

The treatment of MEN1-associated PHPT is controversial.[3] Surgery is recommended in patients with symptomatic disease, severe hypercalcemia (ie, corrected serum calcium >3.0 mmol/L), and/or evidence of end organ damage (eg, renal stones or osteoporosis).[3] The timing and extent of surgery are debated, however, balancing the risks of persistent/recurrent PHPT with those of permanent hypoparathyroidism.[33] Most centers advocate subtotal parathyroidectomy of at least 3.5 glands, which is associated with a reduced risk of permanent hypoparathyroidism (compared with total parathyroidectomy with autotransplantation) but lower persistence/recurrence rates than lesser surgical approaches.[3,33,34] For example, the removal of less than 3 glands is reported to be associated with persistence/recurrence rates of 15% to 70%.[3,33,34] Some studies, however, have reported more favorable short-term to medium-term outcomes for MEN1 patients treated with less extensive surgical approaches (ie, unilateral parathyroidectomy or minimally invasive parathyroidectomy), such that some centers advocate this approach in young MEN1 patients, accepting the likely need for future surgery but avoiding the immediate risks of permanent hypoparathyroidism.[35] In those undergoing subtotal parathyroidectomy, concurrent bilateral transcervical thymectomy is recommended to remove parathyroid tumors that may be embedded within the thymus. Calcimimetics (eg, cinacalcet) have been used to reduce or normalize serum calcium in MEN1 patients with PHPT in whom surgery has either failed or is contraindicated. Screening for PHPT in MEN1 patients with annual albumin-corrected serum calcium and PTH is recommended from age 5 years.[3]

Molecular Genetics

MEN1 is an autosomal dominant disorder due to loss-of-function germline variants of the *MEN1* gene.[3,10,36] The *MEN1* gene is located on chromosome 11q13 and encodes the multifunctional protein menin. Menin is predominantly a nuclear protein that acts as a molecular scaffold, facilitating the formation of several larger regulatory protein complexes involved in transcriptional and epigenetic regulatory activities as well as modulating multiple cellular signaling pathways (eg, Wnt/β-catenin and hedgehog) in a cell-type and context-specific manner.[37] In endocrine tissues, menin acts as a tumor suppressor protein, with MEN1-associated tumors, including parathyroid tumors, typically demonstrating biallelic *MEN1* inactivation (ie, germline mutation of 1 *MEN1* allele and somatic inactivation of the second allele).[3]

More than 1200 germline *MEN1* mutations have been reported to date (approximately 600 different mutations) and occur throughout the *MEN1* coding region.[36,38,39]

De novo *MEN1* mutations are reported in 10% of cases. Disease-causing *MEN1* mutations include frameshift, nonsense, splice site, and missense mutations, and no clear genotype-phenotype correlation has been established. Approximately 10% of patients with MEN1 do not have a mutation within the coding region of the *MEN1* gene, and some of these cases have large-scale *MEN1* deletions or genetic alterations involving noncoding regions, whereas a minority have pathogenic *CDKN1B* variants (see MEN4).[13,40] Approximately 35% of sporadic parathyroid adenomas reveal biallelic somatic inactivation of the *MEN1* gene, further supporting the central role of the *MEN1* gene in parathyroid tumorigenesis.[41]

Multiple Endocrine Neoplasia Type 2A

Definition/epidemiology

MEN2A is an autosomal dominant disorder with a reported incidence of approximately 1/80,000 live births, characterized by the occurrence of MTC in association with pheochromocytoma and parathyroid tumors.[8,12] In contrast to MEN1 a clear genotype-phenotype correlation is observed, such that the timing of MTC onset and likelihood of other clinical manifestations are related to the specific *RET* mutation.[8]

Primary hyperparathyroidism: clinical features and management. PHPT occurs in fewer than 30% of patients with MEN2A and typically presents in the third to fourth decades.[8,42–44] The risk of PHPT in MEN2A, however, is related to the *RET* mutation. For example, 10% to 30% of patients with codon Cys634 mutations develop PHPT by 35 years to 40 years of age, with carriers of the Cys634Arg *RET* variant at the highest risk.[45–47] The age of onset of PHPT is variable and has been reported as young as 2 years of age.[8] MEN2 patients with PHPT frequently are asymptomatic with mild hypercalcemia.[8] The extent of parathyroid involvement varies from single gland involvement to synchronous or asynchronous involvement of multiple glands, with histologic appearances ranging from mild enlargement with hyperplasia to more overt abnormalities indistinguishable from parathyroid adenomas.[7] The treatment of PHPT in MEN2A typically involves the removal of the enlarged/diseased parathyroid glands with the surgical approach adopted dependent on the timing of diagnosis relative to MTC.[8]

Screening for PHPT in MEN2A is dependent on the specific *RET* mutation and recommended from age 11 years for those with the American Thyroid Association high risk variants (eg, affecting codon 634), whereas it can be delayed until age 16 years for those with moderate risk variants (eg, codons 609–620).[8]

Molecular Genetics

MEN2 results from germline mutation of the *RET* proto-oncogene, located at the pericentromeric region of chromosome 10q11.2, which encodes a single-pass transmembrane receptor tyrosine kinase (RTK) involved in neural crest and enteric nervous system development.[48,49] RET signaling modulates the activity of multiple downstream signaling pathways (eg, Ras/MAPK, PI3K/Akt, JNK, and β-catenin/Wnt) that regulate diverse cellular processes, including differentiation, proliferation, and cell migration.[48,49]

More than 50 different germline *RET* mutations have been reported in association with MEN2A.[8] A majority of MEN2A-associated *RET* mutations involve heterozygous nonsynonymous amino acid substitutions of cysteine residues within the cysteine-rich extracellular domain, most frequently affecting codon Cys634, and result in ligand-independent dimerization and receptor activation, whereas MEN2A mutations affecting the intracellular domain (eg, Tyr791, Val804, and Ser891) result in activated monomers with autonomous tyrosine kinase activity.[49]

Multiple Endocrine Neoplasia Type 4

Definition, clinical features, and management

MEN4 is a rare autosomal dominant disorder with a clinical phenotype similar to that of MEN1, resulting from germline inactivating mutations of the CDKN1B gene.[13] MEN4 should be considered in patients with a MEN1-like clinical phenotype in whom no MEN1 mutation is identified,[3] although to date, fewer than 40 MEN4 patients from less than 20 kindreds have been reported.[13] PHPT, together with functioning or nonfunctioning pituitary adenomas, occur in 30% to 40% of patients and pancreatic and gastrointestinal neuroendocrine tumors (NETs) in 5% to 30%, whereas bronchial and cervical NETs, nonfunctional adrenal tumors, papillary thyroid cancer, lipomas, and breast cancer occur less frequently.[13]

Primary hyperparathyroidism clinical features and management

PHPT is reported in a majority (>90%), if not all, individuals identified with MEN4. The PHPT in MEN4 occurs at a relatively young age but at a later age than in MEN1 (typically ≥40 years), although it has been reported as young as 15 years of age.[13] Recurrent/persistent PHPT has been observed, including in patients treated with subtotal parathyroidectomy, indicating the involvement of multiple glands, and, as such, an investigation and treatment approach similar to MEN1 is suggested.[13]

Molecular Genetics

The CDKN1B gene, located at chromosome 12p13, encodes the cyclin-dependent kinase inhibitor (CDKI) protein p27kip, which regulates the G1/S-phase checkpoint by binding to cyclin E/cdk2 to inhibit cell-cycle progression. The observed germline CDKN1B mutations include protein-truncating (ie, nonsense, frameshift, and splice site) and missense variants, the majority resulting in reduced levels of p27^{kip} protein or altered protein function. Loss of heterozygosity is reported in MEN4-associated tumors, including parathyroid adenomas, further supporting a tumor suppressor function. Germline CDKN1B variants have been reported in patients with apparently sporadic parathyroid adenomas, although the relative high background frequency of rare nonsynonymous variants in CDKI genes indicates that some of these variants may represent benign alleles.[50]

Hyperparathyroidism–Jaw Tumor Syndrome

Definition, clinical features, and management

The HPT-JT syndrome is an autosomal dominant disorder characterized by the development of parathyroid tumors in association with ossifying fibromas of the maxilla and/or mandible, due to mutations of the cell-cycle division 73 (CDC73) gene.[14,15,51] In addition, some patients may develop uterine and renal tumors (eg, Wilms tumors and papillary renal cell carcinomas), whereas rare reported manifestations include pancreatic adenocarcinomas, testicular mixed germ cell tumors, hurthle cell thyroid adenomas, and pituitary lactotroph adenomas.[14,15] HPT-JT is associated with a high incidence of PC.[2,14,15,52] The ossifying fibromas in HPT-JT, which are reported in approximately 10% to 30% of patients, may be single or multiple, may be unilateral or bilateral, and typically present in adulthood with treatment usually involving surgical removal.[15] HPT-JT is associated with reduced disease penetrance such that approximately 10% to 35% of germline CDC73 mutation carriers do not manifest overt clinical features.[14,15]

Primary hyperparathyroidism: clinical features and management

PHPT in HPT-JT is reported to occur in 65% to 90% of patients and arises most frequently in early adulthood (median age of diagnosis 30–35 years), although it is reported in children less than 10 years of age.[2,14,15] A large majority (70%–90%) of patients manifest a single parathyroid tumor, with only a minority (10%–30%) having multigland involvement,[7] although long-term follow-up studies indicate that asynchronous multigland involvement is more common. PC is reported in 15% to 20% of cases and has been reported as early as 8 years of age.[53,54] Although HPT-JT–associated parathyroid adenomas may be indistinguishable from sporadic parathyroid adenomas, a higher frequency of cystic change and other distinct morphologic features are reported.[55]

The investigation and treatment of the HPT-JT–associated PHPT is similar to that in sporadic PHPT although early parathyroidectomy is advisable because of the increased occurrence of PC. The possibility of HPT-JT and genetic testing for the presence of CDC73 mutations should be considered in all patients presenting with PC and atypical parathyroid adenomas.[56]

Molecular Genetics

The CDC73 gene, located on chromosome 1q31.2, encodes the tumor suppressor protein parafibromin.[14,15,57] More than 50 different germline heterozygous CDC73 mutations have been reported.[2,14,15] Somatic CDC73 mutations also have been reported in sporadic PC, parathyroid adenomas, and ossifying fibromas. A majority of HPT-JT associated germline CDC73 mutations result in a functional loss of the parafibromin protein. Examination of parathyroid tumor tissue from HPT-JT patients frequently reveals loss of heterozygosity at the CDC73 locus (and loss of parafibromin expression), indicating a tumor suppressor function.[15] Previous studies have demonstrated an over-representation of CDC73 mutations affecting exons 1, 2, and 7.[2,15]

Parafibromin is an evolutionary conserved, predominantly nuclear protein that forms a component of the ubiquitously expressed human RNA polymerase II–associated factor complex, involved in transcription regulation. Parafibromin is an important regulator of several cell signaling pathways, including Wnt, Notch, and hedgehog pathways.[58] Furthermore, parafibromin, located within the cytoplasm, has been reported to control the stability of p53 mRNA, thereby regulating apoptosis, and also is a target of SUMOylation.[59,60]

NONSYNDROMIC FAMILIAL PRIMARY HYPERPARATHYROIDISM
Familial Isolated Hyperparathyroidism

FIHP refers to autosomal dominant familial hyperparathyroidism occurring as an isolated endocrinopathy, in the absence of clinical manifestations associated with other hereditary PHPT syndromes (eg, MEN1 and HPT-JT).[5] Although kindreds with apparent FIHP have been identified to harbor MEN1 and CDC73 mutations, this likely represents incomplete expression of the wider PHPT syndrome and such families should be followed up as for MEN1 and HPT-JT, respectively. Likewise a small number of families with FIHP have been reported to harbor CASR mutations (ie, with a phenotype consistent with PHPT as opposed to FHH). However, most families with hereditary hypercalcemia and an inactivating CASR mutation will have FHH type 1 (see **Table 1**). Thus, diagnosis of FIHP should usually be made only after excluding the presence of mutations associated with other hereditary PHPT tumor syndromes and FHH, and in this context large FIHP kindreds manifesting exclusive PHPT are rare. Recent studies, however, indicate that up to approximately 15% to 20% of FIHP kindreds harbor activating mutations in the GCM2 gene, located on chromosome 6, which encodes the chorion-specific transcription factor GCMb, involved in parathyroid gland development.[16,61] A majority of FIHP-associated GCM2 variants reported to date occur within a C-terminal conserved inhibitory domain and are associated with enhanced transcriptional activity in vitro. Furthermore, an increased prevalence of rare germline missense GCM2 variants has been reported in cohorts of patients with sporadic PHPT, although associated with a low disease penetrance.[27,28,62–64] Recent clinical studies report an increased prevalence of multi-gland parathyroid disease, lesser rates of surgical cure, and increased risk of parathyroid carcinoma in FIHP kindreds harboring GCM2 variants[27,64] The genetic basis of the remaining 80% of FIHP kindreds remains unexplained, although a majority of such kindreds have low numbers of affected individuals, and in some instances may represent the chance occurrence of sporadic disease in multiple family members. To date, genetic investigation of such kindreds has not identified other recurrently mutated genes.

Familial Hypocalciuric Hypercalcemia

Definition/epidemiology

FHH is a genetically heterogeneous disorder, typically characterized by lifelong mild to moderate hypercalcemia associated with inappropriately normal or elevated PTH, thereby mimicking the phenotype of PHPT.[1,7,18,19,22,65] Clinically it is differentiated from PHPT by the finding of a low urinary calcium excretion (eg, calcium-creatinine clearance ratio [CCCR] less than 0.01 or 24-hour urinary calcium less than 2.5 mmol), because approximately 80% of FHH patients are hypocalciuric. There may be considerable biochemical overlap, however, with PHPT, because approximately 20% of FHH patients have a CCCR above this threshold, whereas 10% to 20% of PHPT patients have a CCCR below this cutoff.[1,19,22] Thus, genetic testing increasingly is used in the diagnostic evaluation.[26] To date, 3 variants of FHH are identified each inherited in an autosomal dominant manner: FHH1 represents approximately 65% of cases and is due to loss-of-function mutations of the CASR; FHH2 accounts for fewer than 5% of FHH cases and is due to loss-of-function GNA11 mutations; and FHH3, which accounts for approximately 20% of FHH cases without a CASR mutations, is due to loss-of-function mutations in the AP2S1 gene.[1,19,22] FHH previously was considered a rare disease, although recent population genetic studies indicate a prevalence of 1/1000 to 1/5000.[50,66] The importance of recognizing FHH from PHPT (and other causes of hereditary PHPT) is in the avoidance of unnecessary investigation and/or treatment. Approximately 10% to 25% of patients who have undergone failed neck exploration for apparent PHPT have been reported to have FHH.[18]

Clinical features and management

Although there may be subtle difference in phenotype, each of the recognized forms of FHH generally is indistinguishable. A majority of patients are asymptomatic, although a minority report symptomatic hypercalcemia (eg, fatigue, muscle cramps, and constipation), whereas end organ manifestations are observed in a small percentage of patients (eg, nephrocalcinosis, osteoporosis and/or fractures, chondrocalcinosis, and pancreatitis), although it is unclear if such associations are causative.[18] Although most individuals with FHH1 and FHH2 have a mild phenotype, individuals with FHH3 typically manifest a higher serum calcium and are reported to have an increased likelihood of reduced bone mineral density, osteomalacia, recurrent pancreatitis, and cognitive dysfunction.[1,7,19]

Asymptomatic individuals with FHH typically do not require treatment. For those with symptomatic hypercalcemia or potential complications related to the condition (eg, recurrent pancreatitis), treatment with cinacalcet has been associated with improvement in biochemical parameters (ie, normalization of serum calcium) in each of FHH1, FHH2, and FHH3.[18,19,67] Although the parathyroid glands of patients with FHH may be mildly enlarged with or without hyperplasia, surgery, including subtotal parathyroidectomy, generally is ineffective and should be avoided.[7,18] Parathyroid adenomas have been reported in occasional patients with apparent inactivating *CASR* mutations, where surgery has improved hypercalcemia, although it is unclear whether these associations are causal.[68]

A history of parental FHH may be important for infants in the neonatal period because they may be at risk of calcium-related phenotypes. For example, infants who inherit a paternal FHH mutation and are exposed to normal maternal calcium levels in utero may manifest marked hypercalcemia (eg, manifesting as neonatal hyperparathyroidism [discussed later]), whereas the offspring of affected mothers who do not inherit the FHH mutation may manifest transient neonatal hypoparathyroidism following exposure to relatively high maternal calcium levels during pregnancy.[1,69]

Molecular Genetics

Familial hypocalciuric hypercalcemia 1. FHH1 is an autosomal dominant disorder due to germline heterozygous mutations in *CASR* gene (a small minority result from homozygous *CASR* mutations), located on chromosome 3q13.3-q21.1, that encodes the calcium-sensing receptor (CaSR).[19,22,65] The CaSR is a class C, G protein–coupled receptor, localized to the cell membrane within calcitropic tissues (eg, parathyroid glands, kidney, and bone) and is responsible primarily for regulation of PTH secretion and urinary calcium excretion. Approximately 300 different *CASR* mutations have been reported in FHH1 patients, the majority missense variants (>80%), with the remainder loss-of-function variants.[19,22,65] A majority of missense variants are located within the extracellular domain, having an impact on key functional domains, with the remainder located within the transmembrane domain.[19,22,65] Recent population-based genetic studies suggest FHH1 occurs with a prevalence of approximately 75/100,000 individuals.[66]

Familial hypocalciuric hypercalcemia 2. FHH2 results from germline heterozygous loss-of function variants in the *GNA11* gene, located on chromosome 19p13.3.[19,70] *GNA11* encodes the $G\alpha_{11}$ protein, which forms part of the heterotrimeric G protein complex associated with CaSR signaling. To date, only a small number of FHH2-associated *GNA11* mutations have been reported, including several missense variants and 1 inframe deletion, which impair CaSR signaling by disrupting key functional domains involved in coupling with the CaSR or interacting with downstream effector proteins.[19]

Familial hypocalciuric hypercalcemia 3. FHH3 results from germline loss-of-function mutations of the *AP2S1* gene located on chromosome 19q13.3, which encodes the adaptor protein 2 sigma subunit that forms part of a larger heterotetrameric complex involved in clathrin-mediated endocytosis.[19,71–73] In contrast to FHH1 and FHH2, an overwhelming majority of FHH3-associated mutations affect a single amino acid residue, Arg15, although several different amino acid substitutions have been observed (eg, Arg15Cys, Arg15His, and Arg15Leu). These different Arg15 variants are predicted to disrupt the interaction between the AP2 complex and the CaSR intracellular domain, thereby reducing endocytosis of the receptor and altering cell surface expression and signal transduction.[72,73]

Neonatal Severe Hyperparathyroidism

NSHPT is a rare disorder that typically presents in the postpartum period (median age of diagnosis, 14 days) with severe hypercalcemia (serum calcium typically 3.0–6.0 mmol/L); elevated PTH; skeletal demineralization, leading to fracture; respiratory distress; and failure to thrive; and; if left untreated, potentially is fatal.[1,20,22,74] Infants with NSHPT typically manifest markedly enlarged parathyroid glands with evidence of diffuse chief cell hyperplasia.[7] Most commonly, NSPHT results from homozygous or compound heterozygous loss-of-function *CASR* variants although also

Clinical Evaluation

Patient presenting with PHPT/FHH phenotype:

Identification of patients suitable for genetic testing:

History/evaluation identifies features suggestive of a potential hereditary PHPT syndrome:

eg, pituitary, pancreatic, thymic/bronchial NETs (MEN1/4), ossifying fibroma (HPT-JT), MTC or pheochromocytom (MEN2A)

Early-onset PHPT disease onset:

- All children with PHPT/FHH (including NSHPT/NHPT)
- Consider in adults <40 y of age

Family history of relevant phenotype:

- FDRs with PHPT/FHH
- FDRS with manifestations of hereditary PHPT disorders (eg, MEN1, MEN2A, HPT-JT associated tumours)

Parathyroid-specific features:

- Parathyroid carcinoma/atypical adenoma(s)
- Multi-gland parathyroid adenomas/hyperplasia
- Previous negative neck exploration/non-curative surgery

Consider potential utility of test for patient/wider family

Patient provided with relevant information

Informed consent obtained from patient (or parent/ guardian in pediatric setting)

Genetic Testing

Single gene test

Suitable where clinical features/family history indicate a specific genetic diagnosis:

eg, MEN1 (*MEN1*), HPT-JT (*CDC73*), MEN2A (*RET*)

Disease-targeted gene panel for PHPT and/or FHH

Indicated where differential diagnosis remains broad:

Hereditary PHPT panel: :

- (*CASR*), *CDC73, CDKN1B, GCM2, MEN1, RET*

FHH panel:

- *AP2S1, CASR, GNA11*

DNA sequencing to include all coding exons and splice sites of the relevant gene (for *RET* analysis may be restricted to exons harboring MEN2A-associated variants)

FHH and PHPT panels may be combined into single panel

MLPA recommended for *MEN1/CDC73* where MEN1/HPT-JT suspected but no mutation identifed by DNA sequencing

ACMG guidelines employed for variant interpretation

All genetic testing performed in an accredited clinical genetics laboratory

---

Post-genetic testing

Review results to establish clinical/genetic diagnosis (ie, does clinical phenotype fit with genetic test result?)

Pathogenic/likely pathogenic variant identified

PHPT syndrome (ie, *MEN1, CDKN1B, CDC73, RET* variant)

- commence appropriate management and follow up (eg, regular surveillance for associated manifestations)
- cascade testing of FDRs

FIHP (ie, *GCM2* variant)

- consider cascade testing of FDRs although *GCM2* variants associated with reduced disease penetrance

FHH1-3 (*CASR, GNA11, AP2S1*)

- cascade testing of FDRs
- appropriate management and patient education (eg, avoidance of surgical intervention for hypercalcaemia)

VUS in relevant gene identified

Estbalish potential to acquire additional evidence to support a more definitive classification

Cascade testing of asymptomatic FDRs not usually recommended

Negative genetic test results

Where a high clinical suspicion of a genetic diagnosis persists, discuss with clinical genetics team to determine whether alternate genetic testing strategies appropriate

---

Fig. 1. Illustrative workflow for genetic testing in patients presenting with PHPT/FHH phenotypes. The strategy for genetic testing (ie, single gene testing vs disease-targeted gene panel) will be determined by the clinical presentation and local policies. Variants identified through genetic testing should be classified according to the ACMG guidelines.[77] Where VUSs are identified, it is important to establish whether additional information may be acquired to facilitate a more categorical classification (eg, genetic testing of further affected family members to evaluate for co-segregation of the variant with disease phenotype or additional in vitro/in silico functional analysis). Whether patients harboring VUS require clinical follow-up may depend on the further risk stratification of the variant (eg, hot vs cold VUS classification). Furthermore, variant classification may change over time, such that periodic re-evaluation of variants is recommended. FDRs, first-degree relatives; MLPA, multiplex ligation-dependent probe amplification.

may occur in the setting of heterozygous *CASR* mutations.[20,74] Some centers differentiate between NSPHT and neonatal hyperparathyroidism (NHPT) based on the presence of homozygous/biallelic or heterozygous *CASR* mutations, respectively, and in the latter group, the severity of hypercalcemia typically is less pronounced than in NSHPT and may improve over time to a phenotype consistent with FHH1, without the need for parathyroid surgery[1,20,74] The treatment of NSHPT usually is

Table 2
Potential indications for genetic testing in patients with primary hyperparathyroidism /familial hypocalciuric hypercalcemia

Indication for Genetic Testing	Genetic Testing Strategy
All children/young persons with PHPT phenotype (eg, <21 y of age)	PHPT/FHH panel[c] (including *MEN1/ CDC73/CASR*)
Adults with PHPT <40 y[a] of age	PHPT panel (FHH panel[c])
Multigland PHPT (adenoma or hyperplasia)	PHPT panel (FHH panel[c])
PC	*CDC73 (GCM2*[b]*)*
Atypical parathyroid adenoma(s)	*CDC73 (GCM2*[b]*)*
Clinical diagnosis and/or features consistent with hereditary PHPT syndrome (current or past history of relevant tumors)	Relevant gene(s) or PHPT gene panel
MEN1/4 (eg, PHPT + other MEN1- associated tumor(s))	*MEN1/CDKN1B*
MEN2A (eg, PHPT + MTC and/or pheochromocytoma)	*RET*
HPT-JT (eg, PHPT + ossifying fibroma of mandible/maxilla)	*CDC73*
Family history suggestive of hereditary PHPT syndrome (ie, manifestations consistent with MEN1/4, MEN2A, or HPT-JT)	Relevant gene (PHPT panel)
Family history of PHPT/FHH in first-degree relatives	PHPT/FHH panels
History and biochemistry consistent with FHH (eg, CCCR <0.01)	FHH panel
Previous negative neck exploration/ noncurative surgery	FHH panel (PHPT panel)

This list of indications is not evidence based but rather provided to help highlight patients with a potentially increased risk of hereditary disease. The criteria for referral in any given center depend on local policies and resources.

[a] To date, no clear age-alone cutoff has been established for genetic testing. In some centers, the age cutoff is dependent on the presence of additional risk factors, for example, presence of multigland involvement or positive family history.

[b] Although genetic testing of *CDC73* is recommended in those with PC/atypical parathyroid adenomas, a recent study reports an increased prevalence of PC in those with *GCM2* mutation.

[c] Most centers now adopt the use of disease targeted gene panels for investigation of hereditary PHPT and FHH syndromes. The content of the panels varies by center but typically includes PHPT panel; *CDC73, CDKN1B, MEN1, RET, CASR*, and *GCM2*; and/or FHH panel: *AP2S1, CASR*, and *GNA11*. In some centers, these are combined into a single PHPT/FHH panel. The value of genetic testing for pathogenic variants in *GCM2* has not yet been fully evaluated because such variants are likely to be associated with low disease penetrance.

with urgent parathyroidectomy, with bisphosphonates employed preoperatively to control the hypercalcemia. Cinacalcet also has been used successfully to lower calcium and PTH levels in some NSHPT patients, including those with heterozygous (eg, Arg185Gln) and homozygous (eg, Arg69His) *CASR* mutations, although some mutations are unresponsive to such therapy.[74]

GENETIC TESTING WORKFLOW

The decision to undertake genetic testing should be determined by the potential to improve health outcomes in the patient and/or wider family (**Fig. 1**).[9] For example, establishing a genetic diagnosis of a multiple tumor syndrome, such as MEN1, MEN2A, or HPT-JT, not only facilitates the appropriate investigation and management of the associated clinical features in a patient but also enables predictive testing in family members. Genetic testing also may resolve diagnostic confusion arising from phenocopies (ie, patients manifesting the phenotypic characteristics of a particular genetic disorder but without the relevant gene mutation), which are reported in clinical presentations of MEN1, MEN2A, HPT-JT, and FHH.[3,31,64,75,76] Genetic testing, however, is not without potential harms. For example, uncertain test results or variant misclassification (eg, benign variants reported as pathogenic) may lead to diagnostic confusion and/or inappropriate patient management.

Although several criteria for genetic testing in patients with PHPT have been suggested (**Table 2**), these have not been evaluated systematically. Likewise, the genetic testing strategy employed depends on several factors, although a majority of centers now adopt disease-targeted gene panels to facilitate the simultaneous evaluation of multiple PHPT and/or FHH genes (see **Fig. 1**, **Table 2**). The evaluation of variants identified during genetic testing should be undertaken using standardized methods (eg, American College of Medical Genetics and Genomics [ACMG] guidelines) (see **Fig. 1**),[77] which combine several variant and gene-specific factors to categorize variants into 1 of 5 categories: benign, likely benign, variant of uncertain significance (VUS), likely pathogenic, and pathogenic. This classification system, however, is not absolute, and is dependent on the accuracy of available evidence at the time of assessment (see **Fig. 1**). Furthermore, a high cumulative frequency of rare coding region variation in the background population may hamper variant interpretation and increases the potential to identify VUS variants during gene panel testing.[50]

Following genetic testing, it is important to consider the result in the clinical context of the patient (ie, to establish a clinical-genetic diagnosis). Where a genetic diagnosis is suspected but initial genetic testing is negative, it is important to liaise with the local genetics team to determine whether alternate testing strategies may be helpful. For example, next-generation sequencing methods with increased depth of sequencing have identified *MEN1* mutations in patients in whom prior Sanger genetic testing was negative.[30,76] Finally, following the identification of a positive test result in a patient (ie, pathogenic/likely pathogenic variant), clinical evaluation and predictive testing of family members should be undertaken through the clinical genetics team (see **Fig. 1**).

SUMMARY

Up to 10% of PHPT cases occur in a hereditary context either as part of 1 of several syndromic disorders or as an apparently isolated feature. Differentiating these hereditary causes is important not only to ensure the appropriate management of PHPT but also to identify any coexistent clinical features in patients with hereditary PHPT syndromes as well as allowing the identification of other affected family members.

Germline genetic testing forms a key component of the evaluation of patients with possible hereditary PHPT but should be undertaken only after thorough clinical evaluation.

CLINICS CARE POINTS

- A thorough family history should be acquired in all patients presenting with PHPT, although the absence of any apparent relevant findings does not exclude the possibility of a hereditary disorder.

- Evaluating historic medical records to look for evidence of previously normal albumin-corrected serum calcium levels may help differentiate between PHPT and FHH, with the latter associated with lifelong hypercalcemia

- Close collaborative working between endocrinologists, clinical genetics, and genetic laboratory scientists is required to facilitate the most appropriate genetic testing strategies and to facilitate accurate variant interpretation

- Patients with hereditary PHPT syndromes, including MEN1 and MEN2A, should be managed by multidisciplinary teams with relevant expertise in the management of the respective disorders.

FUNDING STATEMENT

The author holds a Scottish Senior Clinical Fellowship (SCAF/15/01) funded by the Chief Scientist Office (UK), NHS Research Scotland (NRS) and University of Dundee.

DISCLOSURE

The author receives research funding from the Chief Scientist Office. The author has received speaker fees from Ipsen.

REFERENCES

1. Stokes VJ, Nielsen MF, Hannan FM, et al. Hypercalcemic Disorders in Children. J Bone Miner Res 2017;32:2157–70.
2. Cardoso L, Stevenson M, Thakker RV. Molecular genetics of syndromic and non-syndromic forms of parathyroid carcinoma. Hum Mutat 2017;38:1621–48.
3. Thakker RV, Newey PJ, Walls GV, et al. Clinical practice guidelines for multiple endocrine neoplasia type 1 (MEN1). J Clin Endocrinol Metab 2012;97:2990–3011.
4. Marx SJ, Goltzman D. Evolution of Our Understanding of the Hyperparathyroid Syndromes: A Historical Perspective. J Bone Miner Res 2019;34:22–37.
5. Marx SJ. New Concepts About Familial Isolated Hyperparathyroidism. J Clin Endocrinol Metab 2019;104:4058–66.
6. Cetani F, Saponaro F, Borsari S, et al. Familial and Hereditary Forms of Primary Hyperparathyroidism. Front Horm Res 2019;51:40–51.
7. DeLellis RA, Mangray S. Heritable forms of primary hyperparathyroidism: a current perspective. Histopathology 2018;72:117–32.
8. Wells SA Jr, Asa SL, Dralle H, et al. Revised American Thyroid Association guidelines for the management of medullary thyroid carcinoma. Thyroid 2015;25:567–610.
9. Newey PJ. Clinical genetic testing in endocrinology: Current concepts and contemporary challenges. Clin Endocrinol (Oxf) 2019;91:587–607.

10. Brandi ML, Agarwal SK, Perrier ND, et al. Multiple Endocrine Neoplasia Type 1: Latest Insights. Endocr Rev 2021;42:133–70.
11. Al-Salameh A, Cadiot G, Calender A, et al. Clinical aspects of multiple endocrine neoplasia type 1. Nat Rev Endocrinol 2021;17:207–24.
12. Wells SA Jr. Advances in the management of MEN2: from improved surgical and medical treatment to novel kinase inhibitors. Endocr Relat Cancer 2018;25:T1–13.
13. Frederiksen A, Rossing M, Hermann P, et al. Clinical Features of Multiple Endocrine Neoplasia Type 4: Novel Pathogenic Variant and Review of Published Cases. J Clin Endocrinol Metab 2019;104:3637–46.
14. van der Tuin K, Tops CMJ, Adank MA, et al. CDC73-Related Disorders: Clinical Manifestations and Case Detection in Primary Hyperparathyroidism. J Clin Endocrinol Metab 2017;102:4534–40.
15. Newey PJ, Bowl MR, Cranston T, et al. Cell division cycle protein 73 homolog (CDC73) mutations in the hyperparathyroidism-jaw tumor syndrome (HPT-JT) and parathyroid tumors. Hum Mutat 2010;31:295–307.
16. Guan B, Welch JM, Sapp JC, et al. GCM2-Activating Mutations in Familial Isolated Hyperparathyroidism. Am J Hum Genet 2016;99:1034–44.
17. Seabrook AJ, Harris JE, Velosa SB, et al. Multiple Endocrine Tumors Associated with Germline MAX Mutations: Multiple Endocrine Neoplasia Type 5? J Clin Endocrinol Metab 2021;106:1163–82.
18. Lee JY, Shoback DM. Familial hypocalciuric hypercalcemia and related disorders. Best Pract Res Clin Endocrinol Metab 2018;32:609–19.
19. Hannan FM, Babinsky VN, Thakker RV. Disorders of the calcium-sensing receptor and partner proteins: insights into the molecular basis of calcium homeostasis. J Mol Endocrinol 2016;57:R127–42.
20. Marx SJ, Sinaii N. Neonatal Severe Hyperparathyroidism: Novel Insights From Calcium, PTH, and the CASR Gene. J Clin Endocrinol Metab 2020;105.
21. Mayr B, Schnabel D, Dorr HG, et al. GENETICS IN ENDOCRINOLOGY: Gain and loss of function mutations of the calcium-sensing receptor and associated proteins: current treatment concepts. Eur J Endocrinol 2016;174:R189–208.
22. Hannan FM, Kallay E, Chang W, et al. The calcium-sensing receptor in physiology and in calcitropic and noncalcitropic diseases. Nat Rev Endocrinol 2018;15:33–51.
23. Alagaratnam S, Kurzawinski TR. Aetiology, Diagnosis and Surgical Treatment of Primary Hyperparathyroidism in Children: New Trends. Horm Res Paediatr 2015;83:365–75.
24. El Allali Y, Hermetet C, Bacchetta J, et al. Presenting features and molecular genetics of primary hyperparathyroidism in the paediatric population. Eur J Endocrinol 2021;184:347–55.
25. El Lakis M, Nockel P, Gaitanidis A, et al. Probability of Positive Genetic Testing Results in Patients with Family History of Primary Hyperparathyroidism. J Am Coll Surg 2018;226:933–8.
26. Mariathasan S, Andrews KA, Thompson E, et al. Genetic testing for hereditary hyperparathyroidism and familial hypocalciuric hypercalcaemia in a large UK cohort. Clin Endocrinol (Oxf) 2020;93:409–18.
27. Coppin L, Dufosse M, Romanet P, et al. Should the GCM2 gene be tested when screening for familial primary hyperparathyroidism? Eur J Endocrinol 2020;182:57–65.
28. Guan B, Welch JM, Vemulapalli M, et al. Ethnicity of Patients With Germline GCM2-Activating Variants and Primary Hyperparathyroidism. J Endocr Soc 2017;1:488–99.

29. Beijers H, Stikkelbroeck NML, Mensenkamp AR, et al. Germline and somatic mosaicism in a family with multiple endocrine neoplasia type 1 (MEN1) syndrome. Eur J Endocrinol 2019;180:K15–9.

30. Coppin L, Ferriere A, Crepin M, et al. Diagnosis of mosaic mutations in the MEN1 gene by next generation sequencing. Eur J Endocrinol 2019;180:L1–3.

31. Newey PJ, Thakker RV. Role of multiple endocrine neoplasia type 1 mutational analysis in clinical practice. Endocr Pract 2011;17(Suppl 3):8–17.

32. Goudet P, Dalac A, Le Bras M, et al. MEN1 disease occurring before 21 years old: a 160-patient cohort study from the Groupe d'etude des Tumeurs Endocrines. J Clin Endocrinol Metab 2015;100:1568–77.

33. Choi HR, Choi SH, Choi SM, et al. Benefit of diverse surgical approach on short-term outcomes of MEN1-related hyperparathyroidism. Sci Rep 2020;10:10634.

34. Nilubol N, Weinstein LS, Simonds WF, et al. Limited Parathyroidectomy in Multiple Endocrine Neoplasia Type 1-Associated Primary Hyperparathyroidism: A Setup for Failure. Ann Surg Oncol 2016;23:416–23.

35. Kluijfhout WP, Beninato T, Drake FT, et al. Unilateral Clearance for Primary Hyperparathyroidism in Selected Patients with Multiple Endocrine Neoplasia Type 1. World J Surg 2016;40:2964–9.

36. Lemos MC, Thakker RV. Multiple endocrine neoplasia type 1 (MEN1): analysis of 1336 mutations reported in the first decade following identification of the gene. Hum Mutat 2008;29:22–32.

37. Matkar S, Thiel A, Hua X. Menin: a scaffold protein that controls gene expression and cell signaling. Trends Biochem Sci 2013;38:394–402.

38. Marini F, Giusti F, Brandi ML. Multiple endocrine neoplasia type 1: extensive analysis of a large database of Florentine patients. Orphanet J Rare Dis 2018;13:205.

39. Concolino P, Costella A, Capoluongo E. Multiple endocrine neoplasia type 1 (MEN1): An update of 208 new germline variants reported in the last nine years. Cancer Genet 2016;209:36–41.

40. Kooblall KG, Boon H, Cranston T, et al. Multiple Endocrine Neoplasia Type 1 (MEN1) 5'UTR Deletion, in MEN1 Family, Decreases Menin Expression. J Bone Miner Res 2021;36:100–9.

41. Newey PJ, Nesbit MA, Rimmer AJ, et al. Whole-exome sequencing studies of nonhereditary (sporadic) parathyroid adenomas. J Clin Endocrinol Metab 2012; 97:E1995–2005.

42. Machens A, Dralle H. Therapeutic Effectiveness of Screening for Multiple Endocrine Neoplasia Type 2A. J Clin Endocrinol Metab 2015;100:2539–45.

43. Moley JF, Skinner M, Gillanders WE, et al. Management of the Parathyroid Glands During Preventive Thyroidectomy in Patients With Multiple Endocrine Neoplasia Type 2. Ann Surg 2015;262:641–6.

44. Guerin C, Romanet P, Taieb D, et al. Looking beyond the thyroid: advances in the understanding of pheochromocytoma and hyperparathyroidism phenotypes in MEN2 and of non-MEN2 familial forms. Endocr Relat Cancer 2018;25:T15–28.

45. Machens A, Dralle H. Variability in penetrance of multiple endocrine neoplasia 2A with amino acid substitutions in RET codon 634. Clin Endocrinol (Oxf) 2016;84: 210–5.

46. Machens A, Dralle H. Advances in risk-oriented surgery for multiple endocrine neoplasia type 2. Endocr Relat Cancer 2018;25:T41–52.

47. Valdes N, Navarro E, Mesa J, et al. RET Cys634Arg mutation confers a more aggressive multiple endocrine neoplasia type 2A phenotype than Cys634Tyr mutation. Eur J Endocrinol 2015;172:301–7.

48. Plaza-Menacho I. Structure and function of RET in multiple endocrine neoplasia type 2. Endocr Relat Cancer 2018;25:T79–90.

49. Mulligan LM. 65 YEARS OF THE DOUBLE HELIX: Exploiting insights on the RET receptor for personalized cancer medicine. Endocr Relat Cancer 2018;25: T189–200.

50. Newey PJ, Berg JN, Zhou K, et al. Utility of Population-Level DNA Sequence Data in the Diagnosis of Hereditary Endocrine Disease. J Endocr Soc 2017;1:1507–26.

51. Carpten JD, Robbins CM, Villablanca A, et al. HRPT2, encoding parafibromin, is mutated in hyperparathyroidism-jaw tumor syndrome. Nat Genet 2002;32: 676–80.

52. Cetani F, Pardi E, Marcocci C. Parathyroid Carcinoma. Front Horm Res 2019;51: 63–76.

53. Dutta A, Pal R, Jain N, et al. Pediatric Parathyroid Carcinoma: A Case Report and Review of the Literature. J Endocr Soc 2019;3:2224–35.

54. Davidson JT, Lam CG, McGee RB, et al. Parathyroid Cancer in the Pediatric Patient. J Pediatr Hematol Oncol 2016;38:32–7.

55. Gill AJ, Lim G, Cheung VKY, et al. Parafibromin-deficient (HPT-JT Type, CDC73 Mutated) Parathyroid Tumors Demonstrate Distinctive Morphologic Features. Am J Surg Pathol 2019;43:35–46.

56. Cetani F, Marcocci C, Torregrossa L, et al. Atypical parathyroid adenomas: challenging lesions in the differential diagnosis of endocrine tumors. Endocr Relat Cancer 2019;26:R441–64.

57. Newey PJ, Bowl MR, Thakker RV. Parafibromin–functional insights. J Intern Med 2009;266:84–98.

58. Kikuchi I, Takahashi-Kanemitsu A, Sakiyama N, et al. Dephosphorylated parafibromin is a transcriptional coactivator of the Wnt/Hedgehog/Notch pathways. Nat Commun 2016;7:12887.

59. Lamoliatte F, Caron D, Durette C, et al. Large-scale analysis of lysine SUMOylation by SUMO remnant immunoaffinity profiling. Nat Commun 2014;5:5409.

60. Jo JH, Chung TM, Youn H, et al. Cytoplasmic parafibromin/hCdc73 targets and destabilizes p53 mRNA to control p53-mediated apoptosis. Nat Commun 2014;5:5433.

61. Cetani F, Pardi E, Aretini P, et al. Whole exome sequencing in familial isolated primary hyperparathyroidism. J Endocrinol Invest 2020;43:231–45.

62. Garcia-Castano A, Madariaga L, Gomez-Conde S, et al. Five patients with disorders of calcium metabolism presented with GCM2 gene variants. Sci Rep 2021;11:2968.

63. Riccardi A, Aspir T, Shen L, et al. Analysis of Activating GCM2 Sequence Variants in Sporadic Parathyroid Adenomas. J Clin Endocrinol Metab 2019;104:1948–52.

64. El Lakis M, Nockel P, Guan B, et al. Familial isolated primary hyperparathyroidism associated with germline GCM2 mutations is more aggressive and has a lesser rate of biochemical cure. Surgery 2018;163:31–4.

65. Gorvin CM, Frost M, Malinauskas T, et al. Calcium-sensing receptor residues with loss- and gain-of-function mutations are located in regions of conformational change and cause signalling bias. Hum Mol Genet 2018;27:3720–33.

66. Dershem R, Gorvin CM, Metpally RPR, et al. Familial Hypocalciuric Hypercalcemia Type 1 and Autosomal-Dominant Hypocalcemia Type 1: Prevalence in a Large Healthcare Population. Am J Hum Genet 2020;106:734–47.

67. Gorvin CM, Hannan FM, Cranston T, et al. Cinacalcet Rectifies Hypercalcemia in a Patient With Familial Hypocalciuric Hypercalcemia Type 2 (FHH2) Caused by a Germline Loss-of-Function Galpha11 Mutation. J Bone Miner Res 2018;33:32–41.

68. Frank-Raue K, Leidig-Bruckner G, Haag C, et al. Inactivating calcium-sensing receptor mutations in patients with primary hyperparathyroidism. Clin Endocrinol (Oxf) 2011;75:50–5.
69. Dharmaraj P, Gorvin CM, Soni A, et al. Neonatal Hypocalcemic Seizures in Offspring of a Mother With Familial Hypocalciuric Hypercalcemia Type 1 (FHH1). J Clin Endocrinol Metab 2020;105.
70. Nesbit MA, Hannan FM, Howles SA, et al. Mutations affecting G-protein subunit alpha11 in hypercalcemia and hypocalcemia. N Engl J Med 2013;368:2476–86.
71. Nesbit MA, Hannan FM, Howles SA, et al. Mutations in AP2S1 cause familial hypocalciuric hypercalcemia type 3. Nat Genet 2013;45:93–7.
72. Gorvin CM, Rogers A, Hastoy B, et al. AP2sigma Mutations Impair Calcium-Sensing Receptor Trafficking and Signaling, and Show an Endosomal Pathway to Spatially Direct G-Protein Selectivity. Cell Rep 2018;22:1054–66.
73. Gorvin CM. Insights into calcium-sensing receptor trafficking and biased signalling by studies of calcium homeostasis. J Mol Endocrinol 2018;61:R1–12.
74. Gorvin CM. Molecular and clinical insights from studies of calcium-sensing receptor mutations. J Mol Endocrinol 2019;63:R1–16.
75. Lines KE, Nachtigall LB, Dichtel LE, et al. Multiple Endocrine Neoplasia Type 1 (MEN1) Phenocopy Due to a Cell Cycle Division 73 (CDC73) Variant. J Endocr Soc 2020;4:bvaa142.
76. Backman S, Bajic D, Crona J, et al. Whole genome sequencing of apparently mutation-negative MEN1 patients. Eur J Endocrinol 2020;182:35–45.
77. Richards S, Aziz N, Bale S, et al. Standards and guidelines for the interpretation of sequence variants: a joint consensus recommendation of the American College of Medical Genetics and Genomics and the Association for Molecular Pathology. Genet Med 2015;17:405–24.

Parathyroid Carcinoma and Ectopic Secretion of Parathyroid hormone

Filomena Cetani, MD, PhD[a],*, Elena Pardi, MS, PhD[b],
Claudio Marcocci, MD[a,b]

KEYWORDS

- Primary hyperparathyroidism • HPT-JT • PTH • Hypercalcemia • *CDC73*
- Parafibromin • PI3K/AKT/mTOR

KEY POINTS

- Parathyroid carcinoma (PC) is one of the rarest known malignancies and accounts for less than 1% of primary hyperparathyroidism (PHPT).
- Preoperatively, PC cannot be distinguished from benign PHPT, because no disease-specific markers are available and should be suspected in patients with severe hypercalcemia or related PHPT end-organ complications.
- Somatic *CDC73* mutations are found in up 80% of cases and in approximately one-third are germline; thus, testing for germline *CDC73* mutation is strongly recommended in patients with apparently sporadic PC.
- Patients suspected of having PC should have primary radical en bloc surgery performed by an experienced surgeon.
- Ectopic production of parathyroid hormone (PTH) is a rare condition and accounts for less than 1% of malignancy-associated hypercalcemia and is due to the ectopic secretion of PTH by malignant nonparathyroid tumors.

INTRODUCTION

The most common causes of hypercalcemia are primary hyperparathyroidism (PHPT) and malignancy. PHPT occurs mostly in free-living individuals (80%–90%) and hypercalcemia of malignancy in hospitalized patients.[1] The latter condition implies a limited life expectancy whereas PHPT usually has a relatively benign course. Parathyroid carcinoma (PC), causing severe PHPT, is the rarest parathyroid tumor, accounting for less than 1% of all cases of PHPT and approximately 0.005% of all cancer.[2,3] An increased

[a] University Hospital of Pisa, Endocrine Unit 2, Via Paradisa, 2, Pisa 56124, Italy; [b] Department of Clinical and Experimental Medicine, University of Pisa, Via Paradisa, 2, Pisa 56124, Italy
* Corresponding author.
E-mail address: cetani@endoc.med.unipi.it

Endocrinol Metab Clin N Am 50 (2021) 683–709
https://doi.org/10.1016/j.ecl.2021.07.001   **endo.theclinics.com**

incidence of PC (60%) has been reported in the United States for 16 years, from 1988 to 2003.[4] Such a trend also has been observed in Australia and Finland, from 2000 to 2010 and from 2000 to 2013, compared with the previous decade, and from 1955 to 1999, respectively.[5,6] A similar rise of PC incidence over time recently has been reported in South Korea,[7] at variance with benign disease, where women predominate over men, with a ratio of 3 to 4:1, PC occurs are a ratio of 1:1. The age at diagnosis is in the mid-40s or 50s, which is a decade earlier than the typical age of benign disease. PCs typically occur sporadically or as part of hereditary syndromes particularly in hyperparathyroidism–jaw tumor syndrome (HPT-JT), a rare autosomal disorder, in which as many as 37% of patients have malignant parathyroid disease.[8,9] The clinical profile of patients with PC is characterized by bone and renal involvement, and signs and symptoms related to tumor burden occur lately with the development of intractable hypercalcemia, leading to death.[10] In exceptional cases (2% of all PCs), PC is nonfunctioning, that is, characterized by normal serum calcium and parathyroid hormone (PTH) levels, and the presenting symptoms and signs are due to local growth and invasion of adjacent structures.[11–14]

From a clinical perspective, a diagnosis of PC is challenging because the clinical presentation overlaps with that of benign parathyroid tumors, although more severe, and, as a consequence, diagnosis rarely is made preoperatively unless there is evidence of local invasion or metastases.[3] Moreover, the histologic diagnosis of PC sometimes is difficult because some pathologic features overlap with those of atypical parathyroid adenomas, an intermediate form of parathyroid neoplasms of uncertain malignant potential.[15] When clinical, biochemical, and instrumental findings raise suspicion of malignancy, however, a more extensive surgery with en bloc resection of the primary tumor along with the adjacent structures (ie, the ipsilateral thyroid lobe) may facilitate complete tumor resection.[13,16–18] This initial operative approach seems to reduce the risk of recurrence and metastasis, thus allowing for the highest chance of a cure, although in some series mortality or recurrence rates were not affected by the extent of thyroid resection.[13,19–22]

Mutation of the cell division cycle 73 (CDC73) gene (previously known as HRPT2) have been detected in up to 80% of sporadic PCs and in approximately one-third of cases is germline.[3,6] Studies using a next-generation sequencing approach have identified alterations in several genes other than the CDC73, being the most common mutated genes enriched in the phosphatidylinositol 3-kinase/Protein kinase B/mechanistic target of rapamycin (PI3K/AKT/mTOR) signaling pathway.

Ectopic production of PTH by malignant nonparathyroid tumors is a rare condition and accounts for less than 1% of hypercalcemia of malignancy. In this condition, PTH secretion can be considered an aberration in the tissue specificity of gene expression and may involve heterogeneous molecular mechanisms, such as rearrangements of the PTH gene promoter with the cyclin D1 gene and amplification and rearrangement of the 5′ regulatory region of the PTH gene.[23] Surgery represents the most effective treatment, although the control of hypercalcemia in these patients often is difficult.

This review focuses on the more recent advances on PC, in particular its molecular profile, diagnosis, and treatment, and on ectopic production of PTH.

PARATHYROID CARCINOMA
Genetic Profile

The rarity of PC, due to its low prevalence, late diagnosis, and difficult access to tissue banks, has posed particular challenges to define its molecular etiology. Loss-of-function mutations of the CDC73 gene represent the most common genetic alteration underlying HPT-JT (up to 75%) and also have been detected in up to 80% of PC occurring outside the setting of the syndrome.[9,24] The different frequency of CDC73 mutations in sporadic PCs (between 15% and 100%) varies on the basis of case selections, that is, if PCs with local invasion/recurrence and/or metastasis or PCs fulfilling only histologic features were included in the study.[25–29] Nevertheless, in approximately one-third of apparently sporadic PC patients, the mutations are germline, suggesting that a subset of these patients might have the HPT-JT syndrome or a variant. On the contrary, CDC73 mutations rarely are found in sporadic parathyroid adenomas (PAs), indicating a limited, if any, pathogenic role in this neoplasia.[25,29–33]

The mutations detected in PC, mostly nonsense and frameshift, have a high impact on the integrity and function of the CDC73-encoded protein parafibromin, mainly caused by the disruption of its C-terminal domain.[34] The reduction or the complete loss of expression of parafibromin at immunohistochemistry, reflecting the established role of the protein as a tumor suppressor in PC, has been detected with a rate significantly higher in PC than in other parathyroid lesions.[35] The question of whether parafibromin immunostaining has the desirable diagnostic accuracy to be used as a diagnostic marker in daily practice has been debated widely.[35–38] Negative parafibromin staining together with a CDC73 mutation-positive genetic test increases the likelihood of malignancy and might be helpful in predicting the prognosis of PC. A recent systematic review and meta-analysis study based on individual patient data outlined that the presence of a CDC73 mutation was not statistically correlated with recurrence, metastasis or mortality in PCs.[39] Conversely, negative parafibromin staining was more promising in predicting the outcome of PC.[39] The inconsistency between the identification of a CDC73 mutation and parafibromin staining might be due to alternative mechanisms causative of the loss of parafibromin expression, such as mutations outside CDC73 coding regions and epigenetic regulation, such as methylation, histone modifications, or mechanisms of RNA interference.[39] Loss of parafibromin expression could affect 1 or several tumor-suppressive mechanisms.

A comprehensive genomic profiling approach has been used to identify novel PC-associated gene variants. Although PC samples presented a marked intertumoral genetic heterogeneity, several studies have found, besides defects in the CDC73 gene, additional gene variations, detected mostly at a modest to low mutational frequencies, in novel candidate tumor genes.

Whole-genome sequencing of primary PC and 2 different recurrences of the same patient first detected somatic mutations in well-known cancer genes, such as MTOR, KMT2D, CDKN2C, and PIK3CA.[40] PIK3CA mutation was detected in the primary, but not in the recurrences, suggesting a role for this gene in tumor initiation rather than in tumor progression.[40] Pandya and colleagues,[41] pooling their data with the whole-exome sequencing results obtained by Yu and colleagues,[42] found alterations of key genes involved in PI3K/AKT/mTOR pathway in up to 21%, suggesting a oncogenic role for this pathway in PC. Recurrent germline and somatic alterations of PRUNE2 gene identified by Yu and colleagues, consistent with a tumor-suppressive role in PC, were not confirmed by the following studies.[42]

Clarke and colleagues[43] detected alterations in genes associated in MAPK signaling, T-cell receptor signaling, chromosome organization, DNA repair, cell cycle regulations and immune response, and well-known tumor suppressor genes in other cancers, such as TP53, BRAF, and BRCA2. The investigators also identified mutations in NF1 and TSC1 genes, regulators of mTOR, confirming PI3K/AKT/mTOR as a potential major oncogenic pathway in sporadic PC.[43] Several chemotherapeutic agents targeting different interaction partners within the pathway have been developed and some of them are approved for clinical use.[44]

Subsequent studies on advanced or metastatic lesions have confirmed the relevant role of PI3K/AKT/mTOR pathway in the pathogenesis of PC and focused their search for mutant genes to the so-called actionable genes that potentially could benefit from approved targeted therapies.[45–47] Mutations in genes belonging to the Wnt/β-catenin signaling pathway rarely have been detected (APC, FAT3, RNF43, and EP300).

Almost all these studies detected a prevalent recurrence of CDC73 mutations (approximately 40%). Conversely, a lower CDC73 mutation rate was reported by Clarke and colleagues[43] and Kutahyalioglu and colleagues[48] (10.3% and 9%, respectively). Clarke and colleagues excluded insertion/deletions, which represent the most common CDC73 gene defects in PCs, from the analysis. Yu and colleagues also observed the preferential amplification of mutant CDC73 alleles and the loss of wild-type allele.[41] Different studies reported contrasting observations concerning the co-occurrence of CDC73 mutations and mutations in other potentially driver genes, such as PIK3CA.[41,45–47] In particular, Cui and colleagues[45] observed that recurrent mutations in genes mainly enriched in the lysine degradation pathway and mismatch repair pathway were present only in CDC73 mutation-negative samples, whereas CDC73 wild-type samples belonging to the cohort of Hu and colleagues[47] had prevalent mutations in genes involved in the antigen-presenting machinery, allograft rejection, or autoimmune diseases.[45,47] Moreover, Hu and colleagues[47] observed a significant correlation between CDC73 variants and recurrent/metastatic PCs rather than primary tumors, and Cui and colleagues[45] reported a higher frequency of CDC73 mutations in metastatic than in recurrent PC patients.

The question of whether these additional genes would have a pivotal role in the pathogenesis of PC and potentially represent targets of therapeutic interest remains to be experimentally demonstrated.

Epigenetic Profile

A few studies have reported gene expression analysis of PCs.[49–51] cDNA microarray-based analyses have been used mostly to identify the expression profile of different parathyroid lesions. Haven and colleagues[49] comparing parathyroid hyperplasia, PAs, and PCs, either sporadic or familial, first identified a cluster containing CDC73-mutated sporadic and familial PCs (ie, HP-JT and FIHP) together with CDC73-mutated familial benign adenomas, suggesting that the presence of either a germline or somatic CDC73 mutation strongly influences the expression pattern of other genes.[49] They also demonstrated the up-regulation of APP, CDH1, HIF2, AKR1C3, CD24, UCHL1, DDEF1, and LAMB1 and the down-regulation of KIAA1376, SGK, CUL5, and NUCB2 genes in this cluster. APP, CDH1, and UCHL1 have been confirmed as differentially expressed genes in one case of PC compared with a biopsy from the normal parathyroid gland of the same patient.[50] Differential gene expression between PAs and PCs of Chinese population revealed the up-regulation of CD24, HMOX1, VCAM1, and KCNA3 genes in PCs.[51] Recently, Condello and colleagues[52] used NanoString technology to compare the gene expression profiles of PAs, nonmetastatic and metastatic PCs. The results of this study seem to confirm the up-regulation of CDH1 in metastatic PCs compared with PAs. A marked up-regulation of CD24, a molecule involved in cell adhesion and signal transduction, reported either by Haven and colleagues[49] and Zhao and colleagues[51] in PCs also has been confirmed by Condello and colleagues[52] in the metastatic PCs versus both nonmetastatic PCs and PAs. These data endorse the concept that higher CD24 expression levels might be related to tumor invasion and dissemination, an evidence also corroborated by in vivo experiments.[53]

Genome-wide changes in DNA methylation, histone modifications, chromatin remodeling and aberrant expression of noncoding RNAs, influencing gene expression and genomic stability, represent the most common feature of human cancers.

The methylation pattern of PCs was characterized by extremely low levels of 5-hydroxymethylcytosine, a marker of human cancers that seemed to be caused by a deregulated expression of *TET1* and *TET2* mRNA, codifying proteins that catalyze the conversion of 5-methylcytosine to 5-hydroxymethylcytosine.[54,55] Data on promoter *CDC73* hypermethylation are controversial (from 0% to 18% of cases), highly due to small sample size of tumors.[56–58] Hypermethylation of the promoter region of *SFRP1* involved a in the Wnt/β-catenin pathway has also been reported in PC.[59]

Similarly to DNA methylation, post-translational histone modifications, namely acetylation, methylation, phosphorylation, and ubiquitination, have an important role in the modulation of gene transcriptional activity. Histone methylation is mediated by histone methyltransferases and have an indirect influence on the recruitment and binding of regulatory proteins to chromatin. Parafibromin is a component of the Paf1 complex associated with RNA polymerase II and, through the interaction with the histone methyltransferase SUV39H1 and subsequent methylation of H3 K9, functions as a transcriptional repressor.[60] Loss of parafibromin expression cause an improper 3′ cleavage of histone H1 mRNA adding a poly(A) tail, which prevents the degradation of the transcripts.[61] The overexpression of Histone 1 Family 2 was found in *CDC73*-mutated sporadic PCs.[49]

Noncoding RNAs, namely micro-RNA (miRNA), long noncoding RNA (LncRNA), and circular RNA, have an overwhelming role of in biological and pathologic processes, representing an alternative mechanism to the regulation of mRNA transcription. PC has approximately 80% of global miRNA down-regulation compared with normal glands, and miR-296, miR-139, miR-126-5p, miR-26b, and miR-30b were the most significant varied. Conversely, an up-regulation of miR-222, miR-372, miR-503, and miR-517c has been reported.[62–64]

Using an integrated analysis, Zhang and colleagues[65] first explored the lncRNA expression profiles in PCs compared with PAs and found *PVT1* and *GLIS2-AS1* the most up-regulated and down-regulated lncRNAs, respectively, in PCs. These dysregulated lncRNAs potentially were associated with *CDC73* mutation-positive PCs. A coexpression network, discovering putative lncRNA–mRNA interactions, revealed that the ECM-receptor interaction pathway was significantly altered in PCs.[65] Four lncRNAs (LINC00959, lnc-FLT3-2:2, lnc-FEZF2-9:2, and lnc-RP11-1035H13.3.1-2:1), significantly dysregulated in PCs, targeted mRNAs enriched in cancer-related pathways, such as MAPK signaling, small and non–small cell lung cancer, TP53 signaling and cell-cycle pathways.[65,66] Recently, Morotti and colleagues[67] showed a different lncRNAs expression between *CDC73* mutation-positive and mutation-negative PCs; in particular, the former overexpressed the lncRNA *BC200*. The expression profiles of miRNAs differentially expressed between PCs and PAs in circulating exosomes detected a significant up-regulation of hsa-miR-27a-5p in PCs, suggesting that it may be a promising preoperative biomarker for an early diagnosis of PC.[68]

Clinical Features

The clinical manifestations at the time of diagnosis are related to hypercalcemia and markedly elevated serum PTH rather than the local spread of the tumors or distant metastases. The challenge for the clinician is to recognize among patients with PHPT those due to PC from those due to the much more common benign counterpart.[3] To date, no preoperative markers for PC have been identified. Thus, raising the suspicion of PC during the preoperative evaluation is extremely important, because the

---

Box 1
Clinical, biochemical, and instrumental features raising the suspicion of parathyroid malignancy

Clinical features
- Male sex
- Relatively young age
- Neurologic manifestations
- Palpable neck mass and/or laryngeal nerve palsy

Biochemical findings
- Moderate–severe hypercalcemia (generally >14 mg/dL)
- Markedly elevated plasma PTH (3–10 times above the normal values)

Ultrasound characteristics
- >3-cm size
- Presence of calcifications
- Signs of infiltration
- Suspicious vascularity

---

likelihood of definitive cure could depend on the extent of the initial surgery. Clinical features that may raise the suspicion of PC are summarized in **Box 1**.

A subgroup of patients with PC secretes an N-terminal PTH fragment distinct from 1-84 PTH. This fragment is recognized by third-generation but not by second-generation PTH immunoassays; thus, an inverted third-generation to second-generation plasma PTH ratio has been found in a majority of patients with advanced PC.[69] A ratio greater than 1 had a sensitivity and specificity of 83.3% and 100%, respectively, as a marker for PC.[70] Bone-specific alkaline phosphatase also is higher in patients with PC than in those with PA. Serum and urinary levels of hCG and its malignant hyperglycosylated isoform are abnormally elevated in patients with PC but not in those with benign parathyroid tumors.[71] Moreover, elevations of hCG might has been found predictive of hip fracture and death.[71] The clinical implication of PTH ratio and the role of hCG measurement in diagnosis and monitoring of patients with PC requires further investigations.

The combined finding of rather elevated serum calcium levels (greater than 12 mg/dL [>3 mmol/L]) and a large parathyroid lesion (>3 cm) (the so-called >3 + >3 rule, as suggested by Talat and colleagues[16]) should raise the suspicion of a PC. In addition, PC also should be suspected preoperatively in all PHPT patients who have ionized serum calcium greater than 1.77 mmol/L.[6]

Nonfunctioning PC can be diagnosed erroneously at clinical evaluation as thyroid or thymic carcinoma because of local growth and invasion of adjacent structures.[11,12] It occurs mostly in patients in the sixth or seventh decade, although some patients younger than 50 years old also have been reported.[14,72,73]

Imaging studies do not allow to make a definite diagnosis of malignancy, except in cases of local invasion or metastases. Neck ultrasound, the most frequent technique, is used to localize the tumor and some morphologic features can raise the suspicion of malignancy (**Box 1**). Recently, Liu and colleagues[74] showed that the ratio between the lesion's maximum and minimum diameter less than 1.86 was as another predictor of PC. At variance with 18F-fluorodeoxyglucose and 18F-choline PET/CT that have been reported to be helpful in the diagnosis and monitoring of patients with PC, 99mTc-sestamibi scintigraphy is not useful in the characterization of PC.[75,76]

Surgery

Surgical intervention is the mainstay of treatment of PC. Successful surgical approach depends upon preoperative suspicion of PC, intraoperative recognition of malignant lesion and experience of the surgeon.[13] The goal standard treatment is the en bloc resection of the tumor, the ipsilateral thyroid lobe with gross clear margins, and the adjacent involved structures, without spillage of the tumor. If PC is suspected, surgery should be performed by an expert parathyroid surgeon. If the patient has not undergone primary en bloc resection and a diagnosis is made postoperatively at histology, timely further expert parathyroid surgery must be considered.

Surgery is first-line treatment also for recurrent disease and, in selected cases, repeated operations in combination with other systemic treatments may improve the prognosis.[77]

Histopathology

According to World Health Organization criteria, a diagnosis of PC requires unequivocal lymphovascular or perineural invasion, or invasion into adjacent structures, or metastatic disease.[78]

The main challenge in the histologic diagnosis consists of distinguishing PC from atypical adenomas. The latter tumors share some histologic features with PC, such as diffuse growth pattern, fibrous septa, and high mitotic activity, but lack unequivocal histologic signs of malignancy, namely capsular, vascular and/or perineural tumor invasion (**Fig. 1**).[15] Capsular invasion is characterized by a tongue-like protrusion through the collagenous fibers and should be distinguished from pseudoinvasion caused by degeneration and subsequent fibrosis and trapping of tumor cells. The criteria of vascular invasion have been defined differently, according to whether capsular vessels in the surrounding tissues are involved.[79,80] Partial attachment of tumor cells to the wall of the vessel or thrombosis also should be present.

Additional immunohistochemical staining may help to support the diagnosis of PC. Immunohistochemical evaluation of parafibromin, the protein encoded by *CDC73* gene, shows nuclear staining in normal parathyroid cells and most PAs.[36,81,82] Loss of nuclear expression of parafibromin occurs in most but not all PC associated with biallelic *CDC73* inactivation and has been associated with a higher likelihood of recurrence and worst outcome in patients with PC.[27,35,39,83] Gill and colleagues[82] have reported that tumors with loss of parafibromin expression may show subtle morphologic clues, including sheetlike growth, eosinophilic cytoplasm, perinuclear cytoplasmic clearing, and nuclear enlargement. In addition, cyclin D1 and/or galectin-3 overexpression or retinoblastoma loss of expression also has been found in PC.[84–86] Protein gene product 9.5 (PGP9.5) also is overexpressed in the majority of PCs and may have a complementary role to parafibromin immunohistochemical evaluation of *CDC73* mutation, although with lower specificity.[37] The combination of parafibromin immunostaining with a panel of other biomarkers (ie, retinoblastoma, Ki67, E-cadherin, galectin-3, and PGP9.5) may be a better tool to the differential diagnosis between PC and other parathyroid neoplasms.[87,88]

Systemic Treatments and Prognosis

Postoperative radiation therapy has not been adopted widely in the treatment of PC because PC is considered radioresistant. Small case series, however, have shown promising results in terms of lower rate of recurrence.[89–91] Chemotherapy rarely is used because of its low/null efficacy. Radiofrequency ablation alone or in combination with arterial embolization has been used successfully in 2 patients with lung and hepatic metastases with PC, respectively.[92] Cinacalcet, an allosteric agonist of the calcium-sensing receptor (*CASR*) expressed on the surface of parathyroid cells, can be used successfully for the control of hypercalcemia-related symptoms.[93] Moreover, antiresorptive agents, such as bisphosphonates and denosumab, also can be used to

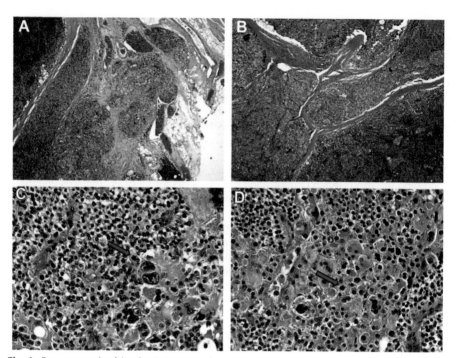

Fig. 1. Representative histologic images of parathyroid carcinoma (hematoxylin-eosin staining). (*A*) This tumor shows invasion of the adjacent soft tissues (original magnification ×4). (*B*) Prominent fibrous bands and solid tumor growth are evident (original magnification ×4). (*C*) The nuclei show marked atypia with focal pleomorphic appearance. In this field, a mitotic figure is present (*red arrow*) (original magnification × 40). (*D*) This tumor shows variation in nuclear size and prominent nucleoli. In this field another mitotic figure is noted (*red arrow*)(original magnification ×40).

lower serum calcium levels.[2,94] Treatment with drugs used in other malignant tumors, directed to mutations of *PIK3CA* or *mTOR* or amplification of *CCND1*, also can be used in PC, because these mutations also are frequent in this neoplasia.[41,45,48] Clinical studies are necessary, however, to validate this option.

Three cases have provided evidence that anti-PTH immunotherapy may control hypercalcemia unresponsive to conventional treatments and primary and metastatic tumor growth.[95–97] In addition, a combination of surgery, radiotherapy, cinacalcet, repeated zoledronic acid infusions, and temozolomide cycles also has resulted in a successful response in an isolated PC case.[98]

Immunotherapy based on the expression of lymphocytes infiltrating the tumor in the microenvironment of PC, makes CD68[+], programmed death-1 (PD-1) and its ligand as potential targets in PC therapies.[99] The PD-1 inhibitor pembrolizumab was recently reported to be effective in decreasing the disease burden in 2 patients with metastatic PC.[100,101]

Prognosis of PC is quite variable. Early identification and complete resection of the tumor at initial surgery carry the best prognosis. The mean time to recurrence usually is 3 years, although intervals of up to 20 years have been reported.[77] Surgery represents the first-line treatment of recurrent disease, but a complete cure is unlikely. Survival rates at 5 years and at 10 years between 77% and 100% and between 49% and 91%, respectively, have been reported.[4,6,7,13,22,27] Negative prognostic factors for survival were simple parathyroidectomy as initial surgery, higher serum calcium at recurrence, numbers of local recurrences, presence of metastases, need of using several calcium-lowering medications, and nonfunctioning PC.

Mortality generally is due to intractable hypercalcemia rather than to direct tumor invasion and distant metastases.

Conclusions

Despite its rarity, in the presence of severe PHPT, large cervical mass, and concomitant renal and skeletal disease, PC should be suspected. Parathyroid surgery remains the mainstay of treatment to be performed in a dedicated endocrine center to improve outcomes and offer the best chance of cure.

ECTOPIC SECRETION OF PARATHYROID HORMONE

Ectopic production of PTH is a rare condition and accounts for less than 1% of malignancy-associated hypercalcemia. It is due to the ectopic secretion of PTH by malignant nonparathyroid tumors. In the past decades, ectopic production of PTH was confounded with malignancy-associated hypercalcemia due to the poor specificity of PTH assays. The identification of PTHrP as the major cause of hypercalcemia of malignancy, the current highly specific immunometric assays for intact PTH combined with molecular biologic approaches led to the definition of the diagnosis of true ectopic PTH syndrome.[102] Since the 1970s, rare cases of patients with malignancies in whom hypercalcemia was associated with elevated PTH secretion by the tumors were reported (**Table 1**). Palmieri and colleagues[103] described the first patient with hypercalcemia and elevated PTH levels, which originated from a squamous cell carcinoma in the lung. Since then, PTH-secreting tumors have been reported in 52 patients with malignant neoplasms mainly located in head and neck, thorax, gastrointestinal tract, and female urogenital system.[23,103–142] (see **Table 1**). These tumors produced PTH mRNA or protein, with or without PTH-related protein (PTHrP) and were associated with hypercalcemia and elevated plasma PTH levels in the absence of documented parathyroid gland tumors.

In patients with clinical evidence of a malignant tumor and a high level of PTH, true ectopic hyperparathyroidism must be considered. It is likely that in such patients intercurrent PHPT is more common than ectopic production of PTH.

Molecular Mechanisms

The ectopic PTH production may be due to different molecular mechanisms. Several reports have documented that various tumor cells expressed the PTH mRNA.[23,113,115,116,120,121,127,130,141] Ectopic hormone production can be considered an aberration in the tissue specificity of gene expression; it usually involves dysregulation of a normal hormone gene product. Wong and colleagues[127] did not find any mutations in the coding region of *PTH* gene, validating the hypothesis that alterations within regulatory sequences of the *PTH* mRNA may account for its high expression. Tissue specificity of gene expression is controlled by positive and negative regulatory DNA elements, called enhancer and silencer, respectively. They often are located in the upstream regulatory region of a hormone gene and interact with DNA-binding proteins characteristic of a specific tissue. The ectopic hormone production in a tumor may be due to an alteration in the DNA-binding protein environment or a change in the enhancer/silencer region adjacent to the hormone structural gene (thereby conferring responsiveness to the DNA-binding proteins typical of the tumor cell type). The chromosomal rearrangement that position the PTH gene promoter upstream the

Table 1
Reported cases with ectopic secretion of parathyroid hormone

Investigators	Ectopic Parathyroid Hormone Origin	Patient Age (y)/Sex	Surgery for Parathyroid Tumors	Serum Parathyroid Hormone	Serum Parathyroid Hormone–related Protein	Parathyroid-Hormone Immunohisto chemistry/ Immunofluorescence in Tumor Cells	mRNA Parathyroid Hormone
Head/neck							
Kandil et al,[134] 2011	Neuroendocrine tumor central compartment	73/F	Parathyroidectomy 42 y before, no data about histology of parathyroid tumor. Neck and carotid sheaths exploration with no abnormal gland	126 pg/mL (NA)	Negative	Positive	NA
Demura et al,[120] 2010	Medullary thyroid carcinoma (lymph node metastasis)	64/M	No	82.7	Negative	Negative	Positive in primary tumor. Very positive in metastasis
Morita et al,[132] 2009	Papillary thyroid carcinoma	59/F	Right superior PA excision	154 pg/mL (10–65)	ND	Positive	ND

Reference	Tumor	Age/Sex		PTH			
Bhattacharya et al,[128] 2006	Cervical paraganglioma	32/M	No	650 pg/mL (12–72)	ND	Positive	ND
Wong et al,[127] 2005	Nasopharyngeal rhabdomyosarcoma	62/M	No	62.22 pmol/L (0.74–5.62)	ND	ND	Positive (negative for PTHrP)
Iguchi et al,[118] 1998	Papillary thyroid carcinoma	72/F	Neck exploration with no abnormal gland	9800 pg/mL (160–520)	26 pmol/L (13–55)	Positive	ND
Samaan et al,[108] 1983	Squamous tonsil carcinoma	49/M	No	0.95 ng/mL (0.05–1.0)	ND	Positive	ND
Hutchinson et al,[107] 1978	Buttock alveolar rhabdomyosarcoma	15/F	No	344 pg/mL (163–347)[a]	ND	ND	ND
	Oropharyngeal rhabdomyosarcoma	12/F	No	318 pg/mL (163–347)[a]			
Thorax							
Weiss et al,[131] 2006	Lung carcinoma	78/F	No	288 pg/mL (10–65)	<0.2 pmol/L (<1.3)	ND	ND
Botea et al,[122] 2003	Small cell lung carcinoma	50/M	No	107 pg/mL (10–65)	ND	Positive	ND
Uchimura et al,[121] 2002	Squamous cell lung carcinoma (liver and other lung metastasis)	74/M	No	180 pg/mL (15–50)[b]	3.09 pmol/L (0.3–0.75)	Positive both in primary and metastasis	Positive

(continued on next page)

Table 1
(continued)

Investigators	Ectopic Parathyroid Hormone Origin	Patient Age (y)/Sex	Surgery for Parathyroid Tumors	Serum Parathyroid Hormone	Serum Parathyroid Hormone-related Protein	Parathyroid-Hormone Immunohisto chemistry/Immunofluorescence in Tumor Cells	mRNA Parathyroid Hormone
Nielsen et al,[117] 1996	Squamous cell lung carcinoma (mediastinal lymph node metastasis)	71/M	Neck exploration with no abnormal gland	150–560 ng/L (10–50)	1.4–2.3 ng/L (<2.9)	Positive in mediastinal metastasis[c]	ND
Rizzoli et al,[116] 1994	Epithelial thymoma	25/M	Neck exploration with no abnormal gland	6.7–8.9 pmol/L (1–6)	ND	Positive	Positive (negative PTHrP mRNA)
Yoshimoto et al,[113] 1989	Small cell lung carcinoma (liver metastasis)	70/M	No	4650 ng/L (230–630)[d] 13,850 ng/L (180–560)[e] 9900 ng/L (<1300)[f]	ND	ND	Positive in liver metastasis
Schmelzer et al,[110] 1985	Lung carcinoma	NA	NA	NA	NA	NA	NA
Palmieri et al,[103] 1974	Three cases of squamous cell carcinoma of lung	NA	NA	ND[g]		2/3 positive (IF), 1/3 ND	ND
	Squamous cell carcinoma of lung (renal metastasis)	NA	NA	ND[g]		Positive in renal metastasis	ND

Gastrointestinal tract

Reference	Tumor	Age/Sex		PTH			
Brun et al,[141] 2021	Rectal adenocarcinoma (bone metastasis)	68/M	No	54.4 pmol/L (1.1–7.5)[h]	Negative	Negative in bone biopsy	Positive (in primary tumor before and after the onset of hypercalcemia, in bone metastasis only after).
Belaid et al,[139] 2020	Bilateral pheochromocytoma in von Hippel–Lindau disease	17/F	No	182 pg/mL (11–62)	ND	ND	ND
Kwon et al,[136] 2018	Combined hepatocellular carcinoma and cholangiocarcinoma (bone metastasis)	44/M	No	3859 pg/mL (15–65)	ND	Negative in primary tumor and metastasis	ND
Doyle and Malcolm,[135] 2014	Pancreatic neuroendocrine tumor (liver metastasis)	28/F	No	24.6–48.2 pmol/L (1.6–9.3)	Negative	Negative in liver metastasis	ND
Nakajima et al,[142] 2013	Gastric carcinoma (liver metastasis)	70/M	No	190 pg/mL (9–39)[i]	3.8 pmol/L (<1.1)	Positive in primary tumor and metastasis (PTHrP >> PTH)	ND
VanHouten et al,[130] 2006	Pancreatic malignancy (liver metastasis)	74/F	Neck exploration with no abnormal gland	399 pg/mL (10–65) 2310 pg/mL (6–40)	11.7 pg/mL (<1.3)	Positive in primary and metastasis	Positive in primary and metastasis (also for PTHrP mRNA)[j]

(continued on next page)

Table 1
(continued)

Investigators	Ectopic Parathyroid Hormone Origin	Patient Age (y)/Sex	Surgery for Parathyroid Tumors	Serum Parathyroid Hormone	Serum Parathyroid Hormone–related Protein	Parathyroid - Hormone Hormone Immunohisto chemistry/ Immunofluorescence in Tumor Cells	mRNA Parathyroid Hormone
Mahoney et al,[129] 2006	Hepatocellular carcinoma	72/M	Neck exploration with no abnormal gland	92 pg/mL (12–65)	<0.7 pg/mL (<1.3)	Negative	ND
Vacher-Coponat et al,[126] 2005	Pancreatic neuroendocrine tumor	58/F	Neck exploration with no abnormal gland	394-1587-8000 pg/mL (8–50)	ND	ND	ND
Koyama et al,[119] 1999	Hepatocellular carcinoma	83/M	No	360 pg/mL (15–50)	18.7 pg/mL (13.8–55.3)	ND	ND
Abe et al,[133] 2011	Hepatocellular carcinoma	73/M	No	99 pg/mL (<60)	Negative	Negative	ND
Arps et al,[111] 1986	Pancreatic neuroendocrine tumor (liver metastasis)	45/M	No	NA	NA	Positive in primary tumor and metastasis	NA
Mayes et al,[109] 1984	Rhabdoid kidney tumor (lumbar paraaortic region and pelvis metastasis)	6 mo/M	No	92 μleq/mL (<10)[k]	NA	Negative in primary tumor Positive in metastases	NA

Palmieri et al,[103] 1974	Gall bladder adenocarcinoma (liver metastasis)	NA	NA	ND^I	NA	Positive in liver metastasis (IF)	NA
	Pancreatic islet cell carcinoma (liver metastasis)	NA	NA	ND^I	NA	Positive in liver metastasis (IF)	NA
Deftos et al,[104] 1976	Gastric carcinoid	27/F	NA	≅3000–4000 pg/mL (NA)	ND	ND	ND
	Pancreatic islet cell carcinoma (liver metastasis)	37/F	NA	≅1000 pg/mL (NA)	ND	Positive in liver metastasis	ND
Robin et al,[106] 1976	Small intestine leiomyosarcoma	NA	NA	NA	NA	NA	NA
Grajower et al,[105] 1976	Esophageal carcinoma	80/M	No	48 µleq/mL (<40)	ND	ND	ND
Pelvis							
Gabriel and Picar,[140] 2020	Large cell neuroendocrine ovarian carcinoma	45/F	No	306.7 pg/mL (15–65)	ND	ND	ND
Deshaies et al,[138] 2019	Endometrioid carcinoma (recurrent carcinosarcoma in the pelvis)	53/F	Neck exploration and cervical thymectomy with no abnormal gland	1100 pg/dL	Negative	Positive in the pelvis mass	ND

(continued on next page)

Table 1
(continued)

Investigators	Ectopic Parathyroid Hormone Origin	Patient Age (y)/Sex	Surgery for Parathyroid Tumors	Serum Parathyroid Hormone	Serum Parathyroid Hormone–related Protein	Parathyroid - Hormone Hormone Immunohisto chemistry/ Immunofluorescence in Tumor Cells	mRNA Parathyroid Hormone
Chen et al,[125] 2005	Small cell ovarian carcinoma	37/F	No	<10–90 pg/mL (10–65.9)	Negative	Positive (30% of tumor cells)	ND
Eid et al,[123] 2004	Transitional cell carcinoma of the bladder (pelvis metastasis)	73/M	Left inferior PA (6 y before). Repeated neck explorations with no abnormal gland. Removal of a normal ectopic parathyroid in the thymus	273–397–423 pg/mL (13–65)	1.6–5.7 pmol/L (0.0–1.5)	Negative in urinary bladder (negative for PTHrP) Positive pelvis metastasis (negative for PTHrP)	ND
Ohira et al,[124] 2004	Non-small cell ovarian carcinoma with admixed endometrioid adenocarcinoma	33/F	No	205 pg/mL (14–66)	Negative	Positive in the neuroendocrine tumor (negative for PTHrP) Negative in the adenocarci noma (negative for PTHrP)	ND

Study	Tumor	Age/Sex	Surgery	PTH			
Buller et al,[114] 1991	Adenosquamous endometrium carcinoma	72/F	No	345 (50–340 pg/mL)[f]	ND	Positive	ND
Nussbaum et al,[23] 1990	Ovarian carcinoma	74/F	Neck exploration with no abnormal gland	325–429 pg/mL (10–60)	ND	ND	Positive (negative for PTHrP)
Abeler et al,[112] 1988	Three cases of ovarian carcinomas	15/F, 24/F, 20/F	NA	ND	ND	Positive all 3 cases	ND
Other sites							
Sardiñas et al,[137] 2018	Penile squamous cell carcinoma (squamous cell carcinoma metastasis in the thigh)	48/M	No	699–761.7–1266 pg/mL (15–65)	18 pg/mL (14–27)	Positive in the metastatic lesion	ND
Strewler et al,[115] 1993	Small cell neuroectodermal malignancy	69/M	Two neck explorations and sternotomy with no abnormal gland	90–290 pg/mL (15–65)	19–20 (<10 ngeq/L)	ND	Positive

(continued on next page)

Table 1
(continued)

Investigators	Ectopic Parathyroid Hormone Origin	Patient Age (y)/Sex	Surgery for Parathyroid Tumors	Serum Parathyroid Hormone	Serum Parathyroid Hormone-related Protein	Parathyroid Hormone Immunohisto chemistry/ Immunofluorescence in Tumor Cells	mRNA Parathyroid Hormone
Palmieri et al,[103] 1974	Malignant melanoma	NA	NA	ND[m]	ND	Negative (IF)	ND

Abbreviations: IF, immunofluorescence; NA, not available; ND, not done; PA, parathyroid adenoma.

Numbers in parenthesis indicate the normal reference range. Please note that also in column PTHrP numbers in parenthesis indicate the normal reference range.

[a] Values within this range were considered normal only when the simultaneously obtained serum calcium level were normal.

[b] PTH was also measured in tissue extracts (>25 pg/g and 4.2 pg/g of wet tissue in lung and liver metastasis, respectively).

[c] Positive for PTH but not PTHrP immunostaining in cultured cells from liver metastasis.

[d] N-terminal PTH.

[e] Midregion PTH (503.5 ng/g wet tissue extracts of liver metastasis, normal range <4.2–5.9).

[f] C-terminal PTH.

[g] PTH positivity was assessed only in tissue extract (liver metastasis).

[h] Systemic PTH level dropped when the lower leg (bone metastasis) was excluded from circulation.

[i] PTH and PTHrP concentrations in the tissue extracts of liver metastasis were 298 pg/mL and 17.2 pmol/L, respectively.

[j] Conditioned media from cultured cells obtained from primary tumor espresse both PTH and PTHrP mRNA.

[k] Radioimmunoassay for the carboxyl terminal sequence of human PTH.

[l] PTH negative in tumor extracts.

[m] PTH level was measured only in tissue extract (18.1 ng/mg).

CCDN1 gene encoding cyclin D1 was detected in a subgroup of PAs and drive overexpression of cyclin D1, suggesting that DNA sequences necessary for tissue-specific expression of the PTH gene reside in the 5' regulatory region of the gene.[143] The molecular etiology of ectopic PTH gene production in a ovarian carcinoma has been proposed by Nussbaum and colleagues,[23] which proposed that the amplification and rearrangement of the 5' regulatory region of the PTH gene might be the cause of the activation of PTH gene transcription. Conversely, 3 different studies found no evidence of such DNA rearrangements through the *PTH* coding gene and upstream its flanking sequences in neuroectodermal, pancreatic, lung, and medullary thyroid carcinomas that ectopically expressed PTH.[113,115,120,130] One of these studies observed instead a pattern of hypomethylation of the *PTH* gene suggestive of activated transcription of *PTH* gene in the nonparathyroid tumor.[130] The investigators did not find detectable expression of specific transcription factors functioning as enhancers of PTH gene transcription and commonly implicated in parathyroid gland development, such as *TBX1* and *GCM2*, in the pancreatic tumor or cultured cells obtained from the primary tumor.[130] Thus, they concluded that none of these transcription factors were likely responsible for *PTH* gene expression in the tumor. The expression of *GCM2* in a nonparathyroid tumor also was investigated by Demura and colleagues.[120] The investigators found the coexpression of *PTH* and *GCM2* mRNA both in the primary and lymph nodes metastases, but the presence of *GCM2* in the adjacent normal thyroid and lymphoblasts from a healthy control, in the absence of PTH expression, strongly suggested that *GCM2* was not responsible for PTH transactivation.[120]

Because no definitive molecular modifications for ectopic PTH expression have been elucidated, additional studies on the transcriptional regulation of the *PTH* gene are warranted.

Conclusions

Ectopic tumoral production of PTH outside parathyroids is a rare event. In the presence of patients with clinical evidence of a malignant tumor and a high level of PTH, this condition must be considered. From a clinical perspective, the control of hypercalcemia in these patients often is difficult and the most effective treatment is the surgical resection of the lesion. The molecular mechanisms underlying the ectopic production of PTH appear to be heterogeneous and in most cases still are unknown.

The recognition of the association between elevated PTH levels and hypercalcemia in the setting of malignancy may prevent unnecessary parathyroid or exploratory neck surgeries and also possibly could lead to the early detection of an undiagnosed malignancy.

CLINICS CARE POINTS

- When a patient has severe PHPT, male sex, age between mid-40 and 50s, a palpable neck mass, and/or HPT-JT–related tumors, suspicion for PC should be raised.

- If PC is suspected, the patient should be referred to an experienced surgeon and an en bloc resection of the tumor should be recommended.

- The presence of a large neck lump in a patient with normal serum calcium and PTH levels might be due to a nonfunctioning PC.

- When a PC specimen tested positive at *CDC73* mutational analysis, the search for germline *CDC73* mutation should be carried out and, if positive, extended to first-degree relatives.

- In a patient with clinical evidence of a nonparathyroid malignant tumor and high levels of PTH, true ectopic hyperparathyroidism must be considered. Intercurrent PHPT, however, can be present.

DISCLOSURE

The authors have nothing to disclose.

ACKNOWLEDGMENTS

This work was supported by Fondi di Ateneo, University of Pisa (to C.M.).

REFERENCES

1. Carroll M, Schade D. A Practical Approach to Hypercalcemia. Am Fam Physician 2003;67(9):1959–66.
2. Marcocci C, Cetani F, Rubin MR, et al. Parathyroid carcinoma. J Bone Miner Res 2008;23(12):1869–80.
3. Cetani F, Pardi E, Marcocci C. Update on parathyroid carcinoma. J Endocrinol Invest 2016;39(6):595–606.
4. Lee PK, Jarosek SL, Virnig BA, et al. Trends in the incidence and treatment of parathyroid cancer in the United States. Cancer 2007;109(9):1736–41.
5. Brown S, O'Neill C, Suliburk J, et al. Parathyroid carcinoma: Increasing incidence and changing presentation. ANZ J Surg 2011;81(7–8):528–32.
6. Ryhänen EM, Leijon H, Metso S, et al. A nationwide study on parathyroid carcinoma. Acta Oncol (Madr) 2017;56(7):991–1003.
7. Kong S, Kim J, Park M, et al. Epidemiology and prognosis of parathyroid carcinoma: real-world data using nationwide cohort. J Cancer Res Clin Oncol 2021. https://doi.org/10.1007/s00432-021-03576-.
8. Chen JD, Morrison C, Zhang C, et al. Hyperparathyroidism-jaw tumour syndrome. J Intern Med 2003;253(6):634–42.
9. Cardoso L, Stevenson M, Thakker RV. Molecular genetics of syndromic and non-syndromic forms of parathyroid carcinoma. Hum Mutat 2017;38(12):1621–48.
10. Bollerslev J, Schalin-Jäntti C, Rejnmark L, et al. Unmet therapeutic, educational and scientific needs in parathyroid disorders: Consensus statement from the first European Society of Endocrinology Workshop (PARAT). Eur J Endocrinol 2019;181(3):P1–19.
11. Fernandez-Ranvier GG, Jensen K, Khanafshar E, et al. Nonfunctioning Parathyroid Carcinoma: Case Report and Review of Literature. Endocr Pract 2007; 13(7):750–7.
12. Wilkins BJ, Lewis JS. Non-functional parathyroid carcinoma: A review of the literature and report of a case requiring extensive surgery. Head Neck Pathol 2009; 3(2):140–9.
13. Harari A, Waring A, Fernandez-Ranvier G, et al. Parathyroid carcinoma: A 43-year outcome and survival analysis. J Clin Endocrinol Metab 2011;96(12):3679–86.
14. Cetani F, Frustaci G, Torregrossa L, et al. A nonfunctioning parathyroid carcinoma misdiagnosed as a follicular thyroid nodule. World J Surg Oncol 2015; 13(1):1–5.
15. Cetani F, Marcocci C, Torregrossa L, et al. Atypical parathyroid adenomas: challenging lesions in the differential diagnosis of endocrine tumors. Endocr Relat Cancer 2019;26(7):R441–64.
16. Talat N, Schulte KM. Clinical presentation, staging and long-term evolution of parathyroid cancer. Ann Surg Oncol 2010;17(8):2156–74.
17. Wei CH, Harari A. Parathyroid carcinoma: Update and guidelines for management. Curr Treat Options Oncol 2012;13(1):11–23.

18. Lenschow C, Schrägle S, Kircher S, et al. Clinical Presentation, Treatment, and Outcome of Parathyroid Carcinoma. Ann Surg 2020. https://doi.org/10.1097/SLA.0000000000004144.

19. Kebebew E, Arici C, Duh QY, et al. Localization and reoperation results for persistent and recurrent parathyroid carcinoma. Arch Surg 2001;136(8):878–85.

20. Busaidy NL, Jimenez C, Habra MA, et al. Parathyroid carcinoma: A 22-year experience. Head Neck 2004;26(8):716–26.

21. Asare EA, Silva-Figueroa A, Hess KR, et al. Risk of Distant Metastasis in Parathyroid Carcinoma and Its Effect on Survival: A Retrospective Review from a High-Volume Center. Ann Surg Oncol 2019;26(11):3593–9.

22. Hu Y, Bi Y, Cui M, et al. The influence of surgical extent and parafibromin staining on the outcome of parathyroid carcinoma: 20-year experience from a single institute. Endocr Pract 2019;25(7):634–41.

23. Nussbaum SR, Gaz RD, Arnold A. Hypercalcemia and ectopic secretion of parathyroid hormone by an ovarian carcinoma with rearrangemnet of the gene for parathyroid hormone. N Engl J Med 1990;323(19):1324–8.

24. Carpten JD, Robbins CM, Villablanca A, et al. HRPT2, encoding parafibromin, is mutated in hyperparathyroidism-jaw tumor syndrome. Nat Genet 2002;32(4):676–80.

25. Howell VM, Haven CJ, Kahnoski K, et al. HRPT2 mutations are associated with malignancy in sporadic parathyroid tumours. J Med Genet 2003;40(9):657–63.

26. Haven CJ, Puijenbroek M Van, Fleuren GJ, et al. Identification of MEN1 and HRPT2 somatic mutations in paraffin-embedded (sporadic) parathyroid carcinomas. Clin Endocrinol (Oxf) 2007;370–6. https://doi.org/10.1111/j.1365-2265.2007.02894.x.

27. Cetani F, Banti C, Pardi E, et al. CDC73 mutational status and loss of parafibromin in the outcome of parathyroid cancer. Endocr Connect 2013;2(4):186–95.

28. Gill AJ. Understanding the genetic basis of parathyroid carcinoma. Endocr Pathol 2014;25(1):30–4.

29. Van Der Tuin K, Tops CMJ, Adank MA, et al. CDC73-related disorders: Clinical manifestations and case detection in primary hyperparathyroidism. J Clin Endocrinol Metab 2017;102(12):4534–40.

30. Cetani F, Pardi E, Borsari S, et al. Genetic analyses of the HRPT2 gene in primary hyperparathyroidism: Germline and somatic mutations in familial and sporadic parathyroid tumors. J Clin Endocrinol Metab 2004;89(11):5583–91.

31. Krebs LJ, Shattuck TM, Arnold A. HRPT2 mutational analysis of typical sporadic parathyroid adenomas. J Clin Endocrinol Metab 2005;90(9):5015–7.

32. Bradley KJ, Cavaco BM, Bowl MR, et al. Parafibromin mutations in hereditary hyperparathyroidism syndromes and parathyroid tumours. Clin Endocrinol (Oxf) 2006;64(3):299–306.

33. Guarnieri V, Battista C, Muscarella LA, et al. CDC73 mutations and parafibromin immunohistochemistry in parathyroid tumors: Clinical correlations in a single-centre patient cohort. Cell Oncol 2012;35(6):411–22.

34. Li Y, Zhang J, Adikaram PR, et al. Genotype of CDC73 germline mutation determines risk of parathyroid cancer. Endocr Relat Cancer 2020;27(9):483–94.

35. Pyo JS, Cho WJ. Diagnostic and prognostic implications of parafibromin immunohistochemistry in parathyroid carcinomaT. Biosci Rep 2019;39(4):1–8.

36. Cetani F, Ambrogini E, Viacava P, et al. Should parafibromin staining replace HRTP2 gene analysis as an additional tool for histologic diagnosis of parathyroid carcinoma? Eur J Endocrinol 2007;156(5):547–54.

37. Howell VM, Gill A, Clarkson A, et al. Accuracy of combined protein gene product 9.5 and parafibromin markers for immunohistochemical diagnosis of parathyroid carcinoma. J Clin Endocrinol Metab 2009;94(2):434–41.

38. Hu Y, Liao Q, Cao S, et al. Diagnostic performance of parafibromin immunohistochemical staining for sporadic parathyroid carcinoma: a meta-analysis. Endocrine 2016. https://doi.org/10.1007/s12020-016-0997-3.

39. Zhu R, Wang Z, Hu Y. Prognostic role of parafibromin staining and CDC73 mutation in patients with parathyroid carcinoma: A systematic review and meta-analysis based on individual patient data. Clin Endocrinol (Oxf) 2020;92(4): 295–302.

40. Kasaian K, Wiseman SM, Thiessen N, et al. Complete genomic landscape of a recurring sporadic parathyroid carcinoma. J Pathol 2013;230:249–60.

41. Pandya C, Uzilov AV, Bellizzi J, et al. Genomic profiling reveals mutational landscape in parathyroid carcinomas. Jci Insight 2017;2(6):1–14.

42. Yu W, McPherson JR, Stevenson M, et al. Whole-exome sequencing studies of parathyroid carcinomas reveal novel PRUNE2 mutations, distinctive mutational spectra related to APOBEC-catalyzed DNA mutagenesis and mutational enrichment in kinases associated with cell migration and invasion. J Clin Endocrinol Metab 2015;100(2):E360–4.

43. Clarke CN, Katsonis P, Hsu T, et al. Comprehensive genomic characterization of parathyroid cancer identifies novel candidate driver mutations & core pathways. J Endocr Soc 2018. https://doi.org/10.1210/js.2018-00043.

44. Jiang N, Dai Q, Su X, et al. Role of PI3K/AKT pathway in cancer: the Framework of malignant Behavior, vol. 47. Springer Netherlands; 2020. https://doi.org/10.1007/s11033-020-05435-1.

45. Cui M, Hu Y, Bi Y, et al. Preliminary exploration of potential molecular therapeutic targets in recurrent and metastatic parathyroid carcinomas. Int J Cancer 2019; 144(3):525–32.

46. Kang H, Pettinga D, Schubert A, et al. Genomic Profiling of Parathyroid Carcinoma Reveals Genomic Alterations Suggesting Benefit from Therapy. Oncologist 2019;24:791–7.

47. Hu Y, Zhang X, Wang O, et al. The genomic profile of parathyroid carcinoma based on whole-genome sequencing. Int J Cancer 2020;147(9):2446–57.

48. Kutahyalioglu M, Nguyen HT, Kwatampora L, et al. Genetic profiling as a clinical tool in advanced parathyroid carcinoma. J Cancer Res Clin Oncol 2019;145(8): 1977–86.

49. Haven C, Howell VM, Eilers PHC, et al. Gene expression of parathyroid tumors: Molecular subclassification and identification of the potential malignant phenotype. Cancer Res 2004;64(20):7405–11.

50. Adam MA, Untch BR, Olson JA Jr. Parathyroid Carcinoma: Current Understanding and New Insights into Gene Expression and Intraoperative Parathyroid Hormone Kinetics. Oncologist 2010;15:61–72.

51. Zhao J, Hu Y, Liao Q, et al. Gene identification of potential malignant parathyroid tumors phenotype in Chinese population. Endocr J 2014;61(6):597–605.

52. Condello V, Cetani F, Denaro M, et al. Gene expression profile in metastatic and non-metastatic parathyroid carcinoma. Endocr Relat 2021;28(2):111–34.

53. Baumann P, Cremers N, Kroese F, et al. CD24 Expression Causes the Acquisition of Multiple Cellular Properties Associated with Tumor Growth and Metastasis. Cancer Res 2005;65(23):10783–94.

54. Barazeghi E, Gill AJ, Sidhu S, et al. 5-Hydroxymethylcytosine discriminates between parathyroid adenoma and carcinoma. Clin Epigenetics 2016;8(1):1–11.

55. Barazeghi E, Gill AJ, Sidhu S, et al. A role for TET2 in parathyroid carcinoma. Endocr Relat Cancer 2017;24(7):329–38.
56. Hewitt KM, Sharma PK, Samowitz W, et al. Aberrant methylation of the HRPT2 gene in parathyroid carcinoma. Ann Otol Rhinol Laryngol 2007;116(12):928–33.
57. Hahn MA, Howell VM, Gill AJ, et al. CDC73/HRPT2 CpG island hypermethylation and mutation of 5′-untranslated sequence are uncommon mechanisms of silencing parafibromin in parathyroid tumors. Endocr Relat Cancer 2010;17(1): 273–82.
58. Sulaiman L, Haglund F, Hashemi J, et al. Genome-Wide and Locus Specific Alterations in CDC73/HRPT2-Mutated Parathyroid Tumors. PLoS One 2012; 7(9):1–11.
59. Sulaiman L, Juhlin CC, Nilsson I-L, et al. Global and gene-specific promoter methylation analysis in primary hyperparathyroidism. Epigenetics 2013;8(6): 646–55.
60. Yang YJ, Han JW, Youn HD, et al. The tumor suppressor, parafibromin, mediates histone H3 K9 methylation for cyclin D1 repression. Nucleic Acids Res 2010; 38(2):382–90.
61. Farber LJ, Kort EJ, Wang P, et al. The tumor suppressor parafibromin is required for posttranscriptional processing of histone mRNA. Mol Carcinog 2010;49(3): 215–23.
62. Corbetta S, Vaira V, Guarnieri V, et al. Differential expression of microRNAs in human parathyroid carcinomas compared with normal parathyroid tissue. Endocr Relat Cancer 2010;17(1):135–46.
63. Rahbari R, Holloway AK, He M, et al. Identification of differentially expressed microRNA in parathyroid tumors. Ann Surg Oncol 2011;18(4):1158–65.
64. Vaira V, Elli F, Forno I, et al. The microRNA cluster C19MC is deregulated in parathyroid tumours. J Mol Endocrinol 2012;49(2):115–24.
65. Zhang X, Hu Y, Wang M, et al. Profiling analysis of long non-coding RNA and mRNA in parathyroid carcinoma. Endocr Relat Cancer 2019;26(2):163–76.
66. Jiang T, Wei BJ, Zhang DX, et al. Genome-wide analysis of differentially expressed lncRNA in sporadic parathyroid tumors. Osteoporos Int 2019;30(7): 1511–9.
67. Morotti A, Forno I, Verdelli C, et al. The oncosuppressors MEN1 and CDC73 are involved in lncRNAs deregulation in human parathyroid tumors. J Bone Miner Res 2020;35(12):2423–31.
68. Wang J, Wang Q, Zhao T, et al. Expression profile of serum-related exosomal miRNAs from parathyroid tumor. Endocrine 2020. https://doi.org/10.1007/s12020-020-02535-7.
69. Cavalier E, Daly AF, Betea D, et al. The ratio of parathyroid hormone as measured by third- and second-generation assays as a marker for parathyroid carcinoma. J Clin Endocrinol Metab 2010;95(8):3745–9.
70. Caron P, Simonds WF, Maiza J, et al. Non-Truncated Amino-Terminal PTH Overproduction in Two Patients with Parathyroid Carcinoma: A Possible Link to HRPT2 Gene Inactivation. Clin Endocrinol 2011;74(6):694–8.
71. Rubin MR, Bilezikian JP, Birken S, et al. Human chorionic gonadotropin measurements in parathyroid carcinoma. Eur J Endocrinol 2008;159(4):469–74.
72. Ordoñez N, Ibañez M, Samaan N, et al. Immunoperoxidase study of uncommon parathyroid tumors. Report of two cases of nonfunctioning parathyroid carcinoma and one intrathyroid parathyroid tumor-producing amyloid. Am J Surg Pathol 1983;7(6):535–42.

73. Wang L, Han D, Chen W, et al. Non-functional parathyroid carcinoma: a case report and review of the literature. Cancer Biol Ther 2015;16(11):1569–76.

74. Liu R, Xia Y, Chen C, et al. Ultrasound combined with biochemical parameters can predict parathyroid carcinoma in patients with primary hyperparathyroidism. Endocrine 2019;66(3):673–81.

75. Evangelista L, Sorgato N, Torresan F, et al. FDG-PET/CT and parathyroid carcinoma: Review of literature and illustrative case series. World J Clin Oncol 2011; 2(10):348.

76. Deandreis D, Terroir M, Al Ghuzlan A, et al. 18Fluorocholine PET/CT in parathyroid carcinoma: a new tool for disease staging? Eur J Nucl Med Mol Imaging 2015;42(12):1941–2.

77. Cetani F, Pardi E, Marcocci C. Parathyroid carcinoma: a clinical and genetic perspective. Minerva Endocrinol 2018;43(2):144–55.

78. DeLellis R, Larsson C, Arnold A, et al. Tumors of the parathyroid glands. In: Lloyd R, Osamura R, Kloppel G, et al, editors. WHO Classification of tumors of endocrine organs, vol. 2017, 4th edition. Lyon: IARC; 2017. p. 145–59.

79. DeLellis RA. Challenging lesions in the differential diagnosis of endocrine tumors: Parathryoid carcinoma. Endocr Pathol 2008;19(4):221–5.

80. DeLellis R. Parathyroid adenoma and variants. In: Rosai J, DeLellis R, Carcangiu M, et al, editors. Tumors of the thyroid and parathyroid glands. Armed Forces Institute of Pathology; Atlas of tumor Patology 4th series. Silverspring (MD): American Registry of Pathology ARP Press; 2014. p. 513–42.

81. Tan MH, Morrison C, Wang P, et al. Loss of parafibromin immunoreactivity is a distinguishing feature of parathyroid carcinoma. Clin Cancer Res 2004;10(19): 6629–37.

82. Gill AJ, Lim G, Cheung VKY, et al. Parafibromin-deficient (HPT-JT Type, CDC73 Mutated) Parathyroid Tumors Demonstrate Distinctive Morphologic Features. Am J Surg Pathol 2019;43(1):35–46.

83. Witteveen JE, Hamdy NA, Dekkers OM, et al. Downregulation of CASR expression and global loss of parafibromin staining are strong negative determinants of prognosis in parathyroid carcinoma. Mod Pathol 2011;24:688–97.

84. Cetani F, Pardi E, Viacava P, et al. A reappraisal of the Rb1 gene abnormalities in the diagnosis of parathyroid cancer. Clin Endocrinol (Oxf) 2004;60(1):99–106.

85. Bergero N, De Pompa R, Sacerdote C, et al. Galectin-3 expression in parathyroid carcinoma: immunohistochemical study of 26 cases. Hum Pathol 2005; 36(8):908–14.

86. Zhao L, Sun LH, Liu DM, et al. Copy number variation in CCND1 gene is implicated in the pathogenesis of sporadic parathyroid carcinoma. World J Surg 2014;38(7):1730–7.

87. Silva-Figueroa AM, Bassett R, Christakis I, et al. Using a Novel Diagnostic Nomogram to Differentiate Malignant from Benign Parathyroid Neoplasms. Endocr Pathol 2019;30(4):285–96.

88. Davies M, Evans T, Tahir F, et al. Parathyroid cancer: A systematic review of diagnostic biomarkers. Surg 2021. https://doi.org/10.1016/j.surge.2021.01.011.

89. Rasmuson T, Kristoffersson A, Boquist L. Positive effect of radiotherapy and surgery on hormonally active pulmonary metastases of primary parathyroid carcinoma. Eur J Endocrinol 2000;143(6):749–54.

90. Munson ND, Foote RL, Northcutt RC, et al. Parathyroid Carcinoma: Is There a Role for Adjuvant Radiation Therapy? Cancer 2003;98(11):2378–84.

91. Tan AHK, Kim HK, Kim MY, et al. Parathyroid carcinoma presenting as a hyperparathyroid crisis. Korean J Intern Med 2012;27(2):229–31.

92. Mellagui Y, Jabi R, Haouli I, et al. Hypercalcemia of Malignancy Revealing a Parathyroid Carcinoma with Hepatic Metastasis: A Case Report and Literature Review. Case Rep Surg 2020;2020:1–5.

93. Silverberg SJ, Rubin MR, Faiman C, et al. Cinacalcet hydrochloride reduces the serum calcium concentration in inoperable parathyroid carcinoma. J Clin Endocrinol Metab 2007;92(10):3803–8.

94. Fountas A, Andrikoula M, Giotaki Z, et al. The emerging role of denosumab in the long-term management of parathyroid carcinoma-related refractory hypercalcemia. Endocr Pract 2015;21(5):468–73.

95. Betea D, Bradwell AR, Harvey TC, et al. Hormonal and biochemical normalization and tumor shrinkage induced by anti-parathyroid hormone immunotherapy in a patient with metastatic parathyroid carcinoma. J Clin Endocrinol Metab 2004;89(7):3413–20.

96. Horie I, Ando T, Inokuchi N, et al. First Japanese patient treated with parathyroid hormone peptide immunization for refractory hypercalcemia caused by metastatic parathyroid carcinoma. Endocr J 2010;57(4):287–92.

97. Sarquis M, Marx SJ, Beckers A, et al. Long-term remission of disseminated parathyroid cancer following immunotherapy. Endocrine 2020;67(1):204–8.

98. Storvall S, Ryhänen E, Bensch FV, et al. Recurrent Metastasized Parathyroid Carcinoma-Long-Term Remission After Combined Treatments With Surgery, Radiotherapy, Cinacalcet, Zoledronic Acid, and Temozolomide. JBMR Plus 2019;3(4):e10114.

99. Verdelli C, Vaira V, Corbetta C. Parathyroid tumor Microenvironment. In: Birbrair A, ed. Advances in Experimental Medicine and Biology - Tumor Microenvironments in Organs. vol. 1226; 2020:37-50. doi: 10.1007/978-3-030-36214-0_3.

100. Park D, Airi R, Sherman M. Microsatellite instability driven metastatic parathyroid carcinoma managed with the anti-PD1 immunotherapy, pembrolizumab. BMJ Case Rep 2020;13(9):1–3.

101. Lenschow C, Fuss CT, Kircher S, et al. Abdominal Lymph Node Metastases of Parathyroid Carcinoma: Diagnostic Workup, Molecular Diagnosis, and Clinical Management. Front Endocrinol (Lausanne) 2021;12. https://doi.org/10.3389/fendo.2021.643328.

102. Sherwood L. Ectopic hormone syndromes. In: DeGroot L, editor. Endocrinology. 2nd edition. Philadelphia: Saunders; 1989. p. 2550–99.

103. Palmieri GMA, Nordquist RE, Omenn GS. Immunochemical localization of parathyroid hormone in cancer tissue from patients with ectopic hyperparathyroidism. J Clin Invest 1974;53(6):1726–35.

104. Deftos LJ, McMillan PJ, Sartiano GP, et al. Simultaneous ectopic production of parathyroid hormone and calcitonin. Metabolism 1976;25(5):543–50.

105. Grajower M, Barzel US. Ectopic hyperparathyroidism (pseudohyperparathyroidism) in esophageal malignancy. Report of a case and a review of the literature. Am J Med 1976;61(1):59–63.

106. Robin N, Siegel L, Hawker C, et al. Hypercalcemia and metastatic intestinal leiomyosarcoma: a case of ectopic parathyroid hormone production. Conn Med 1976;40(9):609–11.

107. Hutchinson R, Shapiro S, Raney R. Elevated parathyroid hormone levels in association with rhabdomyosarcoma. J Pediatr 1978;(May):780.

108. Samaan N, Ordonez N, Ibanez M, et al. Ectopic Parathyroid Hormone Production by a Squamous Carcinoma of the Tonsil. Arch Otolaryngol 1983;109:91–4.

109. Mayes LC, Kasselberg AG, Roloff JS, et al. Hypercalcemia associated with immunoreactive parathyroid hormone in a malignant rhabdoid tumor of the kidney (Rhabdoid Wilms' tumor). Cancer 1984;54(5):882, 884.

110. Schmelzer H, Hesch R, Mayer H. Parathyroid hormone and PTHmRNA in a human small cell lung cancer. Recent Results Cancer Res 1985;99:88–93.

111. Arps H, Dietel M, Schulz A, et al. A Pancreatic endocrine carcinoma with ectopic PTH-production and paraneoplastic hypercalcaemia. Virchows Arch 1986;(1986):497–503.

112. Abeler V, Kjørstad KE, Nesland JM. Small cell carcinoma of the ovary: A report of six cases. Int J Gynecol Pathol 1988;7(4):315–29.

113. Yoshimoto K, Yamasaki R, Sakai H. Ectopic Production of Parathyroid Hormone by Small Cell Lung Cancer in a Patient with Hypercalcemia. J Clin Endocrinol Metab 1989;68(5):976–81.

114. Buller R, Taylor K, Burg AC, et al. Paraneoplastic hypercalcemia associated with adenosquamous carcinoma of the endometrium. Gynecol Oncol 1991; 40(1):95–8.

115. Strewler G, Budayr A, Clark O, et al. Production of parathyroid hormone by a malignant nonparathyroid tumor in a hypercalcemic patient. J Clin Endocrinol Metab 1993;76(5):1373–5.

116. Rizzoli R, Pache J-C, Didierjean L, et al. A Thymoma as a Cause of True Hyperparathyroidism. J Clin Endocrinol Metab 1994;79(3):912–5.

117. Nielsen P, Rasmussen A, Feldt-Rasmusse U, et al. Ectopic Production of intact Parathyroid Hormone by a squamous cell lung carcinoma in vivo and in vitro. J Cell Mol Med 1996;81(10):3793–6.

118. Iguchi H, Miyagi C, Tomita K, et al. Hypercalcemia Caused by Ectopic Production of Parathyroid Hormone in a Patient with Papillary Adenocarcinoma of the Thyroid Gland. J Clin Endocrinol Metab 1998;83(8):2653–7.

119. Koyama Y, Ishijima H, Ishibashi A, et al. Intact PTH-producing hepatocellular carcinoma treated by transcatheter arterial embolization. Abdom Imaging 1999;146:144–6.

120. Demura M, Yoneda T, Wang F, et al. Ectopic Production of Parathyroid Hormone in a Patient with Sporadic Medullary. Thyroid Cancer 2010;57(2):161–70.

121. Uchimura K, Mokuno T, Nagasaka A, et al. Lung cancer associated with hypercalcemia induced by concurrently elevated parathyroid hormone and parathyroid hormone-related protein levels. Metabolism 2002;51(7):871–5.

122. Botea V, Edelson GW, Munasinghe RL. In a patient with small cell carcinoma demonstrating positive immunostain for parathyroid hormone. Endocr Pract 2003;9(1):40–4.

123. Eid W, Wheeler T, Sharma M. Recurrent hypercalcemia due to ectopic production of parathyroid hormone-related protein and intact parathyroid hormone in a single patient with multiple malignancies. Endocr Pract 2004;10(2):125–8.

124. Ohira S, Itoh K, Shiozawa T, et al. Ovarian non-small cell neuroendocrine carcinoma with paraneoplastic parathyroid hormone-related hypercalcemia. Int J Gynecol Pathol 2004;23(4):393–7.

125. Chen L, Dinh TA, Haque A. Small cell carcinoma of the ovary with hypercalcemia and ectopic parathyroid hormone production. Arch Pathol Lab Med 2005; 129(4):531–3.

126. Vacher-Coponat H, Opris A, Denizot A, et al. Hypercalcaemia induced by excessive parathyroid hormone secretion in a patient with a neuroendocrine tumour. Nephrol Dial Transpl 2005;20(12):2832–5.

127. Wong K, Tsuda S, Mukai R, et al. Parathyroid hormone expression in a patient with metastatic nasopharyngeal rhabdomyosarcoma and hypercalcemia. Endocrine 2005;27(1):83–6.
128. Bhattacharya A, Mittal BR, Bhansali A, et al. Cervical paraganglioma mimicking a parathyroid adenoma on Tc-99m sestamibi scintigraphy. Clin Nucl Med 2006; 31(4):234–6.
129. Mahoney EJ, Monchik JM, Donatini G, et al. Life-threatening hypercalcemia from a hepatocellular carcinoma secreting intact parathyroid hormone: localization by sestamibi single-photon emission computed tomographic imaging. Endocr Pract 2006;12(3):302–6.
130. Vanhouten JN, Yu N, Rimm D, et al. Hypercalcemia of Malignancy due to Ectopic Transactivation of the Parathyroid Hormone Gene. J Clin Endocrinol Metab 2006;91:580–3.
131. Weiss ES, Doty J, Brock MV, et al. A case of ectopic parathyroid hormone production by a pulmonary neoplasm. J Thorac Cardiovasc Surg 2006;131(4): 923–4.
132. Morita SY, Brownlee NA, Dackiw APB, et al. Case Report An Unusual Case of Recurrent Hyperparathyroidism and Papillary Thyroid Cancer. Endocr Pract 2009;15(4):349–52.
133. Abe Y, Makiyama H, Fujita Y, et al. Severe hypercalcemia associated with hepatocellular carcinoma secreting intact parathyroid hormone: A case report. Intern Med 2011;50(4):329–33.
134. Kandil E, Noureldine S, Khalek MA, et al. Ectopic secretion of parathyroid hormone in a neuroendo- crine tumor: a case report and review of the literature. Int J Clin Exp Med 2011;4(3):234–40.
135. Doyle M-A, Malcolm J. An unusual case of malignancy-related hypercalcemia. Int J Gen Med 2014;7:21–7.
136. Kwon HJ, Kim JW, Kim H, et al. Combined hepatocellular carcinoma and neuroendocrine carcinoma with ectopic secretion of parathyroid hormone: A case report and review of the literature. J Pathol Transl Med 2018;52(4):232–7.
137. Sardiñas Z, Suazo S, Kumar S, et al. Ectopic Parathyroid Hormone Secretion by A Penile Squamous Cell Carcinoma. AACE Clin Case Rep 2018;4(1):9–12.
138. Deshaies D, Hariri N, Dyer B, et al. Life-threatening hypercalcemia due to ectopic intact parathyroid hormone secretion from a poorly differentiated endometrioid carcinoma. Am Surg 2019;85(1):E45–6.
139. Belaid R, Oueslati I, Chihaoui M, et al. A Case of Von Hippel – Lindau Disease with Bilateral Pheochromocytoma and Ectopic Hypersecretion of Intact Parathyroid Hormone in an Adolescent Girl. Case Rep Endocrinol 2020;2020:1–5.
140. Gabriel FGC, Picar RE. A rare case of hypercalcemic encephalopathy from ectopic secretion of parathyroid hormone. Clin Case Rep 2020;8(3):423–5.
141. Brun VH, Knutsen E, Stenvold H, et al. Severe hypercalcemia caused by parathyroid hormone in a rectal cancer metastasis: a case report. BMC Endocr Disord 2021;21(1):1–6.
142. Nakajima K, Tamai M, Okaniwa S, et al. Humoral hypercalcemia associated with gastric carcinoma secreting parathyroid hormone : a case report and review of the literature. Endocr J 2013;60(5):557–62.
143. Brewer K, Costa-Guda J, Arnold A. Molecular genetic insights into sporadic primary hyperparathyroidism. Endocr Relat Cancer 2019;26(2):R53–72.

Endocrine Disorders with Parathyroid Hormone-Independent Hypercalcemia

Jo Krogsgaard Simonsen, MD*, Lars Rejnmark, PhD, DMSc

KEYWORDS

- Hypercalcemia • Hyperthyroidism • Adrenal insufficiency • Pheochromocytoma
- Vasoactive intestinal polypeptide • Parathyroid hormone-independent
- Endocrine disorders

KEY POINTS

- Consider hyperthyroidism, adrenal insufficiency, pheochromocytoma and VIPoma as possible causes of nonparathyroid hypercalcemia due to endocrine disturbances.
- Measure albumin corrected or ionized calcium in order to account for whether albumin levels are low – of specific importance in the hyperthyroid patient.
- Consider possible effects of altered bone metabolism in patients with endocrine hormonal disorders regardless of the possible association between any individual disorder and hypercalcemia.

INTRODUCTION

Hypercalcemia is a relatively common finding. The prevalence of hypercalcemia, defined as serum calcium of at least 11.0 mg/dL and at least 11.1 mg/dL in a health screening was 3.9% and 1.1%, respectively.[1] The most common causes of hypercalcemia are primary hyperparathyroidism and malignancy, accounting for 80% to 90% of cases, with hyperparathyroidism being most frequent in free-living individuals, whereas malignant etiology is more common in the hospital.[2] Although less common, some endocrine disorders have been associated with nonparathyroid hypercalcemia, and it is important to keep these in mind as a possible differential diagnosis when encountering the hypercalcemic patient. This article looks at hypercalcemia in relation to endocrine disorders connected to thyroid hormone, cortisol, growth hormone, prolactin, gonadal dysfunction, diabetes, pheochromocytoma, and vasoactive intestinal polypeptide (VIPoma). The genetic disorder, familial hypocalciuric hypercalcemia, is not addressed in this article.

Department of Endocrinology and Internal Medicine, Aarhus University Hospital, Palle Juul-Jensens Boulevard 165, Aarhus N 8200, Denmark
* Corresponding author.
E-mail address: josimo@rm.dk

Endocrinol Metab Clin N Am 50 (2021) 711–720
https://doi.org/10.1016/j.ecl.2021.07.002
0889-8529/21/© 2021 Elsevier Inc. All rights reserved.

HYPERTHYROIDISM

Hypercalcemia is well reported in relation to hyperthyroidism, and several studies have found increased mean total, corrected, or ionized serum calcium levels compared with healthy controls.[3–8] Others have reported no significant difference in total S-calcium but a significantly higher level of ionized S-calcium.[9] In addition, hyperthyroid patients have also been found to exhibit an increased excretion of calcium by the kidneys.[7,8,10]

The reported prevalence of overt hypercalcemia in hyperthyroid patients varies considerably whether total, corrected, or ionized calcium is measured and depending on the applied threshold for hypercalcemia. Studies reporting hypercalcemia based on total S-calcium tend to relate a lower prevalence, typically ranging from 15.6% to 27%[3–5,7] compared with corrected and ionized calcium where the reported prevalence is as high as 47% to 51.1%.[5,7] One study reported a lower prevalence of hypercalcemia in hyperthyroid patients, with a prevalence based on total calcium of 3.2% and a prevalence based on corrected calcium of 5.7% to 8.5% depending on applied method for correction.[11] Nonetheless, this study still found a significantly higher mean total and corrected calcium levels in the hyperthyroid patient compared with both after treatment and healthy controls. The generally higher prevalence of hypercalcemia reported based on corrected and ionized calcium may in part be due to the lower level of serum albumin measured in hyperthyroid patients.[3,4,11] However, 1 study suggested that a conventional formula for corrected calcium might overestimate the level in hyperthyroid patients.[11]

It remains uncertain whether there is a correlation between severity of thyrotoxicosis and degree of hypercalcemia. Although some studies report a positive correlation between corrected S-calcium and S-thyroxine,[7] S-triiodothyronine,[8] S-triiodothyronine uptake,[7] and free thyroxine index,[7] others report a poor correlation between ionized S-calcium and S-thyroxine.[4,5]

The most supported cause of increased calcium in hyperthyroid patients is the theory of increased bone turnover. Increased levels of the bone markers C-terminal telopeptides of type I collagen (CTx), serum alkaline phosphatase (s-AP), diphosphonate retention (WBR_{100}), and clearance corrected serum osteocalcin (s-OCxCl) were reported in hyperthyroid patients,[12,13] while a decreased level of tartrate-resistant acid phosphatase (TRAP) was reported in 1 study.[12] In addition, increased urinary excretion of the collagen metabolites hydroxylysyl glucosides was reported in hyperthyroid patients.[14] Histomorphometric bone changes were described in bone biopsies before and after treatment, suggesting increased bone turnover in hyperthyroid patients as a possible contributor to development of hypercalcemia, where an increase in both bone resorption and formation was reported.[8,10,15,16] One study found a significantly lower volume of trabecular bone,[16] while others reported significantly higher cortical porosity in hyperthyroid patients compared with controls.[8,15,16]

Another cause of hypercalcemia in hyperthyroid patients has been suggested. One study reported increased PTHrP levels positively correlated with ionized calcium in hyperthyroid patients with simultaneously decreased levels of parathyroid hormone (PTH), suggesting an involvement of PTHrP in the pathogenesis of hypercalcemia.[6] However, PTHrP-related hypercalcemia has been associated with malignancy and has in even apparently benign diseases been associated with short overall survival.[17]

The previously mentioned studies report hyperthyroidism in general based on serum levels of thyroid hormone, and few studies have analyzed the importance of goiter type. One study found that 8 of 9 hyperthyroid patients had nodular goiters with 1 or multiple nodules, while 1 patient was oversubstituted after thyroidectomy;[18] however, further studies are required in order to determine the role of goiter type.

HYPOTHYROIDISM

Hypothyroidism is sometimes mentioned as a possible cause of hypercalcemia; however, studies related to this are few, and episodes of hypercalcemia are mostly related to concomitant supplementation with calcium.[19] Changes in bone metabolism in hypothyroid patients have been described as opposite that of hyperthyroidism, with low bone turnover and reduced osteoclastic activity in cortical bone.[20] Decreased excretion of hydroxylysyl glycosides in urine was reported.[14] Although no significant difference in bone markers was reported in hypothyroid patients, a tendency to subnormal levels of serum OCxCl was observed.[13] Accordingly, available data do not exclude that patients with hypothyroidism are more prone to develop hypercalcemia when treated with calcium supplements, which may be associated with a low bone turnover, lowering the ability of bone to incorporate additional calcium. However, further large-scale studies are needed to test this hypothesis.

CORTISOL

Hypercalcemia has been reported on several occasions in relation to adrenal insufficiency. One study on primary adrenocortical insufficiency including 54 patients reported hypercalcemia in 41%,[21] while another study on 108 patients observed hypercalcemia in only 6%.[22] In both studies, hypercalcemia regressed after treatment. A study on children with congenital adrenal hyperplasia reported elevated calcium on at least 1 occasion in 82.5% of children, while 53% had elevated calcium levels on 2 or more occasions.[23] Meanwhile, a study of 112 patients in a critical care setting with relative adrenal insufficiency defined as cortisol below 25 μg/dL found no significant difference in calcium compared to patients without relative adrenal insufficiency. The authors observed no hypercalcemic patients in the group with relative adrenal insufficiency.[24]

Case reports have described patients with adrenal insufficiency and associated hypercalcemia in whom normalization of electrolyte disturbances was seen after treatment.[25–27] Others have described hypercalcemia associated with adrenal insufficiency presenting with normal saline levels.[28] Overall, the precise mechanism causing hypercalcemia in adrenal insufficiency is yet to be fully elucidated.[29] Volume depletion and decreased glomerular filtration[27,30] seem to be of importance, as well as an increased calcium mobilization from bone, although the mechanism remains unclear.[26] Other theorized but uncertain explanations mentioned in the literature are increased intestinal calcium absorption caused by decreased cortisol levels, as cortisol normally acts as a vitamin D antagonist.[31]

Idiopathic adrenal insufficiency has been associated with other diseases related to hypercalcemia where concurrent thyrotoxicosis was reported in 10% of patients in 1 study.[22] Furthermore, in studies mentioned previously on adrenal insufficiency, tuberculous etiology accounted for 17% to 33% of cases,[21,22] and tuberculosis in itself was associated with hypercalcemia.[32] Thus, both concomitant thyrotoxicosis and tuberculosis are possible contributors to the development of hypercalcemia in these patients.

Cushing syndrome is not directly associated with hypercalcemia, although hypercalcemia has been observed after adrenalectomy in 3 of 5 symptomatic patients after operation in 15 patients.[28] Glucocorticoid treatment is associated with osteoporosis because of inhibited bone formation and enhanced bone resorption in addition to a decreased intestinal calcium resorption and an increased renal calcium excretion.[33]

PHEOCHROMOCYTOMA

Several cases of hypercalcemia in relation to pheochromocytoma have been reported with normalization of calcium levels after surgical removal of the catecholamine-secreting tumors.[34–41] Some suggested that a direct effect of catecholamines on bone tissue could be the cause.[41] However, the idea that hypercalcemia is a direct effect of increased catecholamines was disputed by a study of 12 patients with pheochromocytoma in which hypercalcemia in 2 patients was caused by concomitant hyperplastic parathyroid glands. In the remaining 10 patients with increased catecholamines, serum PTH was normal, and no patient had hypercalcemia.[42] It should be remembered that pheochromocytoma is part of the MEN syndrome, where 50% and 20% to 30% of patients with MEN2A develop pheochromocytoma and parathyroid tumors, respectively.[43] Reports have suggested pheochromocytoma may cause high or inappropriately increased levels of serum PTH.[34,38] Tumor production of a substance activating PTH receptors[36] and PTH-like activity in tumor tissue has been presented,[39] while increased PTHrP was identified as the cause of hypercalcemia in another patient.[40] Nevertheless, a recent case described pheochromocytoma with hypercalcemia and hypercortisolism but low levels of intact PTH and PTHrP in serum.[35] This suggests that more than 1 cause of hypercalcemia in patients with pheochromocytoma might be found.

VASOACTIVE INTESTINAL POLYPEPTIDE

The neuroendocrine tumors secreting VIPoma are rare ,with an incidence of 0.05 to 0.1 cases per 100,000 population per year.[44] VIPomas are associated with watery diarrhea, hypokalemia, and hypochlorhydria. Hypercalcemia has been reported in patients with VIPoma,[45–47] one of whom had a variant of unknown significance in the MEN1 gene. One report of 18 patients with VIPoma found hypercalcemia in 9 patients, among whom 2 patients had MEN1,[48] although VIPoma is a rare finding in MEN1 patients.[49] Possible causes are altered bone metabolism,[50] hyperparathyroidism as part of the MEN1 syndrome,[51] or dehydration.

GROWTH HORMONE

Excess growth hormone (GH) is associated with altered bone metabolism[52] although it is not generally associated with hypercalcemia. One study reported normal mean corrected serum calcium in acromegalic patients with no change after treatment,[53] while another study reported mild hypercalcemia in 3 out of 27 untreated patients with acromegaly. Another 2 patients were excluded from this study because of hyperthyroidism, as both had increased levels of calcium and PTH.[54] PTH in other studies has been reported within normal range in acromegalic patients with no significant change after treatment, while a significant decrease in 1,25-dihydroxyvitamin D has been observed in patients with acromegaly after treatment, suggesting an association between acromegaly and active vitamin D.[53,55]

Several studies have reported increased calcium levels in patients receiving GH therapy as part of burn treatment in addition to standard conservative therapy compared with patients receiving conservative therapy without GH therapy.[56,57] A study of GH administration for 6 months in adults with GH deficiency found a nonsignificant tendency toward increased calcium levels in adults after 1 month, after which calcium levels returned to pretreatment levels.[58] In another study, administration of GH to healthy subjects resulted in significantly increased corrected serum calcium after 2 weeks, while administration of IGF-1 did not change calcium levels.[59]

Consequently, although GH administration might affect calcium levels in some patient subgroups, there is no evidence of increased prevalence of hypercalcemia in acromegalic patients.

GONADAL DYSFUNCTION

Premature menopause and primary or secondary amenorrhea in women and primary or secondary hypogonadism in men are all associated with increased risk of osteoporotic fractures,[60] but gonadal dysfunction is not by itself associated with hypercalcemia.

HYPERPROLACTINEMIA

Hyperprolactinemic amenorrhea is associated with lower bone mineral density,[61] but changes in prolactin levels are not traditionally associated with hypercalcemia. One study found a normal but significantly higher mean calcium level in lactating women compared to controls, while patients with pituitary adenomas did not differ from controls. Both lactating women and patients with pituitary adenoma had significantly higher levels of PTHrP.[62] A role of PTHrP in lactation has been suggested,[63] with possible systemic effects when reaching the maternal circulation.[64] However, further investigation is needed to determine whether there is a relation between prolactin, PTHrP, and calcium levels in lactating women.

DIABETES

Although diabetes mellitus has been associated with low bone turnover[65] and increased risk of fracture,[66] it has to the authors' knowledge not been associated with hypercalcemia.

DISCUSSION

Although all the examined endocrinological disorders are in some way associated with altered bone metabolism, nonparathyroid hypercalcemia is observed in only a few endocrinological disorders, of which the most well described is hyperthyroidism (**Box 1**). Studies report significantly higher serum calcium levels in hyperthyroid patients, and increased bone turnover is the most supported cause. Contrary to this, hypercalcemia in hypothyroid patients is described in only a limited number of reports, where it is suggested that hypothyroid patients are more prone to develop hypercalcemia upon receiving calcium supplements. Further investigation is needed to examine this.

Several studies and case reports find hypercalcemia in patients with adrenal insufficiency; however, the etiology remains unclear, and other contributing causes of hypercalcemia are seen in some of the reported studies. Furthermore, hypercalcemia is described in both patients with pheochromocytoma and VIPoma, although the literature is sparse and primarily consisting of case reports. This is likely because of the low incidence of these endocrine disorders, making larger-scale studies difficult to carry out. Other endocrine disorders, including acromegaly, hyperprolactinemia, gonadal dysfunction, and diabetes, are not associated with hypercalcemia.

Several of the examined endocrine disorders are associated with the MEN syndrome, which should be kept in mind as a possible undiagnosed underlying cause of hypercalcemia in patients with endocrine disorders and concomitant increased PTH. Primary hyperparathyroidism, VIPoma, and anterior pituitary adenomas secreting prolactin, GH, and more rarely TSH, in addition to the more uncommon

Box 1
Nonparathyroid disorders associated with hypercalcemia

Nonparathyroid endocrine hypercalcemia

Disorders associated with hypercalcemia
  Hyperthyroidism
  Adrenal insufficiency
  Pheochromocytoma
  VIPoma

Disorders possibly associated with hypercalcemia
  Hypothyroidism

Disorders not associated with hypercalcemia
  Acromegaly
  Mb Cushing
  Diabetes
  Hyperprolactinemia
  Gonadal dysfunction

pheochromocytoma, are all associated with MEN1, while medullary thyroid carcinoma, primary hyperparathyroidism and pheochromocytoma are associated with MEN2A.[43]

Hypercalcemia in both hyperthyroidism and pheochromocytoma was associated with PTHrP.[6,40] As previously mentioned, this hormone is associated with malignancy, and is even in apparent benignant diseases related to short-term survival[17] Detection of PTHrP in patients should therefore elicit a thorough examination in order to exclude malignancy.

One endocrine cause of hypercalcemia, familiar hypocalciuric hypercalcemia, is not addressed in this article. This genetic disease is another relevant differential diagnosis of hypercalcemia. Other possible causes of hypercalcemia not previously mentioned include, but are not limited to, drug-induced hypercalcemia, granulomatous disease, immobilization, and renal failure. Many of the addressed reports and studies in this article did not fully exclude these differential diagnoses, and other contributing causes of hypercalcemia in the examined patients cannot be excluded.

SUMMARY

The most common causes of hypercalcemia are primary hyperparathyroidism and malignancy, constituting 80% to 90% of all cases. Although much less common, several nonparathyroid endocrine disorders are associated with hypercalcemia. The most well described is hyperthyroidism, although the reported prevalence of hypercalcemia in hyperthyroid patients varies considerably depending on applied method for measuring serum calcium levels. Also, adrenal insufficiency, pheochromocytoma, and VIPoma are associated with hypercalcemia. These are important differential diagnoses when assessing the hypercalcemic patient in whom the most common causes have been excluded. Further investigation is needed regarding hypothyroidism, while acromegaly, hyperprolactinemia, gonadal dysfunction, and diabetes are not associated with hyperthyroidism.

CLINICS CARE POINTS

- Nonparathyroid endocrine hypercalcemia is associated with hyperthyroidism, adrenal insufficiency, pheochromocytoma, and VIPoma.

- Further studies are needed to determine whether hypothyroid patients are more prone to develop hypercalcemia in connection with calcium administration.
- Acromegaly, hyperprolactinemia, gonadal dysfunction, and diabetes are not associated with hypercalcemia.

DISCLOSURE

The authors have no disclosures.

REFERENCES

1. Christensson T, Hellström K, Wengle B, et al. Prevalence of hypercalcaemia in a health screening in Stockholm. Acta Med Scand 1976;200(1–2):131–7.
2. Lafferty FW. Differential diagnosis of hypercalcemia. J bone mineral Res 1991; 6(Suppl 2):S51–9 [Discussion S61].
3. Baxter JD, Bondy PK. Hypercalcemia of thyrotoxicosis. Ann Intern Med 1966; 65(3):429–42.
4. Gordon DL, Suvanich S, Erviti V, et al. The serum calcium level and its significance in hyperthyroidism: a prospective study. Am J Med Sci 1974;268(1):31–6.
5. Burman KD, Monchik JM, Earll JM, et al. Ionized and total serum calcium and parathyroid hormone in hyperthyroidism. Ann Intern Med 1976;84(6):668–71.
6. Giovanella L, Suriano S, Keller F, et al. Evaluation of serum parathyroid hormone-related peptide in hyperthyroid patients. Eur J Clin Invest 2011;41(1):93–7.
7. Mosekilde L, Christensen MS. Decreased parathyroid function in hyperthyroidism: interrelationships between serum parathyroid hormone, calcium-phosphorus metabolism and thyroid function. Acta endocrinologica 1977;84(3): 566–75.
8. Jastrup B, Mosekilde L, Melsen F, et al. Serum levels of vitamin D metabolites and bone remodelling in hyperthyroidism. Metab Clin Exp 1982;31(2):126–32.
9. Frizel D, Malleson A, Marks V. Plasma levels of ionised calcium and magnesium in thyroid disease. Lancet 1967;1(7504):1360–1.
10. Lalau JD, Sebert JL, Marie A, et al. Effect of thyrotoxicosis and its treatment on mineral and bone metabolism. J Endocrinol Invest 1986;9(6):491–6.
11. Daly JG, Greenwood RM, Himsworth RL. Serum calcium concentration in hyperthyroidism at diagnosis and after treatment. Clin Endocrinol 1983;19(3):397–404.
12. Minisola S, Dionisi S, Pacitti MT, et al. Gender differences in serum markers of bone resorption in healthy subjects and patients with disorders affecting bone. Osteoporos Int 2002;13(2):171–5.
13. Hyldstrup L, Clemmensen I, Jensen BA, et al. Non-invasive evaluation of bone formation: measurements of serum alkaline phosphatase, whole body retention of diphosphonate and serum osteocalcin in metabolic bone disorders and thyroid disease. Scand J Clin Lab Invest 1988;48(7):611–9.
14. Askenasi R, Demeester-Mirkine N. Urinary excretion of hydroxylysyl glycosides and thyroid function. J Clin Endocrinol Metab 1975;40(2):342–4.
15. Mosekilde L, Melsen F. Effect of antithyroid treatment on calcium-phosphorus metabolism in hyperthyroidism. II: bone histomorphometry. Acta Endocrinol 1978;87(4):751–8.
16. Mosekilde L, Melsen F, Bagger JP, et al. Bone changes in hyperthyroidism: interrelationships between bone morphometry, thyroid function and calcium-phosphorus metabolism. Acta Endocrinol 1977;85(3):515–25.

17. Donovan PJ, Achong N, Griffin K, et al. PTHrP-mediated hypercalcemia: causes and survival in 138 patients. J Clin Endocrinol Metab 2015;100(5):2024–9.

18. Szabó ZS, Ritzl F. Hypercalcemia in hyperthyroidism. Role of age and goiter type. Klin Wochenschr 1981;59(6):275–9.

19. Lowe CE, Bird ED, Thomas WC Jr. Hypercalcemia in myxedema. J Clin Endocrinol Metab 1962;22:261–7.

20. Mosekilde L, Melsen F. Morphometric and dynamic studies of bone changes in hypothyroidism. Acta Pathol Microbiol Scand A 1978;86(1):56–62.

21. De Rosa G, Corsello SM, Cecchini L, et al. A clinical study of Addison's disease. Exp Clin Endocrinol 1987;90(2):232–42.

22. Nerup J. Addison's disease–clinical studies. A report fo 108 cases. Acta endocrinologica 1974;76(1):127–41.

23. Schoelwer MJ, Viswanathan V, Wilson A, et al. Infants with congenital adrenal hyperplasia are at risk for hypercalcemia, hypercalciuria, and nephrocalcinosis. J Endocr Soc 2017;1(9):1160–7.

24. Kromah F, Tyroch A, McLean S, et al. Relative adrenal insufficiency in the critical care setting: debunking the classic myth. World J Surg 2011;35(8):1818–23.

25. Leeksma CH, De Graeff J, De Cock J. Hypercalcaemia in adrenal insufficiency. Acta Med Scand 1957;156(6):455–8.

26. Montoli A, Colussi G, Minetti L. Hypercalcaemia in Addison's disease: calciotropic hormone profile and bone histology. J Intern Med 1992;232(6):535–40.

27. Muls E, Bouillon R, Boelaert J, et al. Etiology of hypercalcemia in a patient with Addison's disease. Calcified Tissue Int 1982;34(6):523–6.

28. Jorgensen H. Hypercalcemia in adrenocortical insufficiency. Acta Med Scand 1973;193(3):175–9.

29. Horwitz MJ, Hodak SP, Stewart AF. Non-Parathyroid Hypercalcemia. In: Rosen CJ, editor. Primer on the Metabolic Bone Diseases and Disorders of Mineral Metabolism. 8. Ames, IA: Wiley-Blackwell; 2013. p. 562–71.

30. Ahn SW, Kim TY, Lee S, et al. Adrenal insufficiency presenting as hypercalcemia and acute kidney injury. Int Med Case Rep J 2016;9:223–6.

31. Walser M, Robinson BH, Duckett JW Jr. The hypercalcemia of adrenal insufficiency. J Clin Invest 1963;42(4):456–65.

32. Lind L, Ljunghall S. Hypercalcemia in pulmonary tuberculosis. Upsala J Med Sci 1990;95(2):157–60.

33. Lukert BP, Raisz LG. Glucocorticoid-induced osteoporosis: pathogenesis and management. Ann Intern Med 1990;112(5):352–64.

34. Kukreja SC, Hargis GK, Rosenthal IM, et al. Pheochromocytoma causing excessive parathyroid hormone production and hypercalcemia. Ann Intern Med 1973; 79(6):838–40.

35. Edafe O, Webster J, Fernando M, et al. Phaeochromocytoma with hypercortisolism and hypercalcaemia. BMJ Case Rep 2015;2015. http://dx.doi.org/10.1136/bcr-2014-208657.

36. Stewart AF, Hoecker JL, Mallette LE, et al. Hypercalcemia in pheochromocytoma. Evidence for a novel mechanism. Ann Intern Med 1985;102(6):776–9.

37. Swinton NW Jr, Clerkin EP, Flint LD. Hypercalcemia and familial pheochromocytoma. Correction after adrenalectomy. Ann Intern Med 1972;76(3):455–7.

38. Ghose RR, Winsey HS, Jemmett J, et al. Phaeochromocytoma and hypercalcaemia. Postgrad Med J 1976;52(611):593–5.

39. Fairhurst BJ, Shettar SP. Hypercalcaemia and phaeochromocytoma. Postgrad Med J 1981;57(669):459–60.

40. Kimura S, Nishimura Y, Yamaguchi K, et al. A case of pheochromocytoma producing parathyroid hormone-related protein and presenting with hypercalcemia. J Clin Endocrinol Metab 1990;70(6):1559–63.
41. Finlayson JF, Casey JH. Letter: hypercalcaemia and multiple pheochromocytomas. Ann Intern Med 1975;82(6):810–1.
42. Miller SS, Sizemore GW, Sheps SG, et al. Parathyroid function in patients with pheochromocytoma. Ann Intern Med 1975;82(3):372–5.
43. Brandi ML, Gagel RF, Angeli A, et al. Guidelines for diagnosis and therapy of MEN type 1 and type 2. J Clin Endocrinol Metab 2001;86(12):5658–71.
44. Dimitriadis GK, Weickert MO, Randeva HS, et al. Medical management of secretory syndromes related to gastroenteropancreatic neuroendocrine tumours. Endocr Relat Cancer 2016;23(9):R423–36.
45. Ghaferi AA, Chojnacki KA, Long WD, et al. Pancreatic VIPomas: subject review and one institutional experience. J Gastrointest Surg 2008;12(2):382–93.
46. Lubinski SM, Hendrix T. Images in clinical medicine. VIPoma. N Engl J Med 2004; 351(8):808.
47. Acosta-Gualandri A, Kao KT, Wong T, et al. Perioperative hypotensive crisis in an adolescent with a pancreatic VIPoma and MEN1-gene variant. Horm Res Paediatr 2019;91(4):285–9.
48. Smith SL, Branton SA, Avino AJ, et al. Vasoactive intestinal polypeptide secreting islet cell tumors: a 15-year experience and review of the literature. Surgery 1998; 124(6):1050–5.
49. Tonelli F, Giudici F, Fratini G, et al. Pancreatic endocrine tumors in multiple endocrine neoplasia type 1 syndrome: review of literature. Endocr Pract 2011; 17(Suppl 3):33–40.
50. Lerner UH, Persson E. Osteotropic effects by the neuropeptides calcitonin generelated peptide, substance P and vasoactive intestinal peptide. J Musculoskelet Neuronal Interact 2008;8(2):154–65.
51. Cavalli T, Giudici F, Santi R, et al. Ventricular fibrillation resulting from electrolyte imbalance reveals vipoma in MEN1 syndrome. Fam Cancer 2016;15(4):645–9.
52. Mazziotti G, Biagioli E, Maffezzoni F, et al. Bone turnover, bone mineral density, and fracture risk in acromegaly: a meta-analysis. J Clin Endocrinol Metab 2015;100(2):384–94.
53. Bijlsma JW, Nortier JW, Duursma SA, et al. Changes in bone metabolism during treatment of acromegaly. Acta Endocrinol 1983;104(2):153–9.
54. Ezzat S, Melmed S, Endres D, et al. Biochemical assessment of bone formation and resorption in acromegaly. J Clin Endocrinol Metab 1993;76(6):1452–7.
55. Lund B, Eskildsen PC, Lund B, et al. Calcium and vitamin D metabolism in acromegaly. Acta Endocrinol 1981;96(4):444–50.
56. Singh KP, Prasad R, Chari PS, et al. Effect of growth hormone therapy in burn patients on conservative treatment. Burns 1998;24(8):733–8.
57. Knox JB, Demling RH, Wilmore DW, et al. Hypercalcemia associated with the use of human growth hormone in an adult surgical intensive care unit. Arch Surg 1995;130(4):442–5.
58. Binnerts A, Swart GR, Wilson JH, et al. The effect of growth hormone administration in growth hormone deficient adults on bone, protein, carbohydrate and lipid homeostasis, as well as on body composition. Clin Endocrinol 1992;37(1):79–87.
59. Bianda T, Hussain MA, Glatz Y, et al. Effects of short-term insulin-like growth factor-I or growth hormone treatment on bone turnover, renal phosphate reabsorption and 1,25 dihydroxyvitamin D3 production in healthy man. J Intern Med 1997;241(2):143–50.

60. Kanis JA. Diagnosis of osteoporosis and assessment of fracture risk. Lancet 2002;359(9321):1929–36.
61. Schlechte J, Walkner L, Kathol M. A longitudinal analysis of premenopausal bone loss in healthy women and women with hyperprolactinemia. J Clin Endocrinol Metab 1992;75(3):698–703.
62. Kovacs CS, Chik CL. Hyperprolactinemia caused by lactation and pituitary adenomas is associated with altered serum calcium, phosphate, parathyroid hormone (PTH), and PTH-related peptide levels. J Clin Endocrinol Metab 1995; 80(10):3036–42.
63. Budayr AA, Halloran BP, King JC, et al. High levels of a parathyroid hormone-like protein in milk. Proc Natl Acad Sci U S A 1989;86(18):7183–5.
64. Grill V, Hillary J, Ho PM, et al. Parathyroid hormone-related protein: a possible endocrine function in lactation. Clin Endocrinol 1992;37(5):405–10.
65. Hygum K, Starup-Linde J, Harsløf T, et al. Mechanisms in endocrinology: diabetes mellitus, a state of low bone turnover - a systematic review and meta-analysis. Eur J Endocrinol 2017;176(3):R137–57.
66. Shah VN, Shah CS, Snell-Bergeon JK. Type 1 diabetes and risk of fracture: meta-analysis and review of the literature. Diabet Med 2015;32(9):1134–42.

Hypercalcemia of Malignancy

Mimi I. Hu, MD

KEYWORDS

- Cancer • Hypercalcemia • Evaluation • Etiology • Antiresorptive therapy
- Refractory

KEY POINTS

- Hypercalcemia of malignancy (HCM) is the most common paraneoplastic syndrome in the cancer patient.
- Humoral hypercalcemia of malignancy mediated by tumoral secretion of parathyroid hormone-related protein accounts for 80% of HCM.
- Osteoclast-mediated bone resorption is the common factor mediating HCM.
- Further investigation is needed into novel therapies for patients with HCM refractory to standsard therapies, such as fluid resuscitation and bone-modifying agents.

INTRODUCTION

Hypercalcemia of malignancy (HCM), the most common paraneoplastic syndrome, occurs in 2% to 2.8% of all cancer patients in the United States.[1] It can increase to up to 20% to 30% of patients at some point with advanced stages of cancer.[2] While it has been associated with almost all cancer subtypes, the most common cancers associated with hypercalcemia include breast cancer, lung cancer, and multiple myeloma. Squamous cell carcinoma of the head and neck and renal cell, ovarian, colorectal, and prostate cancers can also be associated with HCM to a lesser extent. Multiple myeloma patients have the highest rates of HCM (7.5%–10.2%), with prostate cancer patients having the lowest rates (1.4%–2.1%) based on a retrospective review of a US large oncology database of laboratory values between 2009 and 2013.[1]

HCM is associated with a spectrum of symptoms including nausea, vomiting, anorexia, abdominal pain, constipation, polyuria, hypotension, bone pain, fatigue, and confusion. Renal failure or coma can occur; thus, HCM is considered an oncologic emergency. HCM is a poor prognostic indicator for cancer patients. Historically, the estimated median survival in cancer patients with hypercalcemia was 30 days regardless of active treatment.[3] A more recent analysis of US cancer patients reported a

Department of Endocrine Neoplasia & Hormonal Disorders, The University of Texas MD Anderson Cancer Center, 1515 Holcombe Boulevard, Unit 1461, Houston, TX 77030, USA
E-mail address: mhu@mdanderson.org

Endocrinol Metab Clin N Am 50 (2021) 721–728
https://doi.org/10.1016/j.ecl.2021.07.003
0889-8529/21/© 2021 Elsevier Inc. All rights reserved.
endo.theclinics.com

median survival after cancer diagnosis of 11 months in hypercalcemic patients compared with 14 months in normocalcemic patients (*P*<.001) with a mortality hazard ratio (HR) of 4.9 (95% confidence interval [CI] 4.29–5.48, *P*<.0001).[1] The availability of more effective treatments, such as bone-modifying and antineoplastic agents, may have contributed to longer survival over the last few decades.

The definitive method to control HCM is to treat the underlying cancer with systemic chemotherapy, surgical resection or targeted radiation as appropriate to the clinical setting. However, severe hypercalcemia that compromises renal or cardiovascular function can preclude the implementation of such antitumoral treatments, and consequently decrease chance of survival. As HCM is most often associated with increased osteoclast-mediated bone resorption, bone-modifying agents (eg, calcitonin, zoledronic acid, or denosumab) are the cornerstones for managing hypercalcemia to reduce symptom burden and improve performance status, enabling patients to tolerate essential cancer-specific treatments. This article describes the clinical presentation and pathogenic mechanisms mediating HCM. As the strategies for managing HCM are thoroughly described in a different article, this article will highlight the management of refractory hypercalcemia.

CLINICAL VIGNETTE

A 63-year-old woman with metastatic breast cancer involving lung and bones presented to the emergency center with 4 days of nausea, vomiting, constipation, and delirium according to her caretaker. She was treated with fulvestrant and monthly zoledronic acid (ZA) for bone metastases. She started having hypercalcemia with corrected serum Ca (CSC) >10.2 mg/dL after 6 doses of ZA, with persistent and worsening hypercalcemia, with average CSC levels of 12.0 mg/dL. Most recent ZA was administered 3 weeks prior to this acute presentation. On physical examination, her blood pressure was low, at 105/55; heart rate was 116 beats per minute (sinus rhythm), and her respiratory rate was 24. She was arousable and oriented to name and place and groaning in discomfort. She had dry mucus membranes, diminished breath sounds on her right lung base, consistent with a pleural effusion, with diminished bowel sounds, diffuse abdominal tenderness, and skin tenting. Laboratory testing results were remarkable for the following: calcium 13.1 mg/dL [reference range (RR) 8.4–10.2], phosphorus 2.4 mg/dL (RR 2.5–4.5), albumin 4.4 gm/dL (normal: 3.5–4.7), intact parathyroid hormone 4 pg/mL (RR 9–80), blood urea nitrogen 46 mg/dL (RR 8–20), creatinine 2.1 mg/dL (RR 0.6–1.0; patient's baseline 0.8). Last month, her parathyroid hormone-related protein (PTHrP) was elevated at 3.1 pmol/L (RR<2.0). She was admitted and given continuous normal saline intravenously and calcitonin subcutaneously every 12 hours for 4 doses. The next day, her CSC was 12.1 mg/dL, and she received denosumab 120 mg subcutaneously.

DEFINITION AND PRESENTATION OF HYPERCALCEMIA OF MALIGNANCY

In general, mild hypercalcemia is considered to be levels at which a patient is asymptomatic or has mild symptoms, typically with CSC less than 12 mg/dL, moderate hypercalcemia between 12 to 13.9 mg/dL, and severe hypercalcemia at levels ≥14.0 mg/dL.[2] According to the Common Terminology Criteria for Adverse Events (CTCAE, version 5.0), which provide a standardized method of reporting severity of disorders in clinical trials, the grading of hypercalcemia is

Grade 1 CSC between upper limits of normal – 11.5 mg/dL (up to 2.9 mmol/L)
Grade 2 CSC greater than 11.5 to 12.5 mg/dL (>2.9–3.1 mmol/L)

Grade 3 CSC greater than 12.5 to 13.5 mg/dL (>3.1–3.4 mmol/L)

Grade 4 CSC greater than 13.5 mg/dL (>3.4 mmol/L)[4]

Patients with primary hyperparathyroidism (PHPT) typically will have mildly elevated serum calcium levels found on routine laboratory testing that may remain stable or slowly increase over years. In contrast, HCM presents more acutely, with a relatively sudden development of hypercalcemia (grade 1 or higher) after a period of normocalcemia, and serum calcium levels can rise quickly over weeks to months. Although PHPT, particularly that caused by a parathyroid adenoma, can be present in patients with active cancer, clinical features such as severity of symptoms and acuteness of hypercalcemia development should raise the suspicion of malignancy-related hypercalcemia. Patients with HCM will often have gastrointestinal symptoms (eg, constipation, nausea, vomiting, loss of appetite, or abdominal discomfort), bone pain, polydipsia, polyuria, fatigue, weakness, and mental fogginess. With more severe hypercalcemia, patients can become hypotensive and tachycardic from dehydration, develop renal failure or ileus, and have severe neurologic changes such as delirium or coma. For these patients, hospitalization and urgent management are required.

PATHOPHYSIOLOGY OF HYPERCALCEMIA OF MALIGNANCY

Hypercalcemia associated with cancer can be attributed to 1 of 4 mechanisms that lead to a shared outcome of stimulating osteoclast-mediated bone resorption releasing calcium out of the skeleton into the serum (**Table 1**). Humoral hypercalcemia of malignancy (HHM) is the most common mechanism, accounting for more than 80% of HCM cases, characterized by cancer cells secreting PTH-rP. HHM is typically associated with cancers of squamous cell origin (eg, lung, head and neck, esophagus, skin, or cervix) and adenocarcinomas of the breast, kidney, prostate or bladder. There may be little to no bone metastasis evident.[2] In 1987, PTH-rP was isolated and mapped to the parathyroid hormone-like hormone (*PTHLH*) gene on the short arm of chromosome 12.[5–7] Portions of the *PTH* and the *PTHLH* genes, which encode the amino-terminal regions of secreted natural PTH and PTH-rP proteins, respectively, are homologous. Thus, PTH-rP binds and activates the same type I PTH/PTHrP receptor (PTHR1) as PTH and mimics its actions on increasing osteoclastic bone resorption, causing hypercalcemia.[8] Similar to PTH, PTH-rP also increases calcium reabsorption and inhibits phosphate reabsorption by the kidney, thereby exacerbating hypercalcemia and causing hypophosphatemia and phosphaturia. PTH-rP differs from PTH in 2 ways. First, PTH-rP does not stimulate renal 1-alpha-hydroxylase activity as PTH does; thus, serum 1,25-dihydroxyvitamin D (calcitriol) levels are not elevated with HHM. Second, unlike PTH, which stimulates osteoclast and osteoblast activity, PTH-rP stimulates osteoclast activity but suppresses osteoblast formation.

The second mechanism for HCM, accounting for approximately 20% of cases of hypercalcemia, is caused by local osteolysis mediated by osteoclast-activating cytokines (eg, macrophage inflammatory protein-1 alpha, interleukin-1, interleukin-6, receptor activator of nuclear factor-kappaB ligand [RANKL], tumor necrosis factor-alpha, transforming growth factors, or prostaglandin E2) secreted by malignant cells present in the bone marrow.[2,9] Local osteolysis is most commonly associated with multiple myeloma, breast cancer, and leukemia and lymphoma. It is often characterized by a significant burden of bone metastases. There exists a perpetual relationship between tumor cell activity and bone destruction characterized as a vicious circle of osteolytic metastases, where metastatic cells, most commonly breast cancer, secrete PTH-rP and other osteoclast-activating cytokines that upregulate osteoclast activity,

Table 1
Mechanisms of hypercalcemia of malignancy and clinical findings

Features	Humoral Hypercalcemia of Malignancy	Local Osteolysis	Calcitriol Mediated	Ectopic Authentic PTH Production
Incidence	80%	20%	1%	Rare
Extent of bone metastases	Absent – minimal	Extensive	Variable	Variable
Causative factor	PTH-rP	Osteoclast-activating cytokines	1,25(OH)$_2$D	PTH
Phosphorus	Low	High	High	Low
PTH	Low	Low	Low	High
PTH-rP	High	Low	Low	Low
25(OH)D	Variable	Variable	Variable	Low
1,25(OH)2D	Low	Variable	High	High
Osteoblast activity	Reduced	Reduced	Variable	Increased

Abbreviations: 25(OH)D, 25-hydroxyvitamin D; 1,25(OH)$_2$D, 1,25-dihydroxyvitamin D, also known as calcitriol; PTH, parathyroid hormone; PTH-rP, parathyroid hormone-related peptide.

thereby releasing growth factors from the bone into the marrow space, further increasing tumor growth and PTH-rP production.[10]

A less common mechanism of HCM is the ectopic production of the active form of vitamin D, 1,25-dihydroxyvitamin D (or calcitriol), almost exclusively seen with lymphomas, leading to increased absorption of calcium and phosphorus from the intestinal tract and osteoclast-mediated bone resorption. A recent retrospective study of non-Hodgkin lymphoma patients with hypercalcemia found that worse progression-free survival correlated with higher calcitriol levels, a possible surrogate marker for more advanced disease.[11] Interestingly, a significant number of patients in this study (61.1%) did not have elevations of either calcitriol nor PTH-rP when both were collected. There has been 1 case report of vitamin D-mediated hypercalcemia in a patient with metastatic pancreatic neuroendocrine tumor.[12]

An even more rarely reported cause of HCM is the ectopic production of authentic PTH by tumoral cells of various types (eg, ovarian, thyroid-papillary type, nasopharyngeal rhabdomyosarcoma, gastric, small cell lung, and bladder).[2,13–18] This topic is discussed earlier in this special issue.

DIAGNOSTIC APPROACH

The most effective manner in understanding the underlying etiology of hypercalcemia in a patient is to determine if it is PTH mediated. If the PTH is inappropriately elevated in the setting of hypercalcemia, the cause is either PHPT (because of a parathyroid adenoma or carcinoma; parathyroid hyperplasia associated with multiple endocrine neoplasia, type 1, 2A, and 4; hyperparathyroidism jaw-tumor syndrome; or familial isolated hyperparathyroidism) or tertiary hyperparathyroidism. When the PTH is appropriately suppressed with hypercalcemia, malignancy should be considered along with other causes such as medications (eg, hydrochlorothiazide, excessive vitamin A or D supplementation, or lithium), granulomatous diseases (eg, sarcoidosis or fungal infections), hyperthyroidism, or immobilization.

The patient's medical history, physical examination findings, and basic laboratory testing results can also help distinguish the underlying etiology of hypercalcemia (see **Table 1**). For example, hypercalcemic patients with low phosphorus levels will either have a PTH- or a PTH-rP mediated process. If the phosphorus is elevated, then a vitamin D-mediated process should be considered, such as oversupplementation of vitamin D, granulomatous disease or increased calcitriol from underlying lymphoma.

TREATMENT STRATEGIES

To date, there are no guidelines available regarding the management of HCM. Beyond treating the underlying malignancy, general practice recommendations are to implement a series of strategies or agents to correct the volume depletion and hypotension caused by calciuresis and polyuria, inhibit osteoclast activity with bone-modifying agents, or inhibit the overproduction of 1,25-dihydroxyvitamin D with glucocorticoids. The management of hypercalcemia is thoroughly discussed later in this special issue; however, it is worth highlighting here the challenging situation of HCM refractory to intravenous bisphosphonates and other treatments. Although many patients benefit from the use of bone-modifying agents, there are patients who continue have severe hypercalcemia or have short duration of control of hypercalcemia.

Denosumab is a fully human monoclonal antibody that binds to RANKL to prevent ligand interaction with RANK receptors on precursor osteoclasts, thus, interfering with osteoclast maturation, function, and survival. Consequently, bone resorption is reduced. It is approved by the Food and Drug Administration (FDA) for the treatment of postmenopausal women and men with osteoporosis, and cancer treatment-related bone loss. It is also FDA-approved for the prevention of skeletal-related events in patients with metastatic bone disease, unresectable giant cell tumor of bone and hypercalcemia of malignancy.

Denosumab was evaluated in a single-arm multicenter, international phase II study for the treatment of patients with bisphosphonate-refractory HCM, as defined by hypercalcemia (CSC >12.5 mg/dL) despite receiving intravenous bisphosphonate (IVBP) treatment greater than 7 and no more than 30 days prior to screening.[19] The primary endpoint was the proportion of patients with a response of CSC of no more than 11.5 mg/dL (CTCAE grade ≤1) by day 10. Thirty-three patients with solid or hematologic malignancies received denosumab 120 mg subcutaneously on day 1 and every 4 weeks afterward (with 2 loading doses on days 8 and 15 to reach steady-state concentrations). By day 10, 64% of the patients responded with a CSC of no more than 11.5 mg/dL, while 33% had a complete response (defined as CSC ≤10.8 mg/dL). During the course of the entire study, 70% met the primary endpoint of a response, and 64% had a complete response. A striking and clinically significant finding in this study was that in this population with aggressive disease and a pre-enrollment median time from last IVBP to severe hypercalcemia of 17 days, denosumab treatment was associated with a median duration of response (time from initial response to last day when CSC ≤11.5 mg/dL) of 104 days.

Denosumab can lead to hypocalcemia, especially in patients with vitamin D deficiency or severe renal impairment (creatinine clearance <30 mL/min), or patients on hemodialysis. It is also associated with osteonecrosis of the jaw (1.8% incidence) similar to that seen with intravenous BPs (1.3%).[20] It does not have nephrotoxic effects or require dose adjustment based on renal function. Thus, in patients with HCM and renal impairment, denosumab would be preferred over intravenous BP.

Cinacalcet, a calcimimetic, binds to the calcium-sensing receptor on parathyroid cells to increase the cell's sensitivity to extracellular calcium concentration. It is approved for management of severe hypercalcemia in patients with PHPT, secondary hyperparathyroidism from chronic kidney disease, and parathyroid carcinoma. Although not approved for HCM, cinacalcet potentially can ameliorate hypercalcemia mediated by PTH-rP in cancer patients. There have been 7 cancer patients (squamous cell carcinoma of lung, nonsmall cell lung cancer, renal cell carcinoma, neuroendocrine tumor, breast cancer) described in the literature in whom cinacalcet was given to control hypercalcemia when refractory to zoledronic acid and/or denosumab.[21] Some of the patients were able to maintain normal to mildly elevated calcium levels for 3 to 18 months even in the setting of continued metastatic disease.

As most HCM is caused by HHM secondary to oversecretion of PTH-rP or osteolysis due to osteoclast-activating factors including PTH-rP, an agent that could antagonize the effects of PTH-rP or inhibit the PTH receptor would be a potential treatment for patients with HCM refractory to bisphosphonates or denosumab. The development of PTH-rP antagonists has not been successful because of rapid drug turnover and poor concentration in bone, but there has been development of novel PTH-rP antagonists fused to an inert bacterial collagen-binding domain (CBD) that helps targets the drugs to the bone environment, PTH(7–33)-CBD and [W2]PTH(1–33)-CBD.[22] The 2 novel agents were studied in mice inoculated with breast cancer cells to assess their effectiveness in reducing breast cancer bone metastases and to prevent osteolysis. Both agents induced PTHR1-dependent apoptosis of breast cancer cells in vitro, and PTH(7–33)-CBD reduced breast cancer tumor burden and osteolytic bone destruction in mice after treatment. A monoclonal antibody designed to inhibit PTH1R reversed hypercalcemia in rats who developed hypercalcemia after infusion of PTH or PTHrP and in mice who developed hypercalcemia after implantation of mouse colon tumor cells.[23] Further clinical investigation of novel treatments targeting PTH-rP, PTH, and the PTH1R are needed to help meet this unmet need of refractory HCM.

SUMMARY

HCM is an oncologic emergency that causes a high burden of debilitating symptoms, conveys a poor prognosis, and can limit the ability to administer necessary antitumoral treatments. Any patient presenting with hypercalcemia should have an intact parathyroid hormone level checked as an important first step in clarifying the underlying etiology. HCM is a common cause of non-PTH mediated hypercalcemia, but other causes of hypercalcemia should be excluded. Although there are various pathogenic mechanisms of HCM, the common pathway that mediates hypercalcemia is the upregulation of osteoclast bone resorption. Longstanding established strategies using aggressive fluid resuscitation, calcitonin, and/or intravenous bisphosphonates to manage the hypercalcemic episodes can be limited by comorbid conditions or sustainability of response. Denosumab, which was approved for HCM in 2014, was a welcome addition to the armamentarium of antiresorptive therapies, with the benefit of not compromising renal function. However, there remain challenges with patients with HCM refractory to bone-modifying agents. Development of agents that can target the PTH receptor or inhibit the actions of PTH-rP are much needed to further expand treatment options for patients. Successful management of HCM can greatly improve a patient's quality of life and bridge the patient so that more effective agents targeting the underlying cancer can be implemented.

CLINICS CARE POINTS

- When monitoring for hypercalcemia, correct the measured calcium level for the albumin level, as the measured calcium is bound to albumin.
- The first diagnostic test to clarify the underlying etiology for hypercalcemia in any patient is to measure the parathyroid hormone level when hypercalcemia is present. If hypercalcemia has resolved, the parathyroid hormone level may be uninformative.
- Patients who present with new symptomatic hypercalcemia over a short period of time (within weeks to months after normocalcemia) should be evaluated for underlying malignancy-associated hypercalcemia.
- Although PTH-rP shares homology with PTH, PTH-rP mediated HCM does not lead to elevated 1,25-dihydroxyvitamin D.

DISCLOSURE

Nothing to disclose.

REFERENCES

1. Gastanaga VM, Schwartzberg LS, Jain RK, et al. Prevalence of hypercalcemia among cancer patients in the United States. Cancer Med 2016;5(8):2091–100.
2. Stewart AF. Clinical practice. Hypercalcemia associated with cancer. N Engl J Med 2005;352(4):373–9.
3. Ralston SH, Gallacher SJ, Patel U, et al. Cancer-associated hypercalcemia: morbidity and mortality. Clinical experience in 126 treated patients. Ann Intern Med 1990;112(7):499–504.
4. Common Terminology Criteria for Adverse events (CTCAE). Available at: https://ctep.cancer.gov/protocoldevelopment/electronic_applications/docs/CTCAE_v5_Quick_Reference_5x7.pdf. Accessed June 6, 2021.
5. Burtis WJ, Wu T, Bunch C, et al. Identification of a novel 17,000-dalton parathyroid hormone-like adenylate cyclase-stimulating protein from a tumor associated with humoral hypercalcemia of malignancy. J Biol Chem 1987;262(15):7151–6.
6. Mangin M, Webb AC, Dreyer BE, et al. Identification of a cDNA encoding a parathyroid hormone-like peptide from a human tumor associated with humoral hypercalcemia of malignancy. Proc Natl Acad Sci U S A 1988;85(2):597–601.
7. Strewler GJ, Stern PH, Jacobs JW, et al. Parathyroid hormonelike protein from human renal carcinoma cells. Structural and functional homology with parathyroid hormone. J Clin Invest 1987;80(6):1803–7.
8. Strewler GJ. The physiology of parathyroid hormone-related protein. N Engl J Med 2000;342(3):177–85.
9. Lee JW, Chung HY, Ehrlich LA, et al. IL-3 expression by myeloma cells increases both osteoclast formation and growth of myeloma cells. Blood 2004;103(6):2308–15.
10. Roodman GD. Mechanisms of bone metastasis. N Engl J Med 2004;350(16):1655–64.
11. Shallis RM, Rome RS, Reagan JL. Mechanisms of hypercalcemia in non-Hodgkin lymphoma and associated outcomes: a retrospective review. Clin Lymphoma Myeloma Leuk 2018;18(2):e123–9.
12. Zhu V, de Las Morenas A, Janicek M, et al. Hypercalcemia from metastatic pancreatic neuroendocrine tumor secreting 1,25-dihydroxyvitamin D. J Gastrointest Oncol 2014;5(4):E84–7.

13. Nussbaum SR, Gaz RD, Arnold A. Hypercalcemia and ectopic secretion of parathyroid hormone by an ovarian carcinoma with rearrangement of the gene for parathyroid hormone. N Engl J Med 1990;323(19):1324–8.
14. Wong K, Tsuda S, Mukai R, et al. Parathyroid hormone expression in a patient with metastatic nasopharyngeal rhabdomyosarcoma and hypercalcemia. Endocrine 2005;27(1):83–6.
15. Nakajima K, Tamai M, Okaniwa S, et al. Humoral hypercalcemia associated with gastric carcinoma secreting parathyroid hormone: a case report and review of the literature. Endocr J 2013;60(5):557–62.
16. Yoshimoto K, Yamasaki R, Sakai H, et al. Ectopic production of parathyroid hormone by small cell lung cancer in a patient with hypercalcemia. J Clin Endocrinol Metab 1989;68(5):976–81.
17. Iguchi H, Miyagi C, Tomita K, et al. Hypercalcemia caused by ectopic production of parathyroid hormone in a patient with papillary adenocarcinoma of the thyroid gland. J Clin Endocrinol Metab 1998;83(8):2653–7.
18. Eid W, Wheeler TM, Sharma MD. Recurrent hypercalcemia due to ectopic production of parathyroid hormone-related protein and intact parathyroid hormone in a single patient with multiple malignancies. Endocr Pract 2004;10(2):125–8.
19. Hu MI, Glezerman IG, Leboulleux S, et al. Denosumab for treatment of hypercalcemia of malignancy. J Clin Endocrinol Metab 2014;99(9):3144–52.
20. XGEVA prescribing information. Amgen Inc; 2015.
21. O'Callaghan S, Yau H. Treatment of malignancy-associated hypercalcemia with cinacalcet: a paradigm shift. Endocr Connect 2021;10(1):R13–24.
22. Ponnapakkam T, Anbalagan M, Stratford RE Jr, et al. Novel bone-targeted parathyroid hormone-related peptide antagonists inhibit breast cancer bone metastases. Anticancer Drugs 2021;32(4):365–75.
23. Choppin A, et al. A novel anti-PTH1R receptor antagonist monoclonal antibody reverses hypercalcemia induced by PTH or PTHrP: a potential treatment of primary hyperparathyroidism and humoral hypercalcemia of malignancy. Endocr Rev 2017;38(3):167–73.

Vitamin D–dependent Hypercalcemia

Karl Peter Schlingmann, MD

KEYWORDS

- Vitamin D • 1α-hydroxylase • CYP27B1 • 24-Hydroxylase • CYP24A1
- Idiopathic infantile hypercalcemia • IIH • Hypervitaminosis D

KEY POINTS

- The differential diagnosis of vitamin D–mediated hypercalcemia includes acquired and genetic disorders.
- Vitamin D intoxication is associated with increased serum levels of 25-hydroxyvitamin D_3.
- Granulomatous diseases are characterized by differentially regulated, extrarenal 1 α-hydroxylase (cytochrome P450 [CYP]27B1).
- Idiopathic infantile hypercalcemia (IIH) is caused either by defective degradation of serum 1,25-dihydroxyvitamin D_3 by 24-hydroxylase (CYP24A1) (IIH1) or by defective renal phosphate conservation via NaPi-IIa (IIH2). The pathophysiology of IIH2 comprises phosphate depletion and down-regulation of fibroblast growth factor 23, leading to dysregulated vitamin D activation.

VITAMIN D METABOLISM

In the human body, vitamin D_3 can be formed by UV-B irradiation of 7-dehydrocholesterol in the skin or can be derived from dietary sources, in the form of vitamin D_3 or vitamin D_2 (**Fig. 1**).[1] Because vitamin D_2 and vitamin D_3 are thought to be activated and function in the same way,[2] this review, for simplicity, focuses on defining the metabolism and mechanism of action of vitamin D_3. Transport of vitamin D from skin to storage tissues or to liver is carried out by a specific vitamin D–binding protein (DBP).[3] Vitamin D_3 is first activated by 25-hydroxylation, a step probably catalyzed by the liver cytochrome P450 (CYP) enzyme 25-hydroxylase (CYP2R1).[4] Thereafter, serum 25-hydroxyvitamin D_3 (25[OH]D_3) is converted to active 1α,25-dihydroxyvitamin D_3 (1,25[OH]$_2D_3$),[5] by the action of the mitochondrial CYP enzyme 1α-hydroxylase (CYP27B1) in proximal tubular epithelial cells in the kidney.[6] Renal CYP27B1 is up-regulated by parathyroid hormone (PTH) as part of a calcium homeostatic loop and down-regulated by fibroblast growth factor 23 (FGF-23) as part of a phosphate homeostatic loop (see **Fig. 1**). Mutations in the *CYP27B1* gene have been identified as underlying vitamin D–dependent rickets type 1 in humans,[7] a disease mirrored in

Department of General Pediatrics, University Children's Hospital, Albert-Schweitzer-Campus 1, Münster 48149, Germany
E-mail address: karlpeter.schlingmann@ukmuenster.de

Endocrinol Metab Clin N Am 50 (2021) 729–742
https://doi.org/10.1016/j.ecl.2021.08.005
0889-8529/21/© 2021 Elsevier Inc. All rights reserved.

endo.theclinics.com

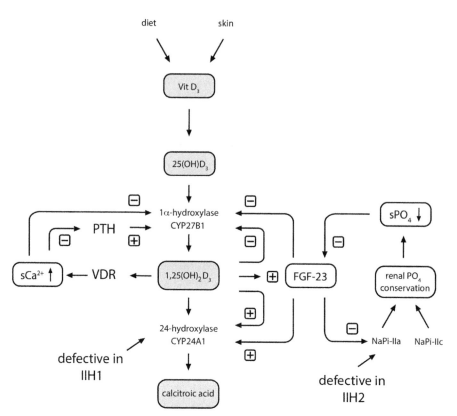

Fig. 1. Vitamin D metabolism interlinked with calcium and phosphate metabolism. The activation of vitamin D to its biologically active form 1,25-$(OH)_2D_3$ by 1α-hydroxylase (CYP27B1) as well as its degradation by 24-hydroxylase (CYP24A1) are tightly controlled by 1,25-$(OH)_2D_3$ itself, serum calcium, and PTH (*left*). The catabolism of active 1,25-$(OH)_2D_3$ to calcitroic acid by CYP24A1 is defective in IIH1. In addition, vitamin D metabolism is critically influenced by phosphate homeostasis via the action of the primary phosphaturic hormone FGF-23 that limits the action of active 1,25$(OH)_2D_3$ by inhibiting 1α-hydroxylase (CYP27B1) and activating 24-hydroxylase (CYP24A1) (*right*). In IIH2, defective renal phosphate conservation via NaPi-IIa causes phosphate depletion and a suppression of FGF-23, thereby disinhibiting vitamin D activation. PO4, phosphate, sCa2+, serum calcium; SPO4, serum phosphate; Vit, vitamin.

Cyp27b1-null mice.[8,9] The CYP27B1 protein also has been detected in extrarenal tissues, which established the concept of extrarenal CYP27B1 catalyzing local production of 1,25$(OH)_2D_3$ from 25$(OH)D_3$ in tissues, such as skin, prostate, intestine, breast, and possibly bone.[10] Granulomatous conditions, such as sarcoidosis involving activated macrophages, are thought to be accompanied by overexpression of extrarenal CYP27B1, resulting in an increased local production of 1,25$(OH)_2D_{3,}$ which may leak out into the general circulation, causing hypercalcemia (discussed later).[11]

Serum 1,25$(OH)_2D_3$ exerts its effects on calcium metabolism through a vitamin D receptor (VDR)-mediated transcriptional mechanism, in which the hormone directly modulates gene expression of a wide variety of vitamin D–dependent genes in target cells.

The inactivation of serum 25$(OH)D_3$ and 1,25$(OH)_2D_3$ is performed by the CYP enzyme CYP24A1, also known as the 24-hydroxylase. CYP24A1 is a multicatalytic enzyme responsible for a 5-step, C-24 oxidation pathway, which inactivates 1,25$(OH)_2D_3$ to water-soluble biliary calcitroic acid (see **Fig. 1**).[12,13] CYP24A1 also is able to directly convert the inactive precursor 25$(OH)D_3$ into inactive 24,25$(OH)_2D_3$ and 25$(OH)D_3$-26,23-lactone.[14] Mutations in human *CYP24A1* gene have been implicated as a cause of idiopathic infantile hypercalcemia (IIH) (discussed later), the symptoms of which resemble those also observed in *Cyp24a1*-knockout mice, confirming the key role of CYP24A1 in vitamin D degradation.[15]

In summary, these CYP enzymes mediating vitamin D activation and degradation comprise an integrated, hormonally regulated endocrine unit closely interlinked with calcium and phosphate homeostatic loops (see **Fig. 1**). Under physiologic conditions, this signaling system establishes a well-balanced equilibrium providing just the appropriate amount of serum 1,25$(OH)_2D_3$ for normal function. This concept is reinforced by the up-regulation of CYP27B1 and 1,25$(OH)_2D_3$ synthesis and down-regulation of CYP24A1 and 1,25$(OH)_2D_3$ catabolism in the vitamin D–deficient animal or VDR-null mouse when vitamin D signaling is inadequate.[16] Contrasting these physiologic adaptations, a relative excess of serum 1,25$(OH)_2D_3$ has been described underlying hypercalcemic states as a result of defective vitamin D degradation or of a dysregulation of vitamin D metabolizing enzymes by primary disturbances in phosphate metabolism. The aim of this article is to illustrate current knowledge on vitamin D–dependent hypercalcemia, describe the resulting phenotypes, and offer therapeutic perspectives for affected patients.

HYPERCALCEMIC STATES INVOLVING ALTERED VITAMIN D METABOLISM
Hypervitaminosis D/Vitamin D Intoxication

Vitamin D toxicity manifesting as hypercalcemia may result from excessive vitamin D intakes producing active metabolites that overwhelm vitamin D metabolism, with an inability of the vitamin D catabolic enzyme CYP24A1 to keep up with vitamin D target cell levels. In this scenario, increased concentrations of an active vitamin D metabolite reach the VDR in the nucleus of target cells and cause exaggerated gene expression. The molecular nature of this active metabolite, however, was a matter of debate. Early animal studies on acute vitamin D toxicity indicated that renal CYP27B1 is effectively turned off, limiting elevations of active 1,25$(OH)_2D_3$ serum levels.[17] Therefore, the focus shifted to other vitamin D metabolites correlated with toxicity, especially 25$(OH)D_3$. The assumption of 25$(OH)D_3$ as the active toxic metabolite was emphasized by the finding that an intoxication of rats with graded doses of vitamin D_3 resulted in micromolar levels of 25$(OH)D_3$ and in marked hypercalcemia.[18] These findings were substantiated by a follow-up study that demonstrated that *Cyp27b1*-knockout mice incapable of the synthesis of 1,25$(OH)_2D_3$ still are susceptible to hypercalcemia, with 25$(OH)D_3$ levels similar to those causing toxicity in wild-type mice.[19] Thus, based on a variety of animal studies, it appears that serum 25$(OH)D_3$ levels associated with toxicity usually exceed 150 ng/mL or 375 nmol/L. Although no systematic studies examining vitamin intoxication in humans have been conducted for ethical reasons, numerous case reports have described accidental vitamin D intoxications.[20–22] In a larger study of 35 hypervitaminotic patients with hypercalcemia resulting from chronic ingestion of overfortified milk,[23] the average serum 25$(OH)D_3$ level was 560 nmol/L (range 140–1490 nmol/L). In an extended family accidently intoxicated with a veterinary vitamin D concentrate, serum 25$(OH)D_3$ levels ranged from 847 nmol/L to 1652 nmol/L in intoxicated family members, whereas serum 1,25$(OH)_2D_3$ values mostly were within the normal range.[24] Earlier, Vieth[25] already had concluded that hypercalcemia only accompanies hypervitaminosis D when 25$(OH)D_3$ levels consistently exceed 375 nmol/L to 500 nmol/L. These data support the assumption that during hypervitaminosis D, elevated levels of 25(OH)D_3 exceed the DBP binding capacity, resulting in a rise of free unbound 25(OH)D in the blood, leading to greater entry into target cells and greater VDR-mediated gene expression. Alternatively, micromolar concentrations of serum 25(OH)D_3 could displace 1,25(OH)$_2$D$_3$ from DBP, resulting in increased levels of free 1,25(OH)$_2$D$_3$ that in turn would become the toxic metabolite.[23]

Granulomatous Conditions, Sarcoidosis, and Tuberculosis

As discussed previously, granulomatous conditions, such as sarcoidosis involving activated macrophages, often are accompanied by overexpression of extrarenal CYP27B1, which can result in excess local production of 1,25(OH)$_2$D$_3$. From these local tissues and cells, the active metabolite may leak out into the general circulation and cause hypercalciuria and hypercalcemia.[11] It was shown that the likely cause of hypercalcemia in sarcoidosis was overproduction of serum 1,25(OH)$_2$D$_3$[26] and that this overproduction was of extrarenal origin.[27] Moreover, in vitro studies demonstrated the ability of cultured pulmonary alveolar macrophages from sarcoidosis patients to make 1,25(OH)$_2$D$_3$.[11] Approximately 10% of sarcoidosis patients develop hypercalcemia, which suggests that the extrarenal synthesis of 1,25(OH)$_2$D$_3$ in granulomatous tissue is poorly regulated. It has been proposed that extrarenal CYP27B1 is up-regulated by inflammatory cytokines, such as interferon-γ.[11]

A similar pathophysiology has been described in tuberculosis associated with hypercalcemia in up to 25% of cases due to overproduction of 1,25(OH)$_2$D$_3$. Here, it was proposed that serum 1,25(OH)$_2$D$_3$ production by monocytes/macrophages could be part of a natural defense mechanism to combat *Mycobacterium tuberculosis*, in which Toll-like receptors trigger the increased expression of CYP27B1 and VDR, resulting in synthesis of serum 1,25(OH)$_2$D$_3$ and increased VDR-mediated gene expression.[28] The monocyte/macrophage CYP27B1 is thought to be not responsive to PTH or FGF-23, but its regulation remains unknown.

Other granulomatous conditions, such as lymphoma, also are associated with hypercalcemia presumably due to mechanisms like those observed in sarcoidosis and tuberculosis.

Idiopathic Infantile Hypercalcemia due to Loss-of-Function CYP24A1 Mutations

Idiopathic infantile hypercalcemia (IIH) first was described in 1952 by Fanconi[29] and by Lightwood and Stapleton.[30] Shortly thereafter, an epidemic occurred in Great Britain, with approximately 200 cases within only 2 years. Affected infants clinically presented with typical symptoms of severe hypercalcemia comprising failure to thrive, vomiting, dehydration, muscular hypotonia, and lethargy. Physiologic studies indicated that the hypercalcemia was due to an increase in intestinal calcium uptake.[31] In addition, a potential connection to vitamin D supplementation given for the prevention of rickets was suspected. Because vitamin D doses were not excessive, Lightwood already suspected an intrinsic sensitivity to vitamin D.[32]

Some children presented with additional syndromic features, including cardiac abnormalities, developmental delay, and an elfin-like facies and were classified as severe cases in contrast to mild cases, with calcium disturbances only.[33] A few years later, Williams and coworkers[34] as well as Beuren and coworkers[35] defined a syndrome comprising supravalvular aortic stenosis, peripheral pulmonary artery stenosis, mental retardation, and peculiar facies. Subsequent observations underscored the assumption that Williams-Beuren syndrome (WBS) and Fanconi-type, severe IIH represented a single medical entity. Finally, the WBS was linked to deletions on chromosome 7q11.23.[36] The etiology of hypercalcemia in WBS still is not understood completely.

The finding of high levels of serum $1,25(OH)_2D_3$ during the hypercalcemic phase clearly implicates a primary disturbance of vitamin D metabolism.[37] Of the at least 15 genes mapped to the WBS deletion interval, the ubiquitously expressed WBS transcription factor encoded by the *BAZ1B* gene has been implicated in vitamin D metabolism.[38] The hypercalcemic phenotype in WBS is transient, with a spontaneous resolution after the first 2 years to 4 years of life.

In contrast, the etiology of the mild or Lightwood variant of IIH remained unknown. The connection to exogenous vitamin D supplementation that was suspected after high doses of vitamin D per day led to the epidemic of IIH in British infants was substantiated by similar observations in other European countries.[39,40] These observations suggested that IIH represented a state of vitamin D intoxication in children especially susceptible to vitamin D.[33,41] Although single familial cases pointed to a genetic background and pedigree analyses indicated a possible autosomal recessive inheritance, it remained unknown if IIH represented a hereditary disease.[42]

Finally, in 2011, recessive loss-of-function mutations in *CYP24A1* gene were described underlying IIH, providing evidence for a vitamin D degradation defect resulting in an accumulation and increased action of serum active $1,25(OH)_2D_3$.[43] The initial patient cohort consisted of 6 children with a common daily vitamin D supplementation of 500 IU and 4 children who received single oral doses of vitamin D2, 600,000 IU. Whereas the first cohort developed symptoms after several months, indicating a critical role of a certain cumulative dose of exogenous vitamin D, the excessive bolus doses in the second cohort resulted in symptoms resembling acute vitamin D toxicity within days to weeks. The laboratory investigation demonstrated elevated serum calcium levels between 3.5 mmol/L and 5.0 mmol/L (14–20 mg/dL), suppressed levels of PTH, and serum $1,25(OH)_2D_3$ between 43 pg/mL and 129 pg/mL (normal range 17–74 pg/mL) in both groups. After acute treatment, serum calcium levels largely normalized but tended to be continuously at the upper end of the normal range or slightly elevated during follow-up. Levels of PTH remained suppressed in a majority of patients and serum $1,25(OH)_2D_3$ persisted mostly within the upper normal range, reflecting a continuous activation of vitamin D metabolism. Renal ultrasound revealed bilateral medullary nephrocalcinosis in all affected patients.[43]

Meanwhile, these initial findings have been substantiated and extended by numerous follow-up studies: several of these studies described typical IIH patients with initial disease manifestation with symptomatic hypercalcemia in infancy,[44–46] mainly confirming the phenotypic and laboratory characteristics of the initial cohort of *CYP24A1* patients. In addition, some of these studies highlighted specific aspects of the disease or report individual therapeutic interventions, such as hemodialysis or bisphosphonate therapy in severe cases.[47,48] These studies described patients with biallelic *CYP24A1* mutations, substantiating the initial assumption of a primarily recessive trait.

In addition to the classic patients presenting during infancy, multiple publications report adolescent and adult patients with biallelic mutations in *CYP24A1*.[45,49,50] Cools and colleagues[51] summarized that more than a third of reported patients with biallelic *CYP24A1* mutations present beyond infancy. These patients usually do not develop symptomatic hypercalcemia but often suffer from borderline hypercalcemia, hypercalciuria, and recurrent episodes of urolithiasis and are at risk for developing a deterioration of renal function.[45,50,51] So far, it remains unclear whether the reported decline in glomerular filtration rate represents a consequence of repeated episodes of urolithiasis, acute kidney injury, and/or urologic interventions or whether it represents a primary complication of the disease itself. Moreover, vascular calcifications have been reported in single adult patients with *CYP24A1* mutations raising the question if increased $1,25(OH)_2D_3$ levels with subsequent changes in calcium metabolism also represent a risk factor for coronary artery disease and arterial occlusive disease.[49] Another interesting aspect of *CYP24A1*-mediated pathology is the observation of disease exacerbation in women during or after pregnancy.[52–54] The reported women developed recurrent episodes of symptomatic hypercalcemia with elevated levels of serum $1,25(OH)_2D_3$ and suppression of PTH. These observations imply that adult patients who are able to limit vitamin D activation under physiologic circumstances may develop symptomatic hypercalcemia if additional risk factors or predisposing conditions emerge, that is, increased vitamin D activation during pregnancy.

Some studies focused especially on the influence of exogenous vitamin D and sunlight exposure for manifestation as well as progression of CYP24A1-associated disease.[50,55] The link between disease manifestation and exogenous vitamin D had been suggested early: (1) moderate doses of supplemental vitamin D led to the development of clinical symptoms usually within months whereas higher doses provoked an acute disease manifestation in the initial study cohort; (2) higher doses of supplemental vitamin D were associated with an increased incidence in countries with higher supplementary vitamin D; and (3) omitting vitamin D supplementation prevented hypercalcemic episodes and the development of nephrocalcinosis in infant with biallelic *CYP24A1* mutations.[43,46] These initial findings already indicated an incomplete penetrance of inherited *CYP24A1* defects and argued for a critical role of a certain cumulative dose of exogenous vitamin D. Therefore, the implementation of prophylactic measures as well as therapeutic strategies in patients with proved *CYP24A1* mutations is of special importance. Recent studies point to an influence of sunlight exposure on the course of disease, as investigators observed a tendency toward higher serum calcium levels, PTH suppression, and higher urinary calcium excretions in patients with biallelic *CYP24A1* mutations during the summer months.[50,55] Therefore, the avoidance of excessive sunlight exposure appears to be indicated at least in patients carrying *CYP24A1* mutations with recurrent disease episodes.

In contrast to the extensive reports on patients with biallelic mutations, the knowledge on the impact of heterozygous *CYP24A1* mutations is more limited. Data on carriers of a single mutated allele are derived mainly from family studies, reporting a significant number of heterozygous relatives with hypercalciuria and nephrolithiasis.[49,51,55,56] Analyses in symptomatic as well as asymptomatic family members revealed increased values for $1,25(OH)_2D_3$ and low levels of PTH, arguing for a milder but detectable biochemical phenotype in carriers of a single mutated *CYP24A1* allele. The penetrance of a partial loss of CYP24A1 function remains largely unresolved due to the design of these studies that investigated family members of patients with biallelic CYP24A1 mutations. The mutational spectrum of *CYP24A1* in patients of European descent comprises mainly a small number of recurrent mutations, including CYP24A1-p.E143del, CYP24A1-p.R396 W, and CYP24A1-p.L409S. All 3 variants have been listed in public exome and genome sequencing databases (ie, Exome Aggregation Consortium [ExAC] and Genome Aggregation Database [gnomAD]), with allele frequencies that add up to 0.35% (gnomAD, European non-Finnish alleles), meaning that 0.7% of the European population, or approximately 5 million Europeans, are heterozygous carriers of 1 of these 3 mutant *CYP24A1* alleles.

IDIOPATHIC INFANTILE HYPERCALCEMIA DUE TO MUTATIONS OF *SLC34A1*/NaPi COTRANSPORTER 2A

In a subset of IIH patients, mutations in *CYP24A1* had been excluded arguing for genetic heterogeneity.[57] Using homozygosity mapping with a subsequent candidate gene approach, mutations in *SLC34A1* were identified as a second genetic cause of IIH.[57] The *SLC34A1* gene encodes sodium-phosphate cotransporter IIa (NaPi-IIa) that is expressed at the apical membrane of proximal tubular epithelial cells. NaPi-IIa, together with its close homologue NaPi-IIc (encoded by *SLC34A3*), is involved in the reabsorption and conservation of filtered phosphate.[58] The expression and cell surface localization of both phosphate cotransporters is negatively regulated by the concerted action of PTH and FGF-23, both acting through their receptors at the basolateral membrane. In vitro studies confirmed the loss-of-function character of identified NaPi-IIa mutants.[57] The presumed pathophysiology involves phosphate deficiency and a down-regulation of FGF-23. Next to its role in phosphate metabolism, FGF-23 is a critical negative regulator of vitamin D metabolism because it inhibits 1α-hydroxylase (CYP27B1) and activates 24-hydroxylase (CYP24A1).[59] Therefore, in the presence of suppressed FGF-23 levels, patients exhibit an augmented vitamin D activation with subsequent hypercalcemia.

The retrospective evaluation of biochemical data of patients with *SLC34A1* mutations revealed hypophosphatemia due to renal phosphate wasting along with hypercalcemia. As in patients with *CYP24A1* defects but contrasting with previous observations in patients with NaPi-IIc defects, who develop hypophosphatemic rickets, there was no detectable bone phenotype. At initial presentation, symptomatic infants with NaPi-IIa defects usually display less severe hypercalcemia, with serum calcium levels at approximately 3.5 mmol/L; the levels of PTH are suppressed similarly as in patients with *CYP24A1* defects, and serum 1,25(OH)$_2$D$_3$ is inappropriately high. Comparable biochemical findings already had been reported in 2 asymptomatic siblings with nephrocalcinosis from an Argentinian family who carried a homozygous *SLC34A1* mutation.[60] Originally, a homozygous mutation in *SLC34A1* had been reported in 2 siblings who presented with renal Fanconi syndrome and hypophosphatemic rickets whereas changes in calcium metabolism were less pronounced.[61] Medullary nephrocalcinosis might be detected early in the neonatal period and has even been described as a differential diagnosis for prenatal hyperechogenic kidneys.[62]

The involvement of *SLC34A1* mutations in IIH was substantiated by various follow-up publications.[63,64] Besides, *SLC34A1* mutations in biallelic as well as heterozygous state were discovered in large patient cohorts with nephrocalcinosis and nephrolithiasis.[65–67] Moreover, nephrolithiasis was identified in a significant number of heterozygous family members of classic IIH patients with biallelic *SLC34A1* mutations.[57] Earlier studies already had linked the clinical and biochemical phenotype of hypophosphatemic nephrolithiasis and osteoporosis to heterozygous *SLC34A1* mutations.[68]

These findings together strongly suggest that the assumption, that a significant subset of patients does not present in infancy with symptomatic hypercalcemia but with nephrocalcinosis and nephrolithiasis in later life, holds true not only for *CYP24A1* defects but even more for *SLC34A1* mutations. This does not take into account a potentially high proportion of asymptomatic carriers of 1 or 2 mutant alleles. On the other hand, publications studying the long-term outcome of *SLC34A1* patients, as for *CYP24A1*, also suggest a significant risk for the development of chronic kidney disease in later life.[69,70] These different disease manifestations associated with *SLC34A1* mutations, ranging from hypophosphatemic rickets over infantile hypercalcemia to kidney stone disease in later life, presumably reflect a continuous spectrum rather than pleiotropy with multiple phenotypic traits.

Pathophysiologic changes comparable to those in patients with NaPi-IIa mutations also are observed in patients with mutations in *SLC34A3* encoding the closely related sodium-phosphate cotransporter NaPi-IIc. Both cotransporters are responsible for proximal tubular phosphate reabsorption. Biallelic *SLC34A3* mutations encoding NaPi-IIc initially were reported in patients with hypophosphatemic rickets with hypercalciuria.[71,72] Meanwhile, clinical presentations with isolated nephrocalcinosis and/or kidney stones have been described in patients with biallelic as well as heterozygous *SLC34A3* mutations.[73] Moreover, as for *SLC34A1*, pathogenic variants in *SLC34A3* have been discovered by next-generation sequencing in a large cohort of pediatric and adult patients with renal calcifications.[65] Although patients with NaPi-IIc defects do not develop symptomatic hypercalcemia, biochemical abnormalities closely resemble those observed in patients with NaPi-IIa defects, including increased serum levels of $1,25(OH)_2D_3$.

In summary, all 3 genetic defects (CYP24A1, SLC34A1, and SLC34A3) provoke a marked disturbance in vitamin D metabolism. The pathophysiology involves a defective vitamin D degradation as well as a dysregulation of CYP27B1 and CYP24A1 by a primary disturbance in phosphate metabolism. The incomplete penetrance, a variable clinical course, ranging from childhood presentation to chronic disease in adulthood, and milder but clinically relevant phenotypes in carriers of heterozygous mutations appear to be characteristic features of all 3 genetic entities. Important questions concerning the influence of nutritional calcium and phosphate, exogenous vitamin D, sunlight, and modifying genetic factors remain to be answered in the future.

THERAPEUTIC APPROACHES TO VITAMIN D–MEDIATED HYPERCALCEMIA

For symptomatic hypercalcemia, acute therapeutic measures aim primarily at lowering serum calcium levels for a rapid relief of clinical symptoms. For this purpose, different pharmacologic approaches have been considered. Before clarification of the underlying etiology, vitamin D supplements should be stopped and, if appropriate, a low-calcium diet can be implemented. A vigorous rehydration usually is performed via the intravenous route. Pharmacologic therapies comprise measures to decrease calcium absorption from the intestine, to promote renal calcium excretion, and to inhibit calcium release from bone.

For the increase of renal calcium elimination, loop diuretics that inhibit passive paracellular calcium reabsorption in the thick ascending limb by blocking transcellular salt reabsorption are widely used. The data concerning their therapeutic efficacy, however, are limited.[74] Due to the risk of worsening volume depletion and thereby aggravating hypercalcemia, the use of furosemide requires careful monitoring, especially in young infants. Moreover, the further increase in renal calcium excretion might augment the risk for calcifications and kidney stone formation.

A fast and effective approach to inhibiting enteral calcium absorption is the administration of glucocorticoids (ie, prednisolone). Next to the intestinal effect, glucocorticoids also inhibit the conversion of serum $25(OH)D_3$ into active $1,25(OH)_2D_3$, an effect that is of special importance in vitamin D–mediated hypercalcemia. Colussi and colleagues,[49] however, studied the therapeutic efficacy in patients with *CYP24A1* defects and reported a failure to lower serum calcium levels and to decrease urinary calcium excretions. These findings might indicate that the therapeutic effect in other disorders, such as granulomatous disease, involves mainly the induction of CYP24A1 rather than the intestinal effect.

Sodium cellulose phosphate (SCP) is a nonabsorbable cation exchange resin used for the removal of excess calcium from the body.[75] It initially was used in patients with so-called absorptive hypercalciuria in order to decrease renal calcium excretions and prevent stone formation.[76] SCP has been used successfully in patients with infantile hypercalcemia.[77] Although long-term therapy with SCP appears to be successful and well tolerated, major concerns involve the risk of developing calcium deficiency and iatrogenic rickets and also the risk of an increased intestinal absorption of oxalate that may aggravate renal calcifications and lead to oxalate kidney stones.

In the acute phase of hypercalcemia, calcitonin may be used because of its prompt effect on serum calcium levels; however, its therapeutic usefulness is limited by its short duration of action due to the development of end-organ resistance.[78] In the presence of intermediate to severe symptomatic hypercalcemia, bisphosphonates, such as pamidronate, that reduce calcium release from bone by inhibiting osteoclasts have been used successfully.[48] If the use of bisphosphonates in the acute setting is considered, it is of special importance to have completed the diagnostic work-up in advance.

A class of drugs that have been applied specifically in vitamin D–mediated hypercalcemia are imidazole derivates, such as ketoconazole.[79] Next to their antifungal effect, they also inhibit mammalian CYP enzymes. Via inhibition of CYP27B1, they are able to lower serum $1,25(OH)_2D_3$ levels effectively and consecutively normalize serum calcium levels. The successful therapeutic use of ketoconazole initially were described in patients with hyperparathyroidism, granulomatous disorders, and hypercortisolism.[80] Several studies evaluated the use of ketoconazole in hypercalcemic patients with *CYP24A1* mutations.[79,81,82] Although the therapeutic efficacy of ketoconazole in these studies was encouraging, use in the long term might be problematic because of its side effects and toxicity.[83] Therefore, less-toxic fluconazole was introduced as a therapeutic alternative. The investigators demonstrated that even low doses produced a significant decline of serum $1,25(OH)_2D_3$ levels and a stabilization of serum calcium levels.[83]

Hypercalcemic patients with NaPi-IIa defects require phosphate supplementation to control vitamin D and calcium metabolism in addition to acute therapeutic measures also applied in patients with *CYP24A1* defects.

CLINICS CARE POINTS

- Diagnosis of vitamin D–mediated hypercalcemia is based on suppressed PTH levels and inappropriately high vitamin D metabolite levels.

- High $25(OH)-D_3$ levels (>200 ng/L) usually indicate overt vitamin D intoxication.

- High $1,25(OH)_2D_3$ levels are observed in IIH but also may originate from extrarenal sources in granulomatous disorders.

- IIH may manifest beyond infancy with recurrent hypercalcemic episodes, long-standing hypercalciuria, renal calcifications, and kidney stones, and patients are at risk for a deterioration of renal function.

- Specific treatment options for vitamin D–mediated hypercalcemia include imidazole derivates that inhibit CYP enzymes.

- A differentiation between *CYP24A1* and *SLC34A1* defects is critical because patients with primary renal phosphate wasting require phosphate supplementation to normalize vitamin D and calcium metabolism

DISCLOSURE

The author has nothing to disclose.

REFERENCES

1. Holick MF. Photobiology of Vitamin D. In: Feldman DPJ, Adams M, editors. Vitamin D. 3rd edition. Amsterdam, The Netherlands: Academic Press; 2011. p. 13–22, chapter 2.

2. Jones G, Strugnell SA, DeLuca HF. Current understanding of the molecular actions of vitamin D. Physiol Rev 1998;78(4):1193–231.

3. Bouillon R. The Vitamin D Binding Protein DBP. In: Feldman DPJ, Adams M, editors. Vitamin D. 3rd edition. Amsterdam, The Netherlands: Academic Press; 2011. p. 57–72, chapter 5.

4. Prosser DE, Jones G. Enzymes involved in the activation and inactivation of vitamin D. Trends Biochem Sci 2004;29(12):664–73.

5. DeLuca HF. Vitamin D: the vitamin and the hormone. Fed Proc 1974;33(11):2211–9.

6. St-Arnaud R, Messerlian S, Moir JM, et al. The 25-hydroxyvitamin D 1-alpha-hydroxylase gene maps to the pseudovitamin D-deficiency rickets (PDDR) disease locus. J Bone Miner Res 1997;12(10):1552–9.

7. Fraser D, Kooh SW, Kind HP, et al. Pathogenesis of hereditary vitamin-D-dependent rickets. An inborn error of vitamin D metabolism involving defective conversion of 25-hydroxyvitamin D to 1 alpha,25-dihydroxyvitamin D. N Engl J Med 1973;289(16):817–22.

8. Panda DK, Miao D, Tremblay ML, et al. Targeted ablation of the 25-hydroxyvitamin D 1alpha -hydroxylase enzyme: evidence for skeletal, reproductive, and immune dysfunction. Proc Natl Acad Sci U S A 2001;98(13):7498–503.

9. Dardenne O, Prud'homme J, Arabian A, et al. Targeted inactivation of the 25-hydroxyvitamin D(3)-1(alpha)-hydroxylase gene (CYP27B1) creates an animal model of pseudovitamin D-deficiency rickets. Endocrinology 2001;142(7):3135–41.

10. Hewison M, Adams JS. Extrarenal 1α-hydroxylase. In: Feldman DPW, Adams JS, editors. Vitamin D. 3rd edition. Amsterdam, The Netherlands: Academic Press; 2011. p. 777–804, chapter 45.

11. Adams JS, Sharma OP, Gacad MA, et al. Metabolism of 25-hydroxyvitamin D3 by cultured pulmonary alveolar macrophages in sarcoidosis. J Clin Invest 1983;72(5):1856–60.

12. Makin G, Lohnes D, Byford V, et al. Target cell metabolism of 1,25-dihydroxyvitamin D3 to calcitroic acid. Evidence for a pathway in kidney and bone involving 24-oxidation. Biochem J 1989;262(1):173–80.

13. Reddy GS, Tserng KY. Calcitroic acid, end product of renal metabolism of 1,25-dihydroxyvitamin D3 through C-24 oxidation pathway. Biochemistry 1989;28(4):1763–9.

14. Jones G, Prosser DE, Kaufmann M. 25-Hydroxyvitamin D-24-hydroxylase (CYP24A1): Its important role in the degradation of vitamin D. Arch Biochem Biophys 2011;523(1):9–18.

15. St-Arnaud R, Arabian A, Travers R, et al. Deficient mineralization of intramembranous bone in vitamin D-24-hydroxylase-ablated mice is due to elevated 1,25-dihydroxyvitamin D and not to the absence of 24,25-dihydroxyvitamin D. Endocrinology 2000;141(7):2658–66.

16. Bouillon R, Carmeliet G, Verlinden L, et al. Vitamin D and human health: lessons from vitamin D receptor null mice. Endocr Rev 2008;29(6):726–76.

17. Littledike ET, Horst RL. Vitamin D3 toxicity in dairy cows. J Dairy Sci 1982;65(5):749–59.

18. Shephard RM, Deluca HF. Plasma concentrations of vitamin D3 and its metabolites in the rat as influenced by vitamin D3 or 25-hydroxyvitamin D3 intakes. Arch Biochem Biophys 1980;202(1):43–53.

19. Deluca HF, Prahl JM, Plum LA. 1,25-Dihydroxyvitamin D is not responsible for toxicity caused by vitamin D or 25-hydroxyvitamin D. Arch Biochem Biophys 2011;505(2):226–30.

20. Down PF, Polak A, Regan RJ. A family with massive acute vitamin D intoxication. Postgrad Med J 1979;55(654):897–902.

21. Jacqz E, Garabedian M, Guillozo H, et al. [Circulating metabolites of vitamin D in 14 children with hypercalcemia]. Arch Fr Pediatr 1985;42(3):225–30.

22. Beşbaş N, Oner A, Akhan O, et al. Nephrocalcinosis due to vitamin D intoxication. Turk J Pediatr 1989;31(3):239–44.

23. Blank S, Scanlon KS, Sinks TH, et al. An outbreak of hypervitaminosis D associated with the overfortification of milk from a home-delivery dairy. Am J Public Health 1995;85(5):656–9.

24. Pettifor JM, Bikle DD, Cavaleros M, et al. Serum levels of free 1,25-dihydroxyvitamin D in vitamin D toxicity. Ann Intern Med 1995;122(7):511–3.

25. Vieth R. The mechanisms of vitamin D toxicity. Bone Miner 1990;11(3):267–72.

26. Bell NH, Stern PH, Pantzer E, et al. Evidence that increased circulating 1 alpha, 25-dihydroxyvitamin D is the probable cause for abnormal calcium metabolism in sarcoidosis. J Clin Invest 1979;64(1):218–25.

27. Adams JS, Singer FR, Gacad MA, et al. Isolation and structural identification of 1,25-dihydroxyvitamin D3 produced by cultured alveolar macrophages in sarcoidosis. J Clin Endocrinol Metab 1985;60(5):960–6.

28. Liu PT, Stenger S, Li H, et al. Toll-like receptor triggering of a vitamin D-mediated human antimicrobial response. Science 2006;311(5768):1770–3.

29. FANCONI G. [Chronic disorders of calcium and phosphate metabolism in children]. Schweiz Med Wochenschr 1951;81(38):908–13.

30. LIGHTWOOD R, STAPLETON T. Idiopathic hypercalcaemia in infants. Lancet 1953;265(6779):255–6.

31. Morgan HG, Mitchell RG, Stowers JM, et al. Metabolic studies on two infants with idiopathic hypercalcaemia. Lancet 16 1956;270(6929):925–31.

32. Lightwood R. [Significance of metabolic disorders in the genesis of marasmus]. Arch Fr Pediatr 1953;10(2):190–3.

33. Fraser D. The relation between infantile hypercalcemia and vitamin D--public health implications in North America. Pediatrics 1967;40(6):1050–61.

34. Williams JC, Barratt-Boyes BG, Lowe JB. Supravalvular aortic stenosis. Circulation 1961;24:1311–8.

35. Beuren AJ, Apitz J, Harmjanz D. Supravalvular aortic stenosis in association with mental retardation and a certain facial appearance. Circulation 1962;26:1235–40.

36. Curran ME, Atkinson DL, Ewart AK, et al. The elastin gene is disrupted by a translocation associated with supravalvular aortic stenosis. Cell 1993;73(1):159–68.

37. Garabedian M, Jacqz E, Guillozo H, et al. Elevated plasma 1,25-dihydroxyvitamin D concentrations in infants with hypercalcemia and an elfin facies. N Engl J Med 1985;312(15):948–52.

38. Kitagawa H, Fujiki R, Yoshimura K, et al. The chromatin-remodeling complex WINAC targets a nuclear receptor to promoters and is impaired in Williams syndrome. Cell 2003;113(7):905–17.

39. Pronicka E, Rowińska E, Kulczycka H, et al. Persistent hypercalciuria and elevated 25-hydroxyvitamin D3 in children with infantile hypercalcaemia. Pediatr Nephrol 1997;11(1):2–6.

40. Misselwitz J, Hesse V. [Hypercalcemia following prophylactic vitamin D administration]. Kinderarztl Prax 1986;54(8):431–8.

41. Weisman Y, Harell A, Edelstein S. Infantile hypercalcemia: a defect in the esterification of 1,25-dihydroxyvitamin D? Med Hypotheses 1979;5(3):379–82.

42. McTaggart SJ, Craig J, MacMillan J, et al. Familial occurrence of idiopathic infantile hypercalcemia. Pediatr Nephrol 1999;13(8):668–71.

43. Schlingmann KP, Kaufmann M, Weber S, et al. Mutations in CYP24A1 and idiopathic infantile hypercalcemia. N Engl J Med 2011;365(5):410–21.

44. Dauber A, Nguyen TT, Sochett E, et al. Genetic Defect in CYP24A1, the Vitamin D 24-Hydroxylase Gene, in a Patient with Severe Infantile Hypercalcemia. J Clin Endocrinol Metab 2012;97(2):E268–74.

45. Dinour D, Beckerman P, Ganon L, et al. Loss-of-function mutations of CYP24A1, the vitamin D 24-hydroxylase gene, cause long-standing hypercalciuric nephrolithiasis and nephrocalcinosis. J Urol 2013;190(2):552–7.

46. Castanet M, Mallet E, Kottler ML. Lightwood syndrome revisited with a novel mutation in CYP24 and vitamin D supplement recommendations. J Pediatr 2013; 163(4):1208–10.

47. Fencl F, Blahova K, Schlingmann KP, et al. Severe hypercalcemic crisis in an infant with idiopathic infantile hypercalcemia caused by mutation in CYP24A1 gene. Eur J Pediatr 2013;172(1):45–9.

48. Skalova S, Cerna L, Bayer M, et al. Intravenous pamidronate in the treatment of severe idiopathic infantile hypercalcemia. Iran J Kidney Dis 2013;7(2):160–4.

49. Colussi G, Ganon L, Penco S, et al. Chronic hypercalcaemia from inactivating mutations of vitamin D 24-hydroxylase (CYP24A1): implications for mineral metabolism changes in chronic renal failure. Nephrol Dial Transplant 2014;29(3): 636–43.

50. Figueres ML, Linglart A, Bienaime F, et al. Kidney function and influence of sunlight exposure in patients with impaired 24-hydroxylation of vitamin D due to CYP24A1 mutations. Am J Kidney Dis 2015;65(1):122–6.

51. Cools M, Goemaere S, Baetens D, et al. Calcium and bone homeostasis in heterozygous carriers of CYP24A1 mutations: A cross-sectional study. Bone 2015; 81:89–96.

52. Dinour D, Davidovits M, Aviner S, et al. Maternal and infantile hypercalcemia caused by vitamin-D-hydroxylase mutations and vitamin D intake. Pediatr Nephrol 2015;30(1):145–52.

53. Shah AD, Hsiao EC, O'Donnell B, et al. Maternal Hypercalcemia Due to Failure of 1,25-Dihydroxyvitamin-D3 Catabolism in a Patient With CYP24A1 Mutations. J Clin Endocrinol Metab 2015;100(8):2832–6.

54. Hedberg F, Pilo C, Wikner J, et al. Three Sisters With Heterozygous Gene Variants of. J Endocr Soc 2019;3(2):387–96.

55. Brancatella A, Cappellani D, Kaufmann M, et al. Do the Heterozygous Carriers of a CYP24A1 Mutation Display a Different Biochemical Phenotype Than Wild Types? J Clin Endocrinol Metab 2021;106(3):708–17.

56. Molin A, Baudoin R, Kaufmann M, et al. CYP24A1 Mutations in a Cohort of Hypercalcemic Patients: Evidence for a Recessive Trait. J Clin Endocrinol Metab 2015; 100(10):E1343–52.

57. Schlingmann KP, Ruminska J, Kaufmann M, et al. Autosomal-Recessive Mutations in SLC34A1 Encoding Sodium-Phosphate Cotransporter 2A Cause Idiopathic Infantile Hypercalcemia. J Am Soc Nephrol 2016;27(2):604–14.

58. Lederer E, Wagner CA. Clinical aspects of the phosphate transporters NaPi-IIa and NaPi-IIb: mutations and disease associations. Pflugers Arch 2019;471(1): 137–48.

59. Quarles LD. Role of FGF23 in vitamin D and phosphate metabolism: implications in chronic kidney disease. Exp Cell Res 2012;318(9):1040–8.

60. Rajagopal A, Debora B, James TL, et al. Exome sequencing identifies a novel homozygous mutation in the phosphate transporter SLC34A1 in hypophosphatemia and nephrocalcinosis. J Clin Endocrinol Metab 2014;99(11):E2451–6.

61. Magen D, Berger L, Coady MJ, et al. A loss-of-function mutation in NaPi-IIa and renal Fanconi's syndrome. N Engl J Med 2010;362(12):1102–9.

62. Hureaux M, Molin A, Jay N, et al. Prenatal hyperechogenic kidneys in three cases of infantile hypercalcemia associated with SLC34A1 mutations. Pediatr Nephrol 2018;33(10):1723–9.

63. Pronicka E, Ciara E, Halat P, et al. Biallelic mutations in CYP24A1 or SLC34A1 as a cause of infantile idiopathic hypercalcemia (IIH) with vitamin D hypersensitivity: molecular study of 11 historical IIH cases. J Appl Genet 2017;58(3):349–53.

64. Demir K, Yildiz M, Bahat H, et al. Clinical Heterogeneity and Phenotypic Expansion of NaPi-IIa-Associated Disease. J Clin Endocrinol Metab 2017;102(12):4604–14.

65. Halbritter J, Baum M, Hynes AM, et al. Fourteen Monogenic Genes Account for 15% of Nephrolithiasis/Nephrocalcinosis. J Am Soc Nephrol 2014;26(3):543–51.

66. Braun DA, Lawson JA, Gee HY, et al. Prevalence of Monogenic Causes in Pediatric Patients with Nephrolithiasis or Nephrocalcinosis. Clin J Am Soc Nephrol 2016;11(4):664–72.

67. Daga A, Majmundar AJ, Braun DA, et al. Whole exome sequencing frequently detects a monogenic cause in early onset nephrolithiasis and nephrocalcinosis. Kidney Int 2018;93(1):204–13.

68. Prie D, Huart V, Bakouh N, et al. Nephrolithiasis and osteoporosis associated with hypophosphatemia caused by mutations in the type 2a sodium-phosphate cotransporter. N Engl J Med 2002;347(13):983–91.

69. Dinour D, Davidovits M, Ganon L, et al. Loss of function of NaPiIIa causes nephrocalcinosis and possibly kidney insufficiency. Pediatr Nephrol 2016;31(12):2289–97.

70. Janiec A, Halat-Wolska P, Obrycki Ł, et al. Long-term outcome of the survivors of infantile hypercalcaemia with CYP24A1 and SLC34A1 mutations. Nephrol Dial Transplant 2020;36(8):1484–92.

71. Bergwitz C, Roslin NM, Tieder M, et al. SLC34A3 mutations in patients with hereditary hypophosphatemic rickets with hypercalciuria predict a key role for the sodium-phosphate cotransporter NaPi-IIc in maintaining phosphate homeostasis. Am J Hum Genet 2006;78(2):179–92.

72. Lorenz-Depiereux B, Benet-Pages A, Eckstein G, et al. Hereditary hypophosphatemic rickets with hypercalciuria is caused by mutations in the sodium-phosphate cotransporter gene SLC34A3. Am J Hum Genet 2006;78(2):193–201.

73. Dasgupta D, Wee MJ, Reyes M, et al. Mutations in SLC34A3/NPT2c are associated with kidney stones and nephrocalcinosis. J Am Soc Nephrol 2014;25(10):2366–75.

74. LeGrand SB, Leskuski D, Zama I. Narrative review: furosemide for hypercalcemia: an unproven yet common practice. Ann Intern Med 2008;149(4):259–63.

75. Mizusawa Y, Burke JR. Prednisolone and cellulose phosphate treatment in idiopathic infantile hypercalcaemia with nephrocalcinosis. J Paediatr Child Health 1996;32(4):350–2.

76. Pak CY. Clinical pharmacology of sodium cellulose phosphate. J Clin Pharmacol 1979;19(8–9 Pt 1):451–7.

77. Huang J, Coman D, McTaggart SJ, et al. Long-term follow-up of patients with idiopathic infantile hypercalcaemia. Pediatr Nephrol 2006;21(11):1676–80.
78. Purdue BW, Tilakaratne N, Sexton PM. Molecular pharmacology of the calcitonin receptor. Receptors Channels 2002;8(3–4):243–55.
79. Nguyen M, Boutignon H, Mallet E, et al. Infantile hypercalcemia and hypercalciuria: new insights into a vitamin D-dependent mechanism and response to ketoconazole treatment. J Pediatr 2010;157(2):296–302.
80. Adams JS, Sharma OP, Diz MM, et al. Ketoconazole decreases the serum 1,25-dihydroxyvitamin D and calcium concentration in sarcoidosis-associated hypercalcemia. J Clin Endocrinol Metab 1990;70(4):1090–5.
81. Nesterova G, Malicdan MC, Yasuda K, et al. 1,25-(OH)2D-24 Hydroxylase (CYP24A1) Deficiency as a Cause of Nephrolithiasis. Clin J Am Soc Nephrol 2013;8(4):649–57.
82. Tebben PJ, Milliner DS, Horst RL, et al. Hypercalcemia, hypercalciuria, and elevated calcitriol concentrations with autosomal dominant transmission due to CYP24A1 mutations: effects of ketoconazole therapy. J Clin Endocrinol Metabr 2012;97(3):E423–7.
83. Sayers J, Hynes AM, Srivastava S, et al. Successful treatment of hypercalcaemia associated with a CYP24A1 mutation with fluconazole. Clin Kidney J 2015;8(4):453–5.

Drug-Related Hypercalcemia

Anne-Lise Lecoq, MD, PhD[a], Marine Livrozet, MD, PhD[b],
Anne Blanchard, MD, PhD[b], Peter Kamenický, MD, PhD[a,c],*

KEYWORDS

- Iatrogenic hypercalcemia • Vitamin D analogues • Recombinant human PTH
- Denosumab • Vitamin a analogues • Tamoxifen • Thiazide diuretics • Lithium

KEY POINTS

- Use of over-the-counter vitamin D supplements has considerably increased over the past years.
- Vitamin D supplements together with the 1α-hydroxylated vitamin D analogues are one of the most frequent causes of drug-related hypercalcemia.
- Vitamin A is classically reported as a cause of hypercalcemia but is actually almost never encountered among patients seen in endocrinology departments and remains very rare in oncologic and hepatologic departments.
- Hypercalcemia in thiazide-treated patients is due to enhanced renal proximal calcium reabsorption that turns preexistent asymptomatic normocalcemic hyperparathyroidism or hyperparathyroidism with intermittent hypercalcemia into the hypercalcemic hyperparathyroidism.
- Lithium has a direct effect on calcium-regulated PTH release from parathyroid glands and causes hypercalcemia mainly by drug-induced hyperparathyroidism.

INTRODUCTION

According to the principal hypercalcemic action, drug-induced hypercalcemia may be either parathyroid hormone (PTH)-independent, associated with suppressed plasma PTH concentrations, or PTH-dependent, accompanied by normal or elevated plasma PTH concentrations. Drug-related hypercalcemia with suppressed parathyroid function results from the altered interplay between intestinal calcium absorption, bone remodeling, and renal calcium excretion. Some medicaments act primarily on parathyroid cells to induce functional hyperparathyroidism. However, this

[a] Assistance Publique-Hôpitaux de Paris (AP-HP), Hôpital de Bicêtre, Service d'Endocrinologie et des Maladies de la Reproduction, Centre de Référence des Maladies Rares du Métabolisme du Calcium et du Phosphate, Filière OSCAR, 78 rue du Général Leclerc, Le Kremlin Bicêtre 94270, France; [b] Assistance Publique-Hôpitaux de Paris (AP-HP), Hôpital Européen Georges Pompidou, Centre d'Investigations Cliniques 1418, 20 Rue Leblanc, Paris 75015, France; [c] Université Paris-Saclay, Inserm, Physiologie et Physiopathologie Endocriniennes, Le Kremlin-Bicêtre 94276, France
* Corresponding author. Hôpital de Bicêtre, Service d'Endocrinologie et des Maladies de la Reproduction, 78 rue du Général Leclerc, Le Kremlin Bicêtre 94270, France.
E-mail address: peter.kamenicky@universite-paris-saclay.fr

Endocrinol Metab Clin N Am 50 (2021) 743–752
https://doi.org/10.1016/j.ecl.2021.08.001
0889-8529/21/© 2021 Elsevier Inc. All rights reserved.

endo.theclinics.com

pathophysiological classification of drug-induced hypercalcemia is a simplification, as in reality several mechanisms contribute in parallel to the increase of serum calcium. This review focuses on commonly prescribed medicaments that can be responsible for hypercalcemia, questions the mechanisms of their hypercalcemic actions, and provides an overview of the optimal medical management.

Calcium Supplements

Oral calcium supplements containing calcium carbonate or calcium citrate are part of the conventional therapy for hypocalcemic disorders such as hypoparathyroidism[1] or pseudohypoparathyroidism.[2] The usual daily intake is 0.5 to 2.0 g of elemental calcium *per* day, divided into 2 to 4 daily doses. This treatment leads to hypercalcemia only when combined with other hypercalcemia-inducing drugs, in particular vitamin D and, more commonly, its 1α-hydroxylated analogues (*vide infra*). Exceptionally, oral calcium supplementation can be hypercalcemic in patients with endogenously increased 1α-hydroxylation of vitamin D, that is, patients with chronic granulomatous disorders such as sarcoidosis, or in patients with decreased 1,25-dihydroxyvitamin D degradation due to mutations in *CYP24A1*.[3]

Vitamin D and Analogues

The use of vitamin D therapies has considerably increased these past years, with numerous studies showing potential beneficial effects in areas beyond bone.[4] Both vitamin D_2 (ergocalciferol) and vitamin D_3 (cholecalciferol) are used in over-the-counter vitamin D supplements.[4] Considering the high prevalence of vitamin D deficiency in Europe, an intake of 400 to 1000 IU *per* day is recommended for children and for adults when sun exposure is inadequate or in particular conditions such as pregnancy, malabsorption, or chronic kidney disease.[4] The highest level of daily vitamin D_3 intake that is considered safe for almost all individuals in the general population is 1000 IU/d in infants ages 0 to 6 months, 1500 IU/d in infants ages 6 to 12 months, 2500 IU/d in children ages 1 to 5 years, 3000 IU/d in children ages 4 to 8 years, and 4000 IU/d in adolescents and adults.[5] Vitamin D stocks can be evaluated with the measurement of serum 25-hydroxyvitamin D, a metabolite that has undergone 25-hydroxylation in the liver. Concentrations of 25-hydroxyvitamin D greater than 250 nmol/L (100 ng/mL) are considered excessive, with concentrations greater than 375 nmol/L (150 ng/mL) being associated with toxicity. The short-term ingestion of up to 10,000 IU/d of vitamin D3 seems to be safe with the maintenance of serum 25-hydroxyvitamin D concentrations less than 125 nmol/L (50 ng/mL).[6] Normal individuals exposed to sunlight for short or long periods of time can have serum 25-hydroxyvitamin D concentrations as high as 163 nmol/L (65 ng/mL) without hypercalcemia.[7] Inversely, doses of more than 50,000 IU/d increase serum levels of 25-hydroxyvitamin D to more than 375 nmol/L (150 ng/mL) and are associated with hypercalcemia and hyperphosphatemia.

There are increasing reports of vitamin D toxicity in the literature that seem to be related to manufacturing errors, prescribing errors, and increasing use of supplemental high-dose products.[8] Manufacturing errors have been reported with fortified foodstuffs and unlicensed over-the-counter supplements. Hypercalcemia induced by overfortification of milk with vitamin D has been described in the United States,[9] but in Europe very few foods are fortified. Regarding dietary supplements, substantial variations can be observed between the stated dose and the actual dose contained in pills, from the same bottle and from separate preparations.[10,11] However, vitamin D toxicity with hypercalcemia due to dietary supplements is always related to ingestion of extremely large doses (often several 100-fold the recommended intake) of vitamin D.[8,12–14]

Rarely, vitamin D toxicity can be encountered when high-dose supplements are taken too frequently due to prescription errors, for example, a 50,000 IU prescription provided daily instead of weekly.[15]

Similarly, all the 1α-hydroxylated vitamin D analogues available for the treatment of secondary hyperparathyroidism in the context of end-stage renal disease, hypoparathyroidism, pseudohypoparathyroidism, and various forms of inherited rickets can cause hypercalcemia when administered in excess. Among them, paricalcitol (19-nor-1,25-dihydroxyergocalciferol), an analogue of the active form of ergocalciferol, seems to be less hypercalcemic than others, such as alfacalcidol (1-hydroxycholecalciferol) and calcitriol.[16]

The clinical symptoms of vitamin D toxicity are as those of hypercalcemia due to any other cause. Although vitamin D intoxication is less likely with cholecalciferol and ergocalciferol than with 1α-hydroxylated vitamin D analogues, when it occurs hypercalcemia is more sustained than with alfacalcidol or calcitriol intoxication.[1] Laboratory findings other than hypercalcemia include hyperphosphatemia and suppressed serum PTH concentrations. Absorptive hypercalciuria is frequently present. Urinary calcium excretion is generally elevated before the development of hypercalcemia in patients with hypervitaminosis D. In most cases, serum 1,25-dihydroxyvitamin D concentrations are normal. The serum 25-hydroxyvitamin D concentration at which an individual develops hypercalcemia is influenced by the amount of dietary calcium intake. However, concentrations of serum 25-hydroxyvitamin D greater than 200 nmol/L (80 ng/mL) in the presence of hypercalcemia and the clinical setting of excessive vitamin D ingestion should raise the suspicion of vitamin D intoxication.

Hypercalcemia induced by vitamin D or vitamin D analogues intoxication results mainly from increased intestinal calcium absorption, but increased bone resorption and renal calcium reabsorption also participate. 25-hydroxyvitamin D, when present in excess, could bind to the vitamin D receptor and induce or repress calcium-regulating genes in target tissues such as the intestine, kidney, and bone. A second possible mechanism could be the endogenous production of vitamin D metabolites that bind to the vitamin D receptor.[5]

The duration of ingestion of vitamin D, the starting serum 25-hydroxyvitamin D concentration before ingestion, and the underlying reason for therapy play a role in the occurrence of hypercalcemia. For example, patients with chronic granulomatous disorders such as sarcoidosis are more sensitive to serum 25-hydroxyvitamin D levels greater than 75 nmol/L (30 ng/mL).[4]

Recombinant Human Parathyroid Hormone

Treatment with the recombinant human PTH(1-34) fragment, teriparatide, or (in some countries) with intact PTH(1-84) is currently the only available anabolic therapy for osteoporosis. Both medicaments act by direct stimulation of osteoblast activity and recruitment as well as stimulation of remodeling, favoring bone formation. They increase bone formation rate in cancellous, endocortical, and periosteal envelopes and augment the thickness of bone packets.[17] This treatment is prescribed for 2 years, with the recommendation to monitor serum calcium every 3 to 6 moths. Hypercalcemia occurs very rarely.

Hypoparathyroidism is conventionally treated with oral calcium supplements and active vitamin D derivates, but in patients not controlled with such treatment, recombinant parathyroid hormone therapy with twice-daily subcutaneous injections of teriparatide or with once-daily intact PTH(1-84) can adequately manage hypocalcemia and improve patients' reported symptoms.[1] In patients receiving PTH replacement therapy, the target serum calcium concentrations (albumin-adjusted total calcium or ionized calcium) are in the lower part of the normal range, which is slightly higher than in patients under conventional therapy, in whom calcium is usually kept at the lower limit of the normal range and even less, provided that the patients has not symptoms of hypocalcemia.[18] Regular monitoring of serum calcium every 3 to 6 months is recommended in patients on PTH replacement therapy.[1] Hypercalcemia can occur because of overtreatment, usually in patients also receiving calcium carbonate and active vitamin D derivates. Decreased renal function and dehydration, for instance during acute infection, can favor the occurrence of transient hypercalcemic episodes. The hypercalcemic effect of PTH is considered mainly related to its renal action.[19] In such situations, PTH replacement therapy should be transiently suspended until the normalization of calcaemia, and hospital admission should be considered according to the severity of hypercalcemia.

Denosumab

Hypercalcemia has been reported after discontinuation of denosumab, both in children and adults[20–22] after prolonged treatment with denosumab (several years), at high doses, for various indications (breast cancer, giant cell tumors of bone, Paget disease). Hypercalcemia occurred at various time (7 weeks to 7 months) after cessation of the treatment. It was often severe, requiring hyperhydration and intravenous bisphosphonate treatment.[20,21,23] Associated osteonecrosis of the jaw and atypical femoral fractures have been reported.[20]

Biologically, serum PTH concentrations are suppressed. Hypercalcemia is associated with an increased bone remodeling due to a rebound of bone resorption and hyperactivation of the RANKL pathway.[24] It is thought to be a feature of skeletally immature children because of the high bone turnover present in this population[20] but this side effect is not restricted to young patients.

Vitamin A Analogues

Vitamin A can be consumed as preformed vitamin A, in the form of retinol found in animal sources (meat, liver, liver oils), some multivitamins and fortified foods (milk, butter, cereals), or as provitamin A carotenoids (α- or β-carotene) found in fruits and vegetables. The cleavage of provitamin A carotenoids to retinal is highly regulated and saturation of intestinal absorption occurs with excessive intake,[25] making vitamin A toxicity from provitamin A sources likely impossible. Preformed vitamin A, on the other hand, can be stored in the liver.[25] With the development of multivitamins and fortified food, an increasing amount of people may ingest more than the recommended dietary allowance for vitamin A (3000 IU in children and 5000 IU in adults or, in retinol activity equivalents, 400–950 μg/d), much of it as preformed vitamin A.[26] However, the risk of achieving toxic levels of vitamin A is theoretically very low with commercial formulations. Toxicity results from the ingestion of high amounts of preformed vitamin for months or years. Daily intakes of greater than 25,000 IU for more than 6 years and greater than 100,000 IU for more than 6 months are considered toxic,[27] but there is important interindividual variability in tolerance to vitamin A intake.[28] Children are particularly sensitive to vitamin A, with daily intakes of 1500 IU/kg body weight reportedly leading to toxicity.[27] Alteration in liver function due to drugs, viral hepatitis, or protein-energy malnutrition increases the risk of vitamin A toxicity.

Hypercalcemia is a very rare complication of vitamin A intoxication and is not usually encountered among patients seen in endocrinology departments. It has been reported in the following groups of patients: those receiving all-trans retinoic acid therapy for treatment of acute promyelocytic leukemia[29,30]; children with high-risk neuroblastoma treated with 13-cis-retinoic acid[31,32]; hemodialysis patients who consume nutritional supplements containing a pharmacologic dosage of vitamin A, sometimes combined with high doses of vitamin D[33]; those who ingest unlicensed over-the-counter supplements containing excessive doses of vitamin A[34]; and those given prolonged enteral feeding.[35] However, even in these groups of patients, vitamin A intoxication remains very rare with only anecdotal reports.

Hypercalcemia can be accompanied by classic features of vitamin A toxicity, including dry skin, cheilitis, alopecia, pruritis, fatigue, anorexia, headache, bone pain, pseudotumour cerebri, and liver toxicity. Serum phosphate is normal, whereas 1,25-dihydroxyvitamin D and parathyroid hormone concentrations are low. Serum retinol is not a good measure of vitamin A status during toxicity. Biomarkers other than plasma retinol (retinoic acid and its metabolites) may be useful in diagnosis of vitamin A intoxication but are not easily available in clinical practice.[36]

It is not clear how vitamin A causes hypercalcemia. Few studies reported increased bone resorption (increased number and size of osteoclasts) and reduced bone formation, resulting in bone loss, associated with spontaneous fractures and cartilage abnormalities (epiphyseal closure and calcification) in rats treated with high doses of vitamin A.[37,38] Vitamin A is thought to have a direct effect on osteoclast formation and stimulation of mature osteoclast activity and inhibit collagen synthesis and growth of osteoblast-like cells.[39–41] Indeed, receptors for retinoic acid are located on both osteoblasts and osteoclasts.[42] Vitamin A could also induce PTH release as shown in vitro in bovine parathyroid cells.[43]

Effects of hypervitaminosis A on bone in humans have been rarely described. Periosteal thickening, ligamentous calcification and enthesopathy, osteophyte development, epiphyseal closure, and decreased bone mineral density have been reported with isotretinoin prescribed for acne.[44] These changes resemble those observed in the disorder known as diffuse idiopathic skeletal hyperostosis. However, hypercalcemia is not associated with these manifestations. Few observational studies have evaluated the bone status in subjects taking vitamin A, and their results are contradictory. Some of them are suggesting an increased risk of osteoporosis and hip fractures with vitamin A supplementation,[45,46] independently of the presence of hypercalcemia.

Tamoxifen

In patients with advanced breast cancer, flare hypercalcemia may seem within the first few weeks of initiation of tamoxifen therapy.[47,48] In all reported cases, the hypercalcemic patients had osteolytic or mixed lytic and blastic bone metastases. There are no specific treatment recommendations for flare hypercalcemia, except tamoxifen withdrawal. After normalization of calcemia, tamoxifen can usually be resumed without relapse of hypercalcemia.

The mechanism is not clearly understood. It may be due to increased osteoclast activity and bone resorption, caused by the release of various factors from tumor cells, such as transforming growth factor alpha and epidermal factors, cytokines (interleukin-1 [IL-1] and IL-6), tumor necrosis factor alpha, or prostaglandin E2. Another mechanism in premenopausal women in whom tamoxifen is associated with gonadotropin-releasing hormone agonists could be the insufficient estrogenic effect of tamoxifen on bone, favoring trabecular and endocortical bone resorption.[48,49]

Thiazide Diuretics

Hypercalcemia associated with thiazide use is a well-known clinical entity. Prevalence of hypercalcemia in subjects on thiazide diuretics has been estimated to be around 2%, nearly 3 times higher than the prevalence of hypercalcemia observed in same-aged subjects in the general population.[50] The overall annual age- and sex-adjusted incidence of hypercalcemia in thiazide-treated subjects is as high as 20 per 100, 000 per year in the United States.[51] This unexpected high incidence contrasts with the absence of effect of thiazide administration on plasma calcium concentration in healthy subjects[52] and in subjects with renal hypercalciuria,[53] suggesting that at least one additional factor is requested to allow hypercalcemia to appear. Accordingly, hypercalcemia persists in 70% of patients after thiazide therapy discontinuation. Similar to patients with primary hyperparathyroidism, subjects with thiazide-associated hypercalcemia are mainly women (about 80%) and of older age.[50,51] A primary hyperparathyroidism was documented in about 70% of subjects in the latter studies.

The high frequency of hypercalcemia in thiazide-treated patients could be explained by enhanced renal proximal calcium reabsorption, turning preexistent asymptomatic normocalcemic hyperparathyroidism or hyperparathyroidism with intermittent hypercalcemia into the classic hypercalcemic hyperparathyroidism. Thiazide diuretics stimulate proximal tubular sodium reabsorption as a compensation of their primary natriuretic action in the distal tubule, resulting in enhanced proximal passive calcium transport.[54]

A direct effect of thiazides on parathyroid glands has also been suggested. Long-term administration of hydrochlorothiazide to dogs not only led to hypercalcemia with hypophosphatemia, but also resulted in parathyroid glands enlargement.[55] Along this line, the frequency of parathyroid hyperplasia in thiazide-associated hyperparathyroidism is 2-fold higher than in sporadic hyperparathyroidism.[51]

The differential diagnosis between PTH-dependent hypercalcemia related to thiazides and familial hypocalciuric hypercalcemia can be difficult due to the stimulatory effect of thiazides on renal tubular reabsorption of calcium, lowering calcium excretion. It is thus recommended to measure 24-hour urine calcium and creatinine after withholding diuretics. After an acute exposure to thiazides for 8 days, calciuria returned to baseline within few days,[53] but after long-term treatment with thiazides these should to be discontinued for a longer period before assessment of calcium excretion. Sequencing of genes involved in familial hypocalciuric hypercalcemia can also facilitate the differential diagnosis between these 2 entities, when surgical approach is envisioned.

Lithium

Lithium is a key treatment to control the bipolar disorder. It requires close monitoring, as its therapeutic index is narrow. Hypercalcemia is one of the well-known complications of lithium treatment and seems mainly related to drug-induced hyperparathyroidism.[56] Cross-sectional studies estimated the incidence of hypercalcemia in lithium-treated patients with bipolar disorder between 8% and 15%,[57,58] whereas the reported frequency of patients with PTH concentrations greater than the upper range of normal, without accompanying hypercalcemia, is between 15% and 47%.[59,60] Lithium-induced hyperparathyroidism increases with treatment duration.[56,61] Hypercalcemia may be reversible on discontinuation of lithium therapy[62]; however, after long-term exposition the chances that parathyroid function normalizes are low.[61]

Lithium has a direct effect on calcium-regulated PTH release. It increases the "set-point" for calcium (i.e., the concentration of serum calcium required for half-maximal inhibition of PTH release) in a dose-dependent manner. In vitro studies in human parathyroid tissue concluded that this effect was related to the extracellular rather than the intracellular concentration of the medicament.[63,64] Lithium interferes with transmembrane signal transduction in the parathyroid cells,[65] in particular in the intracellular signaling pathway of the calcium-sensing receptor.[66] From the histopathological point of view, lithium induces both parathyroid hyperplasia[62] and multiple adenomas. Multiple parathyroid lesions are found in more than 50% of operated patients with lithium-induced hyperparathyroidism,[56,61] far more frequently than in patients with primary hyperparathyroidism.[67,68]

In addition to its action on parathyroid cells, lithium enhances renal reabsorption of calcium in the thick limb of Henle loop.[69] This additional effect on renal tubule explains why lithium-induced hyperparathyroidism biochemically mimics familial hypocalciuric hypercalcemia.

Because lithium-induced hypercalcemia may exacerbate psychiatric symptoms and mimic disorder relapse, worsening of psychiatric symptoms should always lead to serum calcium measurement. In cases of asymptomatic and/or mild hypercalcemia, lithium treatment can be continued when regular monitoring of serum calcium can be guaranteed. Parathyroid surgery should be proposed in cases of severe and/or symptomatic hypercalcemia in patients in whom lithium treatment needs to be continued because of ineffectiveness of other psychopharmacological approaches. Cinacalcet has been used with success in several cases of lithium-induced hyperparathyroidism.[68,70–72]

CLINICS CARE POINTS

- Concentrations of 25-hydroxyvitamin D greater than 250 nmol/L (100 ng/mL) are considered excessive, and concentrations greater than 375 nmol/L (150 ng/mL) being associated with toxicity.

- Patients with chronic granulomatous disorders such as sarcoidosis are more sensitive to serum 25-hydroxyvitamin D concentrations greater than 75 nmol/L (30 ng/mL).

- In patients with hypoparathyroidism receiving recombinant human PTH, transient hypercalcemia can occur because of overtreatment, usually in patients with decreased renal function and dehydration during acute infection.

- To differentiate between hypercalcemia related to thiazides and familial hypocalciuric hypercalcemia it is recommended to measure 24-hour urine calcium and creatinine after withholding diuretics.

- Worsening of psychiatric symptoms in a lithium-treated patient should always lead to serum calcium measurement.

DISCLOSURE

The authors have nothing to disclose.

REFERENCES

1. Gafni RI, Collins MT. Hypoparathyroidism. N Engl J Med 2019;380(18):1738–47.
2. Mantovani G, Bastepe M, Monk D, et al. Diagnosis and management of pseudo-hypoparathyroidism and related disorders: first international Consensus Statement. Nat Rev Endocrinol 2018;14(8):476–500.
3. Schlingmann KP, Kaufmann M, Weber S, et al. Mutations in CYP24A1 and idiopathic infantile hypercalcemia. N Engl J Med 2011;365(5):410–21.
4. Holick MF. Vitamin D deficiency. N Engl J Med 2007;357(3):266–81.
5. Tebben PJ, Singh RJ, Kumar R. Vitamin D-mediated hypercalcemia: mechanisms, diagnosis, and treatment. Endocr Rev 2016;37(5):521–47.
6. Vieth R. Vitamin D supplementation, 25-hydroxyvitamin D concentrations, and safety. Am J Clin Nutr 1999;69(5):842–56.
7. Chel VG, Ooms ME, Popp-Snijders C, et al. Ultraviolet irradiation corrects vitamin D deficiency and suppresses secondary hyperparathyroidism in the elderly. J Bone Miner Res 1998;13(8):1238–42.

8. Taylor PN, Davies JS. A review of the growing risk of vitamin D toxicity from inappropriate practice. Br J Clin Pharmacol 2018;84(6):1121–7.

9. Jacobus CH, Holick MF, Shao Q, et al. Hypervitaminosis D associated with drinking milk. N Engl J Med 1992;326(18):1173–7.

10. LeBlanc ES, Perrin N, Johnson JD, et al. Over-the-counter and compounded vitamin D: is potency what we expect? JAMA Intern Med 2013;173(7):585–6.

11. Andrews KW, Pehrsson PR, Betz JM. Variability in vitamin D content among products for multivitamin and mineral supplements. JAMA Intern Med 2013;173(18):1752–3.

12. Lowe H, Cusano NE, Binkley N, et al. Vitamin D toxicity due to a commonly available "over the counter" remedy from the Dominican Republic. J Clin Endocrinol Metab 2011;96(2):291–5.

13. Araki T, Holick MF, Alfonso BD, et al. Vitamin D intoxication with severe hypercalcemia due to manufacturing and labeling errors of two dietary supplements made in the United States. J Clin Endocrinol Metab 2011;96(12):3603–8.

14. Koutkia P, Chen TC, Holick MF. Vitamin D intoxication associated with an over-the-counter supplement. N Engl J Med 2001;345(1):66–7.

15. Kaur P, Mishra SK, Mithal A. Vitamin D toxicity resulting from overzealous correction of vitamin D deficiency. Clin Endocrinol (Oxf) 2015;83(3):327–31.

16. Martin KJ, González EA. Vitamin D analogues for the management of secondary hyperparathyroidism. Am J Kidney Dis 2001;38(5 Suppl 5):S34–40.

17. Cosman F, Nieves JW, Dempster DW. Treatment sequence matters: anabolic and antiresorptive therapy for osteoporosis. J Bone Miner Res 2017;32(2):198–202.

18. Bollerslev J, Rejnmark L, Marcocci C, et al. European Society of Endocrinology Clinical Guideline: treatment of chronic hypoparathyroidism in adults. Eur J Endocrinol 2015;173(2):G1–20.

19. Gardin JP, Paillard M. Normocalcemic primary hyperparathyroidism: resistance to PTH effect on tubular reabsorption of calcium. Miner Electrolyte Metab 1984;10(5):301–8.

20. Uday S, Gaston CL, Rogers L, et al. Osteonecrosis of the Jaw and Rebound Hypercalcemia in young people treated with denosumab for giant cell tumor of bone. J Clin Endocrinol Metab 2018;103(2):596–603.

21. Setsu N, Kobayashi E, Asano N, et al. Severe hypercalcemia following denosumab treatment in a juvenile patient. J Bone Miner Metab 2016;34(1):118–22.

22. Koldkjær Sølling AS, Harsløf T, Kaal A, et al. Hypercalcemia after discontinuation of long-term denosumab treatment. Osteoporos Int 2016;27(7):2383–6.

23. Sydlik C, Dürr HR, Pozza SB-D, et al. Hypercalcaemia after treatment with denosumab in children: bisphosphonates as an option for therapy and prevention? World J Pediatr 2020;16(5):520–7.

24. Roux S, Massicotte M-H, Huot Daneault A, et al. Acute hypercalcemia and excessive bone resorption following anti-RANKL withdrawal: Case report and brief literature review. Bone 2019;120:482–6.

25. Blomhoff R, Green MH, Berg T, et al. Transport and storage of vitamin A. Science 1990;250(4979):399–404.

26. Allen LH, Haskell M. Estimating the potential for vitamin A toxicity in women and young children. J Nutr 2002;132(9 Suppl):2907S–19S.

27. Hathcock JN, Hattan DG, Jenkins MY, et al. Evaluation of vitamin A toxicity. Am J Clin Nutr 1990;52(2):183–202.

28. Lorenzo M, Nadeau M, Harrington J, et al. Refractory hypercalcemia owing to vitamin A toxicity in a 4-year-old boy. CMAJ 2020;192(25):E671–5.

29. Akiyama H, Nakamura N, Nagasaka S, et al. Hypercalcaemia due to all-trans retinoic acid. Lancet 1992;339(8788):308–9.
30. Cordoba R, Ramirez E, Lei SH, et al. Hypercalcemia due to an interaction of all-trans retinoic acid (ATRA) and itraconazole therapy for acute promyelocytic leukemia successfully treated with zoledronic acid. Eur J Clin Pharmacol 2008;64(10):1031–2.
31. Belden TL, Ragucci DP. Hypercalcemia induced by 13-cis-retinoic acid in a patient with neuroblastoma. Pharmacotherapy 2002;22(5):645–8.
32. Marabelle A, Sapin V, Rousseau R, et al. Hypercalcemia and 13-cis-retinoic acid in post-consolidation therapy of neuroblastoma. Pediatr Blood Cancer 2009; 52(2):280–3.
33. Fishbane S, Frei GL, Finger M, et al. Hypervitaminosis A in two hemodialysis patients. Am J Kidney Dis 1995;25(2):346–9.
34. Vyas AK, White NH. Case of hypercalcemia secondary to hypervitaminosis a in a 6-year-old boy with autism. Case Rep Endocrinol 2011;2011:424712.
35. Bremner NA, Mills LA, Durrani AJ, et al. Vitamin A toxicity in burns patients on long-term enteral feed. Burns 2007;33(2):266–7.
36. Penniston KL, Tanumihardjo SA. The acute and chronic toxic effects of vitamin A. Am J Clin Nutr 2006;83(2):191–201.
37. Clark I, Smith MR. Effects of hypervitaminosis A and D on skeletal metabolism. J Biol Chem 1964;239:1266–71.
38. Binkley N, Krueger D. Hypervitaminosis A and bone. Nutr Rev 2000;58(5):138–44.
39. Scheven BA, Hamilton NJ. Retinoic acid and 1,25-dihydroxyvitamin D3 stimulate osteoclast formation by different mechanisms. Bone 1990;11(1):53–9.
40. Oreffo RO, Teti A, Triffitt JT, et al. Effect of vitamin A on bone resorption: evidence for direct stimulation of isolated chicken osteoclasts by retinol and retinoic acid. J Bone Miner Res 1988;3(2):203–10.
41. Dickson I, Walls J. Vitamin A and bone formation. Effect of an excess of retinol on bone collagen synthesis in vitro. Biochem J 1985;226(3):789–95.
42. Harada H, Miki R, Masushige S, et al. Gene expression of retinoic acid receptors, retinoid-X receptors, and cellular retinol-binding protein I in bone and its regulation by vitamin A. Endocrinology 1995;136(12):5329–35.
43. Chertow BS, Williams GA, Norris RM, et al. Vitamin A stimulation of parathyroid hormone: interactions with calcium, hydrocortisone, and vitamin E in bovine parathyroid tissues and effects of vitamin A in man. Eur J Clin Invest 1977;7(4):307–14.
44. DiGiovanna JJ. Isotretinoin effects on bone. J Am Acad Dermatol 2001;45(5): S176–82.
45. Feskanich D, Singh V, Willett WC, et al. Vitamin A intake and hip fractures among postmenopausal women. JAMA 2002;287(1):47–54.
46. Michaëlsson K, Lithell H, Vessby B, et al. Serum retinol levels and the risk of fracture. N Engl J Med 2003;348(4):287–94.
47. Nikolic-Tomasević Z, Jelic S, Popov I, et al. Tumor "flare" hypercalcemia–an additional indication for bisphosphonates? Oncology 2001;60(2):123–6.
48. Arumugam GP, Sundravel S, Shanthi P, et al. Tamoxifen flare hypercalcemia: an additional support for gallium nitrate usage. J Bone Miner Metab 2006;24(3):243–7.
49. Manolagas SC, O'Brien CA, Almeida M. The role of estrogen and androgen receptors in bone health and disease. Nat Rev Endocrinol 2013;9(12):699–712.
50. Christensson TA. Letter: Lithium, hypercalcaemia, and hyperparathyroidism. Lancet 1976;2(7977):144.
51. Griebeler ML, Kearns AE, Ryu E, et al. Thiazide-Associated Hypercalcemia: Incidence and Association With Primary Hyperparathyroidism Over Two Decades. J Clin Endocrinol Metab 2016;101(3):1166–73.

52. Rejnmark L, Vestergaard P, Heickendorff L, et al. Effects of thiazide- and loop-diuretics, alone or in combination, on calcitropic hormones and biochemical bone markers: a randomized controlled study. J Intern Med 2001;250(2):144–53.

53. Parfitt AM. The interactions of thiazide diuretics with parathyroid hormone and vitamin D. Studies in patients with hypoparathyroidism. J Clin Invest 1972;51(7):1879–88.

54. Nijenhuis T, Vallon V, van der Kemp AWCM, et al. Enhanced passive Ca2+ reabsorption and reduced Mg2+ channel abundance explains thiazide-induced hypocalciuria and hypomagnesemia. J Clin Invest 2005;115(6):1651–8.

55. Pickleman JR, Straus FH, Forland M, et al. Thiazide-induced parathyroid stimulation. Metabolism 1969;18(10):867–73.

56. Meehan AD, Wallin G, Järhult J. Characterization of Calcium Homeostasis in Lithium-Treated Patients Reveals Both Hypercalcaemia and Hypocalcaemia. World J Surg 2020;44(2):517–25.

57. McIntosh WB, Horn EH, Mathieson LM, et al. The prevalence, mechanism and clinical significance of lithium-induced hypercalcaemia. Med Lab Sci 1987; 44(2):115–8.

58. Twigt BA, Houweling BM, Vriens MR, et al. Hypercalcemia in patients with bipolar disorder treated with lithium: a cross-sectional study. Int J Bipolar Disord 2013;1:18.

59. van Melick EJM, Wilting I, Ziere G, et al. The influence of lithium on calcium homeostasis in older patients in daily clinical practice. Int J Geriatr Psychiatry 2014;29(6):594–601.

60. Mallette LE, Eichhorn E. Effects of lithium carbonate on human calcium metabolism. Arch Intern Med 1986;146(4):770–6.

61. Bendz H, Sjödin I, Aurell M. Renal function on and off lithium in patients treated with lithium for 15 years or more. A controlled, prospective lithium-withdrawal study. Nephrol Dial Transpl 1996;11(3):457–60.

62. Mallette LE, Khouri K, Zengotita H, et al. Lithium treatment increases intact and midregion parathyroid hormone and parathyroid volume. J Clin Endocrinol Metab 1989;68(3):654–60.

63. Shen FH, Sherrard DJ. Lithium-induced hyperparathyroidism: an alteration of the "set-point. Ann Intern Med 1982;96(1):63–5.

64. Wallace J, Scarpa A. Similarities of Li+ and low Ca2+ in the modulation of secretion by parathyroid cells in vitro. J Biol Chem 1983;258(10):6288–92.

65. McHenry CR, Lee K. Lithium therapy and disorders of the parathyroid glands. Endocr Pract 1996;2(2):103–9.

66. Riccardi D, Brown EM. Physiology and pathophysiology of the calcium-sensing receptor in the kidney. Am J Physiol Ren Physiol 2010;298(3):F485–99.

67. Varhaug JE. Long-term results of surgery for lithium-associated hyperparathyroidism (Br J Surg 2010; 97:1680-1685). Br J Surg 2010;97(11):1685–6.

68. Dixon M, Luthra V, Todd C. Use of cinacalcet in lithium-induced hyperparathyroidism. BMJ Case Rep 2018;2018. bcr2018225154.

69. Dubovsky SL, Franks RD, Lifschitz ML, et al. Hypocalciuric effect of lithium: a confirmatory study. Psychoneuroendocrinology 1982;7(4):355–9.

70. Szalat A, Mazeh H, Freund HR. Lithium-associated hyperparathyroidism: report of four cases and review of the literature. Eur J Endocrinol 2009;160(2):317–23.

71. Gregoor PS, de Jong GMT. Lithium hypercalcemia, hyperparathyroidism, and cinacalcet. Kidney Int 2007;71(5):470.

72. Sloand JA, Shelly MA. Normalization of lithium-induced hypercalcemia and hyperparathyroidism with cinacalcet hydrochloride. Am J Kidney Dis 2006;48(5):832–7.

Hypercalcemia in Pregnancy

Karel Dandurand, MD, FRCPC, Dalal S. Ali, MD, FRCPI,
Aliya A. Khan, MD, FRCPC, FACP, FACE*

KEYWORDS

- Hypercalcemia • Management • Pregnancy • Primary hyperparathyroidism
- Cinacalcet • Calcitonin • Parathyroidectomy

KEY POINTS

- Primary hyperparathyroidism is the most common cause of hypercalcemia in pregnancy and is the result of a solitary parathyroid adenoma in the majority of cases.
- It is essential to exclude a diagnosis of familial hypocalciuric hypercalcemia, because parathyroidectomy is not indicated.
- Mild primary hyperparathyroidism may be managed conservatively with supportive measures.
- In primary hyperparathyroidism with albumin-adjusted calcium levels of 3.00 mmol/L or more ($\geq$12 mg/dL) in which conservative measures fail, parathyroidectomy in the second trimester is advised.
- Pharmacologic options are limited during pregnancy, with no long-term safety data on any of the treatments available.

INTRODUCTION

Hypercalcemia in a pregnant woman is a rare occurrence that may, however, have serious consequences on both the mother and the fetus. Primary hyperparathyroidism (PHPT) represents the leading cause of hypercalcemia in pregnancy.[1] Other causes of hypercalcemia need to be considered and excluded before confirming a PHPT diagnosis. These include familial hypocalciuric hypercalcemia (FHH), milk–alkali syndrome, parathyroid hormone-related protein (PTHrP)-mediated hypercalcemia of pregnancy, hypercalcemia of malignancy, and abnormal vitamin D metabolism.[2] The physiologic reduction in serum parathyroid hormone (PTH) during pregnancy may render a PHPT diagnosis challenging. Because there are currently no long-term safety data in pregnancy for any of the drugs traditionally used to treat hypercalcemia in nonpregnant patients, medical intervention is limited to adequate hydration and avoidance of drugs that may further increase serum calcium. No randomized controlled trials have been conducted comparing medical management with

Division of Endocrinology and Metabolism, McMaster University, Bone Research and Education Centre, 3075 Hospital Gate, Unit 223, Oakville, ON L6M 1M1, Canada
* Corresponding author.
E-mail address: aliya@mcmaster.com

Endocrinol Metab Clin N Am 50 (2021) 753–768
https://doi.org/10.1016/j.ecl.2021.07.009
0889-8529/21/© 2021 Elsevier Inc. All rights reserved.

endo.theclinics.com

parathyroidectomy (PTX) in pregnancy, and therefore current evidence supporting management strategies is severely limited.

We describe calcium homeostasis during euparathyroid pregnancy and the various causes of hypercalcemia reported in pregnant women. We also provide guidance on the evaluation and optimal management of hypercalcemia during pregnancy.

PHYSIOLOGY OF CALCIUM METABOLISM DURING EUPARATHYROID PREGNANCY
Calcium, Magnesium, and Phosphorus

Unadjusted total serum calcium decreases by nearly 10% during pregnancy, owing to the dilutional effect of intravascular volume expansion on serum albumin.[3] This apparent decrease is artifactual, because albumin-adjusted calcium and ionized calcium both remain stable throughout all trimesters.[3] Serum phosphorus and magnesium both remain stable[4] (**Fig. 1**).

Parathyroid Hormone

PTH is suppressed to low normal or slightly below normal reference range in the first trimester secondary to increases in PTH-rP.[5,6] It then either remains suppressed or increases back to mid normal values toward term.[5,6] In the presence of vitamin D inadequacy or low calcium intake, PTH level may not suppress as expected, representing a state of secondary hyperparathyroidism.[7]

Parathyroid Hormone–Related Protein

PTH-rP is synthesized in the breasts and placenta (**Fig. 2**) and may also be produced in other maternal and fetal tissues (parathyroid, amnion, decidua, myometrium, and umbilical cord[2]). PTH-rP increases as early as the 3rd to 13th weeks of gestation, peaking in the third trimester.[8,9]

Calcitriol

Calcitriol increases in the first trimester and peaks in the third trimester.[7] PTH-rP, along with estrogen, prolactin, and human placental lactogen, seem to be the main factors responsible for renal 1α-hydroxylase upregulation.[2]

Calcidiol

Calcidiol levels remain stable throughout pregnancy, despite the increased conversion into calcitriol and transplacental transfer of $25(OH)D_3$ to the fetus.[7]

Calcitonin

The majority of the data suggest an increase in calcitonin during pregnancy[2]; however, some studies have demonstrated stable[10] or even decreased[6] values.

Calcium Balance

The fractional absorption of calcium from the gut doubles as early as 12 weeks of gestation[10] and is maintained to term, creating a positive calcium balance. Increased calcitriol levels may be responsible for part of that adaptive mechanism; however, prolactin, placental lactogen, and growth hormone may all potentiate the capacity of enterocytes to absorb calcium.[2] Combined with the physiologic increase in the glomerular filtration rate, it leads to absorptive hypercalciuria as early as 12 weeks of gestation.[10] Overall, a positive calcium balance is reached by mid pregnancy,[2,11] and as such bone resorption markers seem to be low in the first trimester. Bone resorption afterward increases by the third trimester.[11]

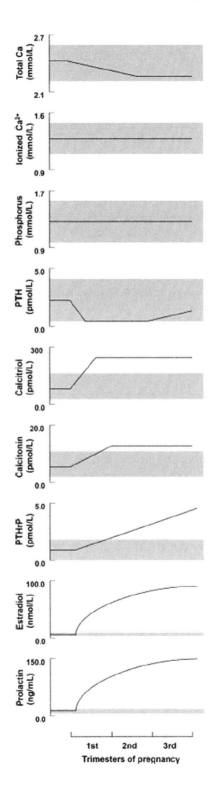

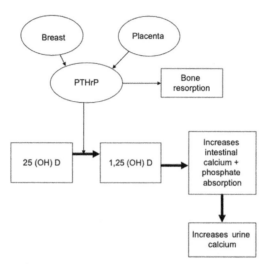

Fig. 2. Role of PTHrP during pregnancy. Schematic illustration demonstrating the role of parathyroid hormone-related protein (PTHrP) during pregnancy. It is produced by the placenta and breast tissue and can result in increase in serum calcium and phosphorus secondary to increased bone resorption and rise in calcitriol. (*From* Khan AA, Clarke B, Rejnmark L, Brandi ML. MANAGEMENT OF ENDOCRINE DISEASE: Hypoparathyroidism in pregnancy: review and evidence-based recommendations for management. Eur J Endocrinol. 2019 Feb 1;180(2):R37-R44.)

CAUSES OF HYPERCALCEMIA IN PREGNANCY
Primary Hyperparathyroidism

PHPT is the most common cause of hypercalcemia in pregnancy, although its exact incidence remains unknown. The incidence of PHPT peaks in female patients 65 to 74 years of age,[12] which makes pregnancy and delivery among women with PHPT an uncommon occurrence. The largest retrospective study to report on prevalence of PHPT in pregnancy examined routine calcium screening of more than 290,000 women aged 20 to 40 years and found PHPT in 0.05% of women of reproductive age, with 0.03% of the cohort conceiving while they had active PHPT.[13] PHPT can present as a solitary adenoma in 85% to 90% of cases, multiglandular hyperplasia in approximately 15% of the cases, or parathyroid carcinoma, which is a very rare occurrence (<1%)[13,14] with only 8 cases reported in pregnancy to date.[15–17] The hereditary causes of PHPT can present as part of syndromes, and include multiple endocrine neoplasia (MEN1, MEN2A, and MEN4) and hyperparathyroidism–jaw tumor syndromes, or occur in isolation as in familial isolated PHPT. Hereditary causes of PHPT tend to occur at a younger age than their sporadic counterparts and are likely to be overexpressed in a population of reproductive aged women. As such, clinical and biochemical screening for associated comorbidities and genetic testing must

Fig. 1. Schematic depiction of longitudinal changes in calcium (Ca), phosphorus, and calciotropic hormone levels during human pregnancy. *Shaded regions* depict the approximate normal ranges. (*From* Kovacs CS. Maternal Mineral and Bone Metabolism During Pregnancy, Lactation, and Post-Weaning Recovery. Physiol Rev. 2016 Apr;96(2):449-547; with permission.)

be considered for patients with PHPT younger than 40 year old (see the Paul Newey's article "Hereditary Primary Hyperparathyroidism").

The physiologic positive calcium balance achieved by midgestation may further exacerbate hypercalcemia and lead to an increased risk of PHPT-related complication (see Signs, Symptoms, and Complications). In contrast, the high transplacental transfer of calcium to the fetus by the end of pregnancy may also confer some protection against increasing serum calcium levels. This finding explains why some cases of hypercalcemic crisis have been described in the immediate postpartum period,[18] when the shunting of excess calcium to the fetus is lost.

Familial Hypocalciuric Hypercalcemia

FHH is a rare autosomal-dominant disorder characterized by life-long, nonprogressive, asymptomatic, mild to moderate hypercalcemia. PTH can either be normal or mildly elevated with relative hypocalciuria.[19] There are 3 identified variants, all leading to abnormal function of the calcium sensing receptor (see Hereditary Primary Hyperparathyroidism). Only 6 cases of FHH in pregnancy have been reported in the literature,[20–22] but the true incidence may be higher because the associated asymptomatic hypercalcemia may go unnoticed if not otherwise detected on routine blood work. Even though the hypercalcemia associated with FHH has traditionally been described to be of mild to moderate severity, in 3 of the reported cases,[20,21] serum calcium reached values or more than 3 mmol/L.

Parathyroid Hormone–Related Protein Mediated Hypercalcemia

Because PTH-rP release by the breasts and placenta seems to be relatively autonomous and independent of serum calcium levels,[2] excess physiologic secretion has been described as a cause of hypercalcemia. Five case reports described the breasts as a source of excessive PTH-rP,[23–25] one of which presented with massive mammary hyperplasia and had to undergo bilateral mastectomy. In the other cases, hypercalcemia resolved with weaning of breastfeeding, but PTH-rP levels remained elevated for many months postpartum.[26] Placental source of excess PTH-rP was also described in a woman who developed hypercalcemic crisis in the third trimester of pregnancy, followed by profound hypocalcemia with undetectable PTH-rP levels hours after emergency cesarean section.[27] In PTH-rP–mediated hypercalcemia cases, it is not possible to ascertain the specific source of the PTH-rP excess until after delivery.

Abnormal 1.25-Dihydroxyvitamin Metabolism

The catabolism of calcitriol to its inactive metabolite $1,24,25(OH)_3D$ is mediated by vitamin D-24-hydroxylase, encoded by Cyp24a1, which also regulates the conversion of $25(OH)D$ to $24,25(OH)_2D$.[2] Homozygous and compound heterozygous loss of function mutation of Cyp24a1 have been described in patients presenting with hypercalcemia, hypercalciuria and low to low-normal PTH levels.[28] Although it may lead to mild hypercalcemia in nonpregnant adults, the physiologic increase in production combined with the pathologic decrease in catabolism of calcitriol has been reported to lead to severe hypercalcemia that may be complicated by nephrolithiasis and pancreatitis in pregnancy.[29–31]

Milk–Alkali Syndrome

Milk–alkali syndrome is defined by the triad of hypercalcemia, metabolic alkalosis, and renal impairment, in association with excessive ingestion of calcium and absorbable alkali. At least a dozen cases of milk–alkali syndrome have been described in pregnant patients.[32–34] Some of these women presented with severe life-threatening hypercalcemia complicated by pancreatitis and eclampsia; it must, therefore not be overlooked as a possible cause of severe hypercalcemia.

Hypercalcemia of Malignancy

Hypercalcemia associated with malignancy has rarely been described in pregnant patients. Pancreatic neuroendocrine tumors,[35,36] metastatic breast cancers,[37,38] ovarian cancer,[39,40] renal cell carcinoma,[41] uterine leiomyoma,[42] and multiple myeloma presenting with hypercalcemia during pregnancy have been described.[43,44] Most of the reported cases seemed to be related to tumoral PTH-rP production and all patients presented with severe hypercalcemia.

Miscellaneous Causes

Other causes of hypercalcemia include granulomatous disease, extrarenal calcitriol production, hyperthyroidism, adrenal insufficiency, pheochromocytoma, immobilization, as well as hypervitaminosis A and D.

CLINICAL PRESENTATION AND MATERNAL–FETAL COMPLICATIONS OF HYPERCALCEMIA

Hypercalcemia in pregnancy is often asymptomatic. In a series of 17 PHPT cases in pregnancy, nearly one-half of them were diagnosed incidentally.[45] When present, symptoms may be nonspecific and easily misdiagnosed as physiologic changes of pregnancy. Symptoms may include malaise, fatigue, constipation, nausea, and vomiting.[46] Hypercalcemia can also present as hyperemesis gravidarum.[47] Polyuria, polydipsia, bone pain, renal colic, and abdominal pain have also been described.[48] Hypercalcemia may be associated with neurocognitive symptoms such as depression, emotional lability, headache, and agitation.[47]

Nephrolithiasis has been described as the most frequent complication of PHPT.[49] PHPT in pregnancy has been consistently reported to be associated with hypertension and preeclampsia[50] with an estimated 25% incidence of preeclampsia.[51] A registry-based study demonstrated a significant association between the presence of a parathyroid adenoma and subsequent preeclampsia, with the risk of preeclampsia remaining increased for up to 5 years after successful intervention.[50] Untreated hypercalcemia in pregnancy may result in end-organ damage, including acute pancreatitis, renal impairment, cardiac arrythmia, peptic ulcer disease, altered mental status, and confusion.[52]

Low bone mass and skeletal fractures have been estimated to occur in less than 10% of pregnant women with PHPT.[53,54] Polyhydramnios has been reported in undiagnosed hypercalcemia of pregnancy and is believed to be related to associated fetal polyuria.[55]

Fetal complications may include neonatal hypocalcemia as a result of fetal parathyroid suppression secondary to maternal hypercalcemia, which can result in seizures and tetany.[56,57] Other reported adverse fetal outcomes include intrauterine growth restriction, preterm labor, stillbirth, and fetal death.[58]

Clinical Presentation and Associated Complications of Familial Hypocalciuric Hypercalcemia

FHH during pregnancy does not seem to pose a risk for the mother, despite the further increases in serum calcium, as noted in published case reports.[20,21] The impact of FHH on the fetus depends on the inherited genotype. Heterozygous transmission is expected to lead to asymptomatic hypercalcemia without adverse outcomes.[20,59] In a fetus not harboring the mutation, maternal hypercalcemia may lead to transient or permanent hypoparathyroidism with subsequent neonatal hypocalcemia.[21,22] Homozygous or compound heterozygous transmission, with the second mutation being inherited from the father, may be associated with severe neonatal hyperparathyroidism.[60]

ASSESSMENT
History and Physical Examination

A detailed history and physical examination should be obtained (**Table 1**), and a familial history is of paramount importance. A positive family history of asymptomatic

Table 1
Evaluation of hypercalcemic disorders in pregnancy

History	Hypercalcemia symptoms: polyuria/polydipsia, nausea, vomiting, constipation, abdominal/flank pain, weakness, confusion/lethargy, depression
	Preeclampsia symptoms: headache, visual disturbance, epigastric pain/upper abdominal pain, altered mental status, dyspnea
	Kidney stones, height loss, fragility fractures
	Previous cancer or irradiation
	Hypertension, stroke or cardiovascular disease
	Granulomatous disease, adrenal insufficiency
	Family history of hypercalcemia and/or clinical entities associated with inherited forms of PHPT (see the Paul Newey's article "Hereditary Primary Hyperparathyroidism")
	Medications: hydrochlorothiazide, lithium, vitamin D supplement, calcium carbonate and other calcium containing antacids
Physical examination	Blood pressure, pulse, height, weight
	Heart, lung, breasts, and abdomen examination
	Neck examination: palpable nodules, surgical incision scar
	Assessment of fetal well-being
Biochemical	Baseline: ionized calcium and/or calcium corrected for albumin[a], iPTH, PO_4, Mg, ALP, vitamin 25(OH)D, creatinine, eGFR, 24-h urine collection for calcium and creatinine, CBC, TSH, CCCR
	PTH-independent hypercalcemia (suppressed iPTH): PTHrP, vitamin $1.25(OH)_2D_3$, serum immunoelectrophoresis, morning cortisol and ACTH
	PTH-dependent hypercalcemia (nonsuppressed or elevated iPTH): DNA analysis of *CaSR, GNa11,* and *AP2S1 genes* if FHH is suspected (see text)
	Preeclampsia panel when clinically indicated
Imaging	Kidney ultrasound examination to exclude renal lithiasis and/or nephrocalcinosis
	Neck ultrasound as preoperative imaging for PHPT

Abbreviations: ACTH, adrenocorticotropic hormone; ALP, alkaline phosphatase; CaSR, calcium sensing receptor; CBC, complete blood count; eGFR, estimated glomerular filtration ratel; iPTH, intact parathyroid hormone; Mg, Magnesium; PO_4, phosphorus; PTHrP, parathyroid hormone-related protein; TSH, thyroid stimulating hormone.

[a] Corrected calcium = measured total calcium (mmol/L) + (40 − serum albumin [g/dL]) × 0.02, Corrected calcium = measured total calcium (mg/dL) + 0.8 × (4 − serum albumin [g/dL]).

Adapted from Khan AA, Kenshole A, Ezzat S, Goguen J, Gomez-Hernandez K, Hegele RA, Houlden R, Joy T, Keely E, Killinger D, Lacroix A, Laredo S, Prebtani APH, Shrayyef MZ, Tran C, Van Uum S, Reardon R, Papageorgiou A, Tays W, Edmonds M. Tools for Enhancement and Quality Improvement of Peer Assessment and Clinical Care in Endocrinology and Metabolism. J Clin Densitom. 2019 Jan-Mar;22(1):125-149.

hypercalcemia, a personal or familial history of failed neck exploration, and a history of hypercalcemia present in childhood or young adulthood are all in favor of FHH.[19]

Laboratory Investigations

Albumin-adjusted serum calcium or ionized calcium should be obtained when evaluating calcium disorders in pregnant women. PHPT is diagnosed in the presence of hypercalcemia along with a nonsuppressed PTH level.[14] The use of lithium and hydrochlorothiazide may lead to elevated serum calcium and PTH levels and should be discontinued for 3 months before confirming a diagnosis of PHPT. Coexisting vitamin D inadequacy may lead to elevated PTH level and should be corrected, aiming for 25(OH)D values between 50 and 125 nmol/L.[1,61]

FHH must be excluded as surgery is not indicated. Calculating the calcium to creatinine clearance ratio (CCCR) is helpful in making the distinction between FHH and PHPT, because it is less than 0.01 in 80% of nonpregnant FHH cases.[19] Approximately 20% of nonpregnant individuals with FHH have a CCCR between 0.01 and 0.02 and can overlap with the values encountered in patients with PHPT. In pregnancy, the absorptive hypercalciuria may further increase the CCCR. A low CCCR is, therefore, of great value in excluding PHPT, but an elevated value may be misleading in the exclusion of FHH. DNA analysis of the *CaSR, GNa11,* and *AP2S1* genes may be warranted to exclude the possibility of FHH, but results may unfortunately not be available in a timely manner, in which case screening of first-degree relatives may prove useful.

Hypercalcemia with an appropriately suppressed PTH level should lead to consideration of PTH-independent causes of hypercalcemia (**Table 2**).

Imaging for Primary Hyperparathyroidism

Preoperative imaging options for PHPT in pregnancy are limited and ultrasound examination remains the safest and first-line imaging technique in pregnancy, with a sensitivity and specificity of 69% and 94%, respectively, at identifying parathyroid adenoma.[62] The sensitivity is lower for multiglandular disease, reported to be 15% to 35%,[63] and ultrasound examination will fail to identify ectopic hyperfunctioning parathyroid tissue.

A recent American College of Obstetricians and Gynecologists committee opinion has stated that fetal exposure of less than 5 mGy is considered safe during pregnancy.[64] A computed tomography scan of the neck is believed to be an examination with very low-dose fetal radiation (0.001–0.01 mGy). 99mTc-MIBI has been shown to cross the placenta in animals[65] and is listed as category C in pregnancy. Very limited data on its use in pregnancy are available, although a prospective registry of more than 100 women exposed to 99mTc scintigraphy, at a dose of less than 5 mGy, during the first trimester did not report increased birth defects or other adverse outcomes.[66]

MANAGEMENT
General Measures, Calcium, and Vitamin D

Adequate hydration should be maintained in all pregnant women with hypercalcemia to avoid further increases in the serum calcium level. Intravenous volume repletion with correction of electrolyte anomalies may be required in severe cases. Furosemide has been used to increase urinary calcium excretion; however, its benefit has been questioned in the nonpregnant population because a recent review failed to report a consistent effect in acutely lowering serum calcium.[67] Furosemide is a category C drug in pregnancy, and although its use does not seem to present a detectable

Table 2
Suggestive clinical features and biochemical profile in hypercalcemic disorders of pregnancy

	Clinical Entities	Suggestive Features	Suggestive Biochemical Profile
PTH-dependent hypercalcemia	PHPT	Previous fracture, height loss or nephrolithiasis/ nephrocalcinosis Personal or familial history of syndromic features of inherited diseases	Nonsuppressed PTH level Hypophosphatemia CCCR >0.02
	FHH	Hypercalcemia dating back to childhood Family history of asymptomatic hypercalcemia Personal/familial history of failed neck exploration	Nonsuppressed PTH level CCCR <0.01 DNA analysis of proband or first-degree relative positive for *CaSR*, *GNA11* or *AP2S1* mutations
PTH-independent hypercalcemia	PTH-rP mediated hypercalcemia of pregnancy	Excessive breast enlargement	Suppressed PTH Elevated PTHrP
	Malignancy-associated hypercalcemia	Previous cancer or radiation Bone pain Constitutional symptoms	Severe hypercalcemia Suppressed PTH May have elevated PTHrP
	Milk–alkali syndrome	Excessive calcium supplements or calcium containing antacids	Suppressed PTH Renal failure Metabolic alkalosis
	1.25OHD impaired catabolism	Previous fracture, height loss or lithiasis Positive family history of hypercalcemic disorder	Elevated 1.25 $(OH)_2D_3$

Abbreviations: PTHrP, parathyroid hormone-related protein.

teratogenic risk, there are concerns related to risk of decreased uteroplacental circulation.[68] It is, therefore, felt that furosemide should be reserved for patients with or at risk of developing congestive heart failure while receiving intravenous hydration.

Calcium supplements should be stopped. Thiazide diuretics and lithium should be avoided if the clinical situation permits, because they can exacerbate the hypercalcemia.

The prevalence of vitamin D inadequacy is higher among patients with PHPT than in the general population and vitamin D supplementation in nonpregnant patients with PHPT has been associated with a mild decrease in PTH levels without increases in serum calcium or urinary calcium levels.[69] It is, therefore, recommended to correct vitamin D inadequacy with supplemental cholecalciferol while closely monitoring serum and urinary calcium excretion, aiming for vitamin D levels of 50 to 125 mmol/L.[70]

Pharmacologic Interventions

Calcitonin decreases calcium levels by directly suppressing bone resorption and promoting urinary calcium excretion. It does not cross the placenta and is a category B medication in pregnancy.[71] It has been used safely during pregnancy at doses 4 to 8 IU/kg given subcutaneously every 12 hours and has been helpful in acutely decreasing calcium levels. However, its continuous use leads to tachyphylaxis that may rapidly blunt its efficacy.

Bisphosphonates cross the placenta and animal studies have suggested that they may be teratogenic at high doses,[72] and therefore are considered category C in pregnancy. Although their use was not reported to cause any serious short term adverse effects on the fetus aside from transient neonatal hypocalcemia and a tendency to low birth weight when used either before or during pregnancy and lactation,[73] long-term data are lacking. As such, their use in pregnancy should be limited to life-threatening situations.

Cinacalcet, a calcimimetic agent, increases the sensitivity of the calcium sensing receptor to activation by extracellular calcium, in turn leading to decreased synthesis and secretion of PTH. It is also classified as category C, but its use has been reported in several cases of PHPT during pregnancy,[74,75] at a dose ranging from 30 mg to 360 mg/d, and animal studies do not suggest adverse fetal outcomes even though it crosses the placenta.[76] Neonatal hypocalcemia has been described with cinacalcet use,; however, it is not known if it was related to maternal hypercalcemia itself.[74]

Denosumab is a category D drug in pregnancy, because its transplacental passage has been shown to increase fetal mortality and cause an osteoporotic-like disorder in animals studies[77] and, therefore, must be avoided in pregnant patients.

Oral phosphate supplementation have been used to decrease calcium levels in PHPT pregnant patients,[78] but owing to limited efficacy[49] and concern for intravascular and extravascular calcifications,[79] its use is not recommended.

Surgical Management of Primary Hyperparathyroidism

Patients with mild hypercalcemia who are relatively asymptomatic can be followed conservatively during pregnancy. However, PTX remains the only curative option for PHPT and should be considered in the presence of severe hypercalcemia (corrected calcium of ≥ 3.0 mmol/L) or in patients with significant symptoms of hypercalcemia. If PTX needs to be performed, it should ideally be carried out in the second trimester of pregnancy, although there are now several reports of successful surgical interventions in the first[80] and third trimesters.[51,81–83]

Different surgical intervention thresholds have been proposed, ranging from 2.7 mmol/L to 3.0 mmol/L.[7,84,85] No randomized trials have compared medical management with PTX in pregnancy. Older series[86,87] have suggested a higher rate of neonatal complications in medically managed compared with surgically treated women with PHPT (53% vs 12.5%) as well as a higher rate of neonatal death (16.0% vs 2.5%). However, it is felt that these represent more severe presentations than the milder cases that are encountered in the modern era. Data from a more recent cohort, in which the majority of patients had mean serum calcium of less than 2.85 mmol/L, did not demonstrate any maternal or late fetal deaths attributable to medically managed women with PHPT.[88] The major morbidity related to medical management compared with surgical intervention seemed to be preeclampsia leading to preterm delivery (30% vs 0%). A large retrospective study by Hirsch and colleagues[13] examined pregnancy outcomes in women with gestational PHPT compared with normocalcemic pregnant women tested during the same time period. The mean calcium levels of the PHPT group was 2.67 ± 0.15 mmol/L. No difference was found in miscarriages rate or any pregnancy-related complications between patients with PHPT and controls, suggesting that mild hypercalcemia does not generally carry an increased risk of obstetric complications.

The bulk of the data available to date favors surgical intervention in the second trimester in the presence of total corrected calcium levels of more than 3.0 mmol/L. Pregnant patients with PHPT who are being followed conservatively with medical management require close postpartum monitoring to avoid a potential abrupt rise in serum calcium following cessation of calcium outflow to the fetus with delivery.

SUMMARY

Hypercalcemia in pregnancy may result in significant maternal and fetal morbidity and requires effective and timely intervention. The nonspecific signs and symptoms of hypercalcemia during pregnancy make the identification of this condition challenging. When considering a diagnosis of PTH-dependent hypercalcemia, it is essential to exclude FHH, because surgical intervention is never indicated for this condition. Appropriate management is determined by the degree of hypercalcemia and the presence of symptoms and complications, as well as the gestational age at presentation. PHPT diagnosed in the first trimester of pregnancy should be managed conservatively if at all possible, until PTX can be offered safely in the second trimester. PHPT in the third trimester requires a careful evaluation of risk and benefits of surgery for both the mother and fetus prior to considering surgical intervention. Close monitoring of the mother and the fetus is of particular importance in the postpartum period to avoid or effectively manage a hypercalcemic crisis in the mother or neonatal tetany.

Currently, the literature is limited to case reports and case series and the quality of evidence on which these recommendations are made is unfortunately very low quality. The optimal management of such complex cases involves the close collaboration of the endocrinologist, obstetrician, and pediatrician.

CLINICS CARE POINTS

- Always use albumin-adjusted serum calcium or ionized calcium, because the unadjusted serum calcium is artefactually decreased in pregnancy.

- Changes in calcium homeostasis and the calcium regulating hormones in pregnancy include suppression of PTH. A nonsuppressed PTH in the presence of hypercalcemia is suspicious for PTH-mediated hypercalcemia.

- A 24-hour urine for calcium and creatinine is recommended for evaluation of hypercalciuria. The spot urine sample may be misleading owing to the development of absorptive hypercalciuria.

- The CCCR in pregnancy may not be as reliable in distinguishing PHPT and FHH. DNA analysis should be considered if FHH is a possible diagnosis.

- PHPT is a biochemical diagnosis. Imaging should only be completed to guide the surgical approach and should not be used as a diagnostic tool.

- PTX in the second trimester of pregnancy should be considered in the presence of significant hypercalcemia (albumin-adjusted calcium of ≥3.0 mmol mmol) owing to PHPT.

- Hypercalcemia should be carefully evaluated with confirmation of the underlying diagnosis and definitive therapy, if possible, before planning a pregnancy.

REFERENCES

1. Khan AA, Hanley DA, Rizzoli R, et al. Primary hyperparathyroidism: review and recommendations on evaluation, diagnosis, and management. A Canadian and international consensus. Osteoporos Int 2017;28(1):1–19.

2. Kovacs CS. Maternal mineral and bone metabolism during pregnancy, lactation, and post-weaning recovery. Physiol Rev 2016;96(2):449–547.
3. Dahlman T, Sjoberg HE, Bucht E. Calcium homeostasis in normal pregnancy and puerperium. A longitudinal study. Acta Obstet Gynecol Scand 1994;73(5):393–8.
4. Cross NA, Hillman LS, Allen SH, et al. Calcium homeostasis and bone metabolism during pregnancy, lactation, and postweaning: a longitudinal study. Am J Clin Nutr 1995;61(3):514–23.
5. Black AJ, Topping J, Durham B, et al. A detailed assessment of alterations in bone turnover, calcium homeostasis, and bone density in normal pregnancy. J Bone Miner Res 2000;15(3):557–63.
6. Moller UK, Streym S, Mosekilde L, et al. Changes in calcitropic hormones, bone markers and insulin-like growth factor I (IGF-I) during pregnancy and postpartum: a controlled cohort study. Osteoporos Int 2013;24(4):1307–20.
7. Kovacs CSCM, El-Hajj Fuleihan G. Disorders of mineral and bone metabolism during pregnancy and lactation. In: Kovacs CSDC, editor. Maternal-fetal and neonatal Endocrinology. Amsterdam, the Netherlands: Elsevier Academic Press; 2020. p. 329–70.
8. Ardawi MS, Nasrat HA, BA'Aqueel HS. Calcium-regulating hormones and parathyroid hormone-related peptide in normal human pregnancy and postpartum: a longitudinal study. Eur J Endocrinol 1997;137(4):402–9.
9. Gallacher SJ, Fraser WD, Owens OJ, et al. Changes in calciotrophic hormones and biochemical markers of bone turnover in normal human pregnancy. Eur J Endocrinol 1994;131(4):369–74.
10. Ritchie LD, Fung EB, Halloran BP, et al. A longitudinal study of calcium homeostasis during human pregnancy and lactation and after resumption of menses. Am J Clin Nutr 1998;67(4):693–701.
11. Moller UK, Vieth Streym S, Mosekilde L, et al. Changes in bone mineral density and body composition during pregnancy and postpartum. A controlled cohort study. Osteoporos Int 2012;23(4):1213–23.
12. Wermers RA, Khosla S, Atkinson EJ, et al. Incidence of primary hyperparathyroidism in Rochester, Minnesota, 1993-2001: an update on the changing epidemiology of the disease. J Bone Miner Res 2006;21(1):171–7.
13. Hirsch D, Kopel V, Nadler V, et al. Pregnancy outcomes in women with primary hyperparathyroidism. J Clin Endocrinol Metab 2015;100(5):2115–22.
14. Pallan S, Rahman MO, Khan AA. Diagnosis and management of primary hyperparathyroidism. BMJ 2012;344:e1013.
15. Palmieri-Sevier A, Palmieri GM, Baumgartner CJ, et al. Case report: long-term remission of parathyroid cancer: possible relation to vitamin D and calcitriol therapy. Am J Med Sci 1993;306(5):309–12.
16. Baretić M, Tomić Brzac H, Dobrenić M, et al. Parathyroid carcinoma in pregnancy. World J Clin Cases 2014;2(5):151–6.
17. Nadarasa K, Bailey M, Chahal H, et al. The use of cinacalcet in pregnancy to treat a complex case of parathyroid carcinoma. Endocrinol Diabetes Metab Case Rep 2014;2014:140056.
18. Nilsson IL, Adner N, Reihner E, et al. Primary hyperparathyroidism in pregnancy: a diagnostic and therapeutic challenge. J Womens Health (Larchmt) 2010;19(6):1117–21.
19. El-Hajj Fuleihan GBE. Familial hypocalciuric hypercalcemia and neonatal severe hyperparathyroidism. In: Bilezikian JPMR, Levine MA, Marcocci C, et al, editors. The parathyroids: basic and clinical concepts. 3rd edition. Amsterdam, the Netherlands: Academic Press; 2014. p. 365–87.

20. Jones AR, Hare MJ, Brown J, et al. Familial hypocalciuric hypercalcemia in pregnancy: diagnostic pitfalls. JBMR Plus 2020;4(6):e10362.
21. Powell BR, Buist NR. Late presenting, prolonged hypocalcemia in an infant of a woman with hypocalciuric hypercalcemia. Clin Pediatr (Phila) 1990;29(4):241–3.
22. Thomas BR, Bennett JD. Symptomatic hypocalcemia and hypoparathyroidism in two infants of mothers with hyperparathyroidism and familial benign hypercalcemia. J Perinatol 1995;15(1):23–6.
23. Morton A. Milk-alkali syndrome in pregnancy, associated with elevated levels of parathyroid hormone-related protein. Intern Med J 2002;32(9–10):492–3.
24. Sato K. Hypercalcemia during pregnancy, puerperium, and lactation: review and a case report of hypercalcemic crisis after delivery due to excessive production of PTH-related protein (PTHrP) without malignancy (humoral hypercalcemia of pregnancy). Endocr J 2008;55(6):959–66.
25. Winter EM, Appelman-Dijkstra NM. Parathyroid hormone-related protein-induced hypercalcemia of pregnancy successfully reversed by a dopamine agonist. J Clin Endocrinol Metab 2017;102(12):4417–20.
26. Lepre F, Grill V, Ho PW, et al. Hypercalcemia in pregnancy and lactation associated with parathyroid hormone-related protein. N Engl J Med 1993;328(9):666–7.
27. Eller-Vainicher C, Ossola MW, Beck-Peccoz P, et al. PTHrP-associated hypercalcemia of pregnancy resolved after delivery: a case report. Eur J Endocrinol 2012; 166(4):753–6.
28. Jacobs TP, Kaufman M, Jones G, et al. A lifetime of hypercalcemia and hypercalciuria, finally explained. J Clin Endocrinol Metab 2014;99(3):708–12.
29. Shah AD, Hsiao EC, O'Donnell B, et al. Maternal hypercalcemia due to failure of 1,25-dihydroxyvitamin-D3 catabolism in a patient with CYP24A1 mutations. J Clin Endocrinol Metab 2015;100(8):2832–6.
30. Kwong WT, Fehmi SM. Hypercalcemic pancreatitis triggered by pregnancy with a CYP24A1 mutation. Pancreas 2016;45(6):e31–2.
31. Hedberg F, Pilo C, Wikner J, et al. Three sisters with heterozygous gene variants of CYP24A1: maternal hypercalcemia, new-onset hypertension, and neonatal hypoglycemia. J Endocr Soc 2019;3(2):387–96.
32. Kolnick L, Harris BD, Choma DP, et al. Hypercalcemia in pregnancy: a case of milk-alkali syndrome. J Gen Intern Med 2011;26(8):939–42.
33. D'Souza R, Gandhi S, Fortinsky KJ, et al. Calcium carbonate intoxication in pregnancy: the return of the milk-alkali syndrome. J Obstet Gynaecol Can 2013; 35(11):976–7.
34. Trezevant MS, Winton JC, Holmes AK. Hypercalcemia-induced pancreatitis in pregnancy following calcium carbonate ingestion. J Pharm Pract 2019;32(2): 225–7.
35. Matsen SL, Yeo CJ, Hruban RH, et al. Hypercalcemia and pancreatic endocrine neoplasia with elevated PTH-rP: report of two new cases and subject review. J Gastrointest Surg 2005;9(2):270–9.
36. Ghazi AA, Boustani I, Amouzegar A, et al. Postpartum hypercalcemia secondary to a neuroendocrine tumor of pancreas; a case report and review of literature. Ir J Med Sci 2011;36(3):217–21.
37. Culbert EC, Schfirin BS. Malignant hypercalcemia in pregnancy: effect of pamidronate on uterine contractions. Obstet Gynecol 2006;108(3 Pt 2):789–91.
38. Illidge TM, Hussey M, Godden CW. Malignant hypercalcaemia in pregnancy and antenatal administration of intravenous pamidronate. Clin Oncol (R Coll Radiol 1996;8(4):257–8.

39. McCormick TC, Muffly T, Lu G, et al. Aggressive small cell carcinoma of the ovary, hypercalcemic type with hypercalcemia in pregnancy, treated with conservative surgery and chemotherapy. Int J Gynecol Cancer 2009;19(8):1339–41.

40. Hwang CS, Park SY, Yu SH, et al. Hypercalcemia induced by ovarian clear cell carcinoma producing all transcriptional variants of parathyroid hormone-related peptide gene during pregnancy. Gynecol Oncol 2006;103(2):740–4.

41. Usta IM, Chammas M, Khalil AM. Renal cell carcinoma with hypercalcemia complicating a pregnancy: case report and review of the literature. Eur J Gynaecol Oncol 1998;19(6):584–7.

42. Tarnawa E, Sullivan S, Underwood P, et al. Severe hypercalcemia associated with uterine leiomyoma in pregnancy. Obstet Gynecol 2011;117(2 Pt 2):473–6.

43. Smith D, Stevens J, Quinn J, et al. Myeloma presenting during pregnancy. Hematol Oncol 2014;32(1):52–5.

44. McIntosh J, Lauer J, Gunatilake R, et al. Multiple myeloma presenting as hypercalcemic pancreatitis during pregnancy. Obstet Gynecol 2014;124(2 Pt 2 Suppl 1):461–3.

45. DiMarco AN, Meeran K, Christakis I, et al. Seventeen cases of primary hyperparathyroidism in pregnancy: a call for management guidelines. J Endocr Soc 2019; 3(5):1009–21.

46. McCarthy A, Howarth S, Khoo S, et al. Management of primary hyperparathyroidism in pregnancy: a case series. Endocrinol Diabetes Metab Case Rep 2019; 2019. https://doi.org/10.1530/EDM-19-0039.

47. Dale AG, Holbrook BD, Sobel L, et al. Hyperparathyroidism in pregnancy leading to pancreatitis and preeclampsia with severe features. Case Rep Obstet Gynecol 2017;2017:6061313.

48. Rey E, Jacob C-E, Koolian M, et al. Hypercalcemia in pregnancy - a multifaceted challenge: case reports and literature review. Clin Case Rep 2016;4(10):1001–8.

49. Carella MJ, Gossain VV. Hyperparathyroidism and pregnancy: case report and review. J Gen Intern Med 1992;7(4):448–53.

50. Hultin H, Hellman P, Lundgren E, et al. Association of parathyroid adenoma and pregnancy with preeclampsia. J Clin Endocrinol Metab 2009;94(9):3394–9.

51. Schnatz PF, Thaxton S. Parathyroidectomy in the third trimester of pregnancy. Obstetrical Gynecol Surv 2005;60(10):672–82.

52. Lee C-C, Chao A-S, Chang Y-L, et al. Acute pancreatitis secondary to primary hyperparathyroidism in a postpartum patient: a case report and literature review. Taiwanese J Obstet Gynecol 2014;53(2):252–5.

53. Kohlmeier L, Marcus R. Calcium disorders of pregnancy. Endocrinol Metab Clin North Am 1995;24(1):15–39.

54. Negishi H, Kobayashi M, Nishida R, et al. Primary hyperparathyroidism and simultaneous bilateral fracture of the femoral neck during pregnancy. J Trauma Acute Care Surg 2002;52(2).

55. Shani H, Sivan E, Cassif E, et al. Maternal hypercalcemia as a possible cause of unexplained fetal polyhydramnion: a case series. Am J Obstet Gynecol 2008; 199(4):410.e1–5.

56. Razavi CR, Charitou M, Marzouk M. Maternal atypical parathyroid adenoma as a cause of newborn hypocalcemic tetany. Otolaryngol Head Neck Surg 2014; 151(6):1084–5.

57. Çakır U, Alan S, Erdeve Ö, et al. Late neonatal hypocalcemic tetany as a manifestation of unrecognized maternal primary hyperparathyroidism. Turk J Pediatr 2013;55(4):438–40.

58. Gokkaya N, Gungor A, Bilen A, et al. Primary hyperparathyroidism in pregnancy: a case series and literature review. Gynecol Endocrinol 2016;32(10):783–6.
59. Ghaznavi SA, Saad NM, Donovan LE. The biochemical profile of familial hypocalciuric hypercalcemia and primary hyperparathyroidism during pregnancy and lactation: two case reports and review of the literature. Case Rep Endocrinol 2016;2016:2725486.
60. Pollak MR, Chou YH, Marx SJ, et al. Familial hypocalciuric hypercalcemia and neonatal severe hyperparathyroidism. Effects of mutant gene dosage on phenotype. J Clin Invest 1994;93(3):1108–12.
61. Bilezikian JP, Brandi ML, Eastell R, et al. Guidelines for the management of asymptomatic primary hyperparathyroidism: summary statement from the fourth international workshop. J Clin Endocrinol Metab 2014;99(10):3561–9.
62. Vitetta GM, Neri P, Chiecchio A, et al. Role of ultrasonography in the management of patients with primary hyperparathyroidism: retrospective comparison with technetium-99m sestamibi scintigraphy. J Ultrasound 2014;17(1):1–12.
63. Sepahdari AR, Bahl M, Harari A, et al. Predictors of multigland disease in primary hyperparathyroidism: a scoring system with 4D-CT imaging and biochemical markers. AJNR Am J Neuroradiol 2015;36(5):987–92.
64. Jain C. ACOG Committee Opinion No. 723: guidelines for diagnostic imaging during pregnancy and lactation. Obstet Gynecol 2019;133(1):186.
65. Gilbert WM, Newman PS, Eby-Wilkens E, et al. Technetium Tc 99m rapidly crosses the ovine placenta and intramembranous pathway. Am J Obstet Gynecol 1996;175(6):1557–62.
66. Schaefer C, Meister R, Wentzeck R, et al. Fetal outcome after technetium scintigraphy in early pregnancy. Reprod Toxicol 2009;28(2):161–6.
67. LeGrand SB, Leskuski D, Zama I. Narrative review: furosemide for hypercalcemia: an unproven yet common practice. Ann Intern Med 2008;149(4):259–63.
68. Kaye AB, Bhakta A, Moseley AD, et al. Review of cardiovascular drugs in pregnancy. J Womens Health (Larchmt) 2019;28(5):686–97.
69. Shah VN, Shah CS, Bhadada SK, et al. Effect of 25 (OH) D replacements in patients with primary hyperparathyroidism (PHPT) and coexistent vitamin D deficiency on serum 25(OH) D, calcium and PTH levels: a meta-analysis and review of literature. Clin Endocrinol (Oxf) 2014;80(6):797–803.
70. Marcocci C, Bollerslev J, Khan AA, et al. Medical management of primary hyperparathyroidism: proceedings of the Fourth International Workshop on the Management of Asymptomatic Primary Hyperparathyroidism. J Clin Endocrinol Metab 2014;99(10):3607–18.
71. Briggs G, Freeman R, Yaffe S. A reference guide to fetal and neonatal risk: drugs in pregnancy and lactation. 5th edition. Philadelphia: Williams and Wilkins; 1998. p. 131–2.
72. Patlas N, Golomb G, Yaffe P, et al. Transplacental effects of bisphosphonates on fetal skeletal ossification and mineralization in rats. Teratology 1999;60(2):68–73.
73. Machairiotis N, Ntali G, Kouroutou P, et al. Clinical evidence of the effect of bisphosphonates on pregnancy and the infant. Horm Mol Biol Clin Investig 2019; 40(2). https://doi.org/10.1515/hmbci-2019-0021.
74. Bashir M, Mokhtar M, Baagar K, et al. A case of hyperparathyroidism treated with cinacalcet during pregnancy. AACE Clin Case Rep 2019;5(1):e40–3.
75. Horton WB, Stumpf MM, Coppock JD, et al. Gestational primary hyperparathyroidism due to ectopic parathyroid adenoma: case report and literature review. J Endocr Soc 2017;1(9):1150–5.

76. SENSIPAR product monograph. 2019. Available at: https://www.amgen.ca/products/~/media/5ed9d5863eab4c34b8c4e973562ecd51.ashx. Accessed February 15, 2021.
77. Boyce RW, Varela A, Chouinard L, et al. Infant cynomolgus monkeys exposed to denosumab in utero exhibit an osteoclast-poor osteoporotic-like skeletal phenotype at birth and in the early postnatal period. Bone 2014;64:314–25.
78. Levy HA, Pierucci L, Stroup P. Oral phosphates treatment of hypercalcemia in pregnancy. J Med Soc N J 1981;78(2):113–5.
79. Vernava AM 3rd, O'Neal LW, Palermo V. Lethal hyperparathyroid crisis: hazards of phosphate administration. Surgery 1987;102(6):941–8.
80. Tachamo N, Timilsina B, Dhital R, et al. Primary hyperparathyroidism in pregnancy: successful parathyroidectomy during first trimester. Case Rep Endocrinol 2018;2018:5493917.
81. Refardt J, Farina P, Hoesli I, et al. Hypercalcemic crisis in third trimester: evaluating the optimal treatment strategy. Gynecol Endocrinol 2018;34(10):833–6.
82. Hui E, Osakwe O, Teoh TG, et al. Three case reports of maternal primary hyperparathyroidism in each trimester and a review of optimal management in pregnancy. Obstet Med 2010;3(1):33–7.
83. Ali D, Divilly P, Prichard R, et al. Primary hyperparathyroidism and Zollinger Ellison syndrome during pregnancy: a case report. Endocrinol Diabetes Metab Case Rep 2021;2021.
84. Schnatz PF, Curry SL. Primary hyperparathyroidism in pregnancy: evidence-based management. Obstet Gynecol Surv 2002;57(6):365–76.
85. Dochez V, Ducarme G. Primary hyperparathyroidism during pregnancy. Arch Gynecol Obstet 2015;291(2):259–63.
86. Kelly TR. Primary hyperparathyroidism during pregnancy. Surgery 1991;110(6):1028–33 [discussion: 1033–4].
87. Kristoffersson A, Dahlgren S, Lithner F, et al. Primary hyperparathyroidism in pregnancy. Surgery 1985;97(3):326–30.
88. Rigg J, Gilbertson E, Barrett HL, et al. Primary hyperparathyroidism in pregnancy: maternofetal outcomes at a quaternary referral obstetric hospital, 2000 through 2015. J Clin Endocrinol Metab 2019;104(3):721–9.

Rare Causes of Hypercalcemia

Federica Saponaro, MD, PhD

KEYWORDS

- Rare hypercalcemia • Hypercalcemia in children • Milk-alkali syndrome
- Immobilization • Williams syndrome

KEY POINTS

- Immobilization hypercalcemia may be associated with low bone mass or osteoporosis and caused by a negative calcium balance.
- Some rare heritable diseases are associated with hypercalcemia in the first years of life, such as Williams-Beuren Syndrome, hypophosphatasia, and Jansen metaphyseal chondrodysplasia (JMC)
- Hypercalcemia can be rarely associated with cosmetic injections.
- Milk-alkali syndrome is caused by the use of calcium pharmaceutical products or absorbable alkali and is characterized by hypercalcemia, metabolic alkalosis, and acute kidney failure.
- Calcium sulfate beads administration, manganese intoxication, postacute kidney failure recovery and Paget disease are other rare causes of hypercalcemia.

INTRODUCTION

Hypercalcemia is generally related to a common endocrine disease such as Primary Hyperparathyroidism, but in less than 10% of cases it can represent the clue of rare diseases. In these cases, it is important to suspect unusual causes and conditions, to prompt the correct diagnosis and treatment. This article will cover rare causes of hypercalcemia.

IMMOBILIZATION HYPERCALCEMIA

Immobilization hypercalcemia was described for the first time by Albright in 1941 and subsequently demonstrated during polio epidemics, accompanying paraplegia.[1] Immobilization hypercalcemia may be associated with low bone mass or osteoporosis and caused by a negative calcium balance. It may occur after fractures (particularly hip fracture), severe burns, stroke, bariatric surgery, and more frequently in patients with

Department of Surgical, Medical, and Molecular Pathology and Critical Care Medicine, University of Pisa, via Roma 55, Pisa 56126, Italy
E-mail address: federica.saponaro@unipi.it

Endocrinol Metab Clin N Am 50 (2021) 769–779
https://doi.org/10.1016/j.ecl.2021.07.004
0889-8529/21/© 2021 Elsevier Inc. All rights reserved.

endo.theclinics.com

spinal cord injury (SCI). It seems to be more frequent in young patients or in those in whom a concurrent cause of high bone turnover is present (eg, myeloma, Paget disease, or cancer with bone metastases).[2] In patients with SCI, immobilization hypercalcemia occurs in 20% to 30% of cases. Risk factors are, in addition to prolonged immobilization, high cervical or complete SCI, age less than 21 years, male gender (probably because of higher bone mass compared with female gender), and tetraplegia more than paraplegia.[3–5] This rare form of hypercalcemia generally presents during the first 4 to 6 weeks after the initial cause of immobilization, but it can arise even months after.[6]

The etiopathogenesis of hypercalcemia caused by immobilization resides in an uncoupling of bone remodeling with an increased bone resorption. Immobilization results in a reduction of mechanical loading stimulus from muscle activity on osteocytes and suppression of bone formation.[6] This is probably mediated by sclerostin, which is increased in rodent models of unloading and in patients with short-term SCI.[7] After injury, bone resorption continues even after remobilization and calcium is excreted, leading to hypercalciuria; when calcium resorption exceeds urinary excretion, hypercalcemia occurs, with PTH suppression and $1,25(OH)_2D$ reduction.[8]

Hypercalcemia caused by immobilization can appear as insidious, without specific symptoms, or even be asymptomatic. Signs or symptoms, when present, include fatigue, lethargy, constipation, anorexia, nausea, vomiting, polydipsia, polyuria, and dehydration. Indeed, the injury itself and being bed ridden are the most suspicious anamnestic features.[9] Serum calcium levels are usually between 11.5 and 12 mg/dL. PTH should be evaluated for differential diagnosis; creatinine, creatinine clearance, blood urea nitrogen (BUN), and urinary calcium excretion should be measured to evaluate a concomitant or subsequent renal function deterioration.

Treatment options are rehabilitation and/or remobilization when possible, hydration with caution in patients with kidney failure, and loop diuretics. Bisphosphonates, such as zoledronic acid, are used, with restoration of normocalcemia within 5 days.[6] Denosumab efficacy in the treatment of immobilization hypercalcemia has been reported in several case reports, but its routine use is still uncertain.[10–12]

HYPERCALCEMIA CAUSED BY HERITABLE DISEASES IN CHILDREN

Hypercalcemia in children is less frequent than in adults. In addition to the same causes of rare hypercalcemia in adults, some rare heritable diseases are associated with hypercalcemia in the first years of life (**Box 1**).

Box 1
Hypercalcemia due to genetic causes in children

Williams-Beuren Syndrome

Hypophosphatasia

Jensen osteodystrophy

Congenital lactase deficiency

Down syndrome

Primary oxalosis

Williams Syndrome

Williams syndrome or Williams-Beuren Syndrome (WBS; OMIM #194050), first described by Williams in 1961, is a rare genetic systemic disorder, with a prevalence of 1 case per 7500 population.[13–15] It is generally a sporadic disease, but it can also present with an autosomal-dominant transmission.[16] It is caused by microdeletions of 26 to 28 genes on human chromosome 7, in q arm, which have been demonstrated in more than 90% of cases. It is known that deletions interest genes encoding for elastin and LIM-kinase (actin-binding kinase that phosphorylates members of the ADF/cofilin family of actin-binding proteins) explaining the cardiovascular and neurologic involvement of patients.[17] Hypercalcemia accompanying WBS was initially thought to depend from calcitonin receptor gene deletion on chromosome 7, which was not confirmed in a small series of patients with WBS.[18]

Patients show the typical elfin-like physiognomy (100%), congenital cardiovascular anomalies (70%-80% of patients) such as supra-vascular aortic stenosis and other arteriopathies, ventricular or atrial septal defects and myxomatous degeneration of aortic or mitral valve, pulmonary stenosis, hypertension, impairment of cognitive and behavioral profile (75%–90%), and skeletal and renal alterations.[17,19,20] Moreover, patients with WBS may present various endocrinopathies and hypercalcemia complicated by hypercalciuria and nephrocalcinosis. The incidence of hypercalcemia is highly variable among the available small series in literature and reported in 0% to 43% of cases.[21,22] In a recent study, Sindhar and colleagues[23] studied 232 patients with WBS and found hypercalcemia in 13% of them, with severe forms only in 6.1%. Generally, hypercalcemia is mild and decreases with growth. The mechanisms leading to hypercalcemia are not fully understood; a combination of gut absorption anomalies and/or decreased renal calcium clearance could be responsible for hypercalcemia. A revision of the 2001 health supervision guidelines for WBS was published in 2020 by the American Academy of Pediatrics; these guidelines suggest monitoring serum calcium levels every 4 to 6 months until 2 years of age and subsequently every 2 years or when a clinical suspicion of hypercalcemia is present.[24] In infants with hypercalcemia, a low calcium diet and hydration are usually enough to normalize serum calcium levels, even if parents should be advised to monitor calcium intake and consult endocrinologist specialists.[25] Vitamin D supplementation should be avoided, at least in early childhood.[13] When hypercalcemia is present, evaluation of circulating levels of PTH, 25OHD, and kidney function and renal ultrasound are recommended. Bone loss, low bone mass, and osteoporosis in adulthood are found in up to 50% of patients with WBS, and bone density should be monitored.[24]

Hypophosphatasia

Hypophosphatasia (OMIM no. 241500, no. 241510, no.146300) is a rare genetic disorder with heterogeneous phenotype ranging from severe forms at birth with seizure, nonmineralized bone, and hypercalcemia to mild variants diagnosed in young adults.[26] Because of its heterogeneous manifestations, the prevalence of the disease is difficult to be established, ranging from 1 case per 297,000 population for the most severe and rarest forms to 1 case per 6370 population for milder forms.[27–29] The genetic cause of the disease was characterized in 1988, when Weiss and colleagues[30] recognized that loss of function mutations in the gene *ALPL* (chromosome 1) encoding for the tissue nonspecific alkaline phosphatase (TNSALP) were pathogenetic. The modality of inheritance can be recessive, because of heterozygous or homozygous mutations or rarely uniparental disomy, or dominant.[31,32] It is possible to identify a genotype-phenotype correlation, with the autosomal-dominant form milder than the recessive form. Currently, more than 300 mutations have been described and characterized.[33,34] TNSALP is an isoenzyme of alkaline phosphatase (ALP) expressed on osteoblasts, crucial for the mineralization mechanism, because it controls the concentration of inorganic pyrophosphate (PPi) and contributes to matrix mineralization in bone. A circulating form also exists.[35] Extraskeletal effects of the disease in patients with hypophosphatasia are caused by the expression of TNSALP also in the liver, kidney, and brain.[36]

From a clinical point of view, it is possible to classify hypophosphatasia according to the presenting symptoms: benign perinatal form presenting during pregnancy, perinatal form severe or lethal, infantile form (symptoms within 6 months from birth), juvenile form, adult form, and odonto-form (only teeth symptoms).[37,38] Symptoms are highly variable depending from the time of onset, including life-threatening impaired bone mineralization, intracranial hemorrhages, deafness, muscle hypotonia, craniosynostosis, recurrent fractures, tooth loss, hypercalcemia with nephrocalcinosis, and kidney failure.[26]

Serum ALP is reduced in hypophosphatasia, and serum ALP levels are inversely correlated with the severity of symptoms. Hypercalcemia is generally present in pediatric forms; the pathophysiology of hypercalcemia resides in the defect of bone matrix mineralization. As a matter of fact, Ca^{++} and phosphate are not normally incorporated in hydroxyapatite and increase in blood, leading to hypercalcemia and hyperphosphatemia. Hypercalcemia is responsible suppression of circulating levels of PTH and $1,25(OH)_2D$ and later on for hypercalciuria and nephrolithiasis.[39]

Treatment depends on the clinical manifestations. Regarding bone metabolism, vitamin D supplementation is not advised, and a low calcium diet (Locasol milk), and oral or enteral hydration should be suggested; bone deformities should be referred to specialized orthopedists.

A milestone in hypophosphatasia treatment was reached in 2015, when the enzyme replacement therapy Asfotase Alfa was approved for severe cases at early onset.[40,41]

Jansen Metaphyseal Chondrodysplasia

Jansen metaphyseal chondrodysplasia (JMC) is a rare skeletal disorder characterized by abnormal growth plate and sclerosis of bones together with biochemical anomalies. It is generally diagnosed in the first years of life, and only rarely it is unrecognized until adulthood. JMC is caused by de novo gain of function mutations of the PTH receptor 1 (PTHR1), the most common being the H223R mutation, which is associated also with severe hypercalcemia.[42]

Radiographic features in these patients include low bone density and demineralization, rickets-like appearance, erosion of the bone cortex, and sclerosis of skull.[43,44] Hypercalcemia is generally severe and at early onset, despite low levels of circulating PTH or PTHrP[42]

COSMETIC HYPERCALCEMIA

Hypercalcemia associated with cosmetic injections is rare. However, because of the increasing spreading of cosmetic surgery worldwide, several cases have been recently described in literature. Fillers containing hyaluronic acid, collagen, and polymethylmethacrylate (PMMA) have been approved by the US Food and Drug Administration (FDA), while silicone injections are not; nevertheless they are frequently used.[45] Silicone can be injected in the site or inserted as silicone implants with an elastomer shell, which may rupture after trauma. The result is that this inorganic material could disperse in the body and form granulomas, reported in 0.02% to 1% of cases of cosmetics injections/administration.[46] Hypercalcemia complication from cosmetics granuloma can occur in these cases, and the physio-pathological hypothesis resides in the overproduction of 1,25(OH)$_2$D from activated macrophages directly in the granuloma, even if 1,25(OH)$_2$D serum levels can be normal.[47,48] The first case of hypercalcemia caused by cosmetic injection was described in 1984.[49] A recent systematic review from the literature reported 23 patients presenting hypercalcemia after cosmetic injections from 20 case report series: they were mainly females (78.3%), with mean age of 49.8 ± 14.7 years, who underwent mainly silicone treatment (43.5%) followed by PMMA and paraffin oil.[50] Hypercalcemia manifested several years after the initial treatment (8.0 ± 7.2 years) and was severe in all cases, with a mean albumin-adjusted serum calcium of 13.7 mg/dL. Other biochemical findings were high serum 1,25(OH)$_2$D levels in most cases and low/suppressed serum 25OHD and PTH levels. Severe hypercalcemia can lead to kidney failure (82.3%) and was fatal in 2 patients from these series.[50,51]

Cosmetics hypercalcemia can be conservatively treated, if mild, with hydration; in severe cases, corticosteroids and bisphosphonates (pamidronate was the most commonly used in the case-report series) are effective.[52] Surgical removal of granulomas, whenever possible, should be performed and may reverse hypercalcemia.[53] Unfortunately, surgery is not always possible, because of the migration of the silicone materials and the infiltrating nature of such granulomas.[50]

MILK-ALKALI SYNDROME

Milk-alkali syndrome (MAS) is caused by the use of calcium pharmaceutical products or absorbable alkali and it is characterized by hypercalcemia, metabolic alkalosis, and acute kidney failure. MAS has been considered a rare disease, but its frequency is recently increased and it is now the third cause of hypercalcemia among hospitalized patients (prevalence 9%–12%) and the first cause among patients with severe hypercalcemia (total serum calcium >14 mg/dL).[54,55] MAS was described for the first time in 1923 as a complication of the Sippy therapy for peptic ulcer, based on heavy alkali administration.[56] The profile of the disease has been changed over time with the recent increase of the use of calcium carbonate in patients with postmenopausal osteoporosis, use of chronic corticosteroid therapies, and availability of nonabsorbable alkali, histamine$_2$ receptor blockers, and proton pump inhibitors, which are all together the major causes of MAS nowadays.[57]

Hypercalcemia arises when the intestinal absorption of calcium is greater than its renal excretion, as it may occur in patients with reduced kidney function. Factors that contribute to the maintenance of hypercalcemia are volume depletion, reduced glomerular filtration rate, and metabolic alkalosis that stimulates renal resorption. Hypercalcemia may arise acutely or can be a chronic complication,[58] and may develop within days or months from the beginning of treatment. The acute form is known as Cope syndrome and the chronic form as Burnett syndrome, but MAS can be considered a spectrum. Symptoms include nausea, vomiting, anorexia, and confusion in the early phase, which may hesitate in psychosis; polyuria and ectopic calcification (keratopathy, nephrocalcinosis, and subcutaneous, periarticular, and brain calcifications) are seen in the chronic phase.[57] When hypercalcemia is severe, MAS may present as life-threatening condition that immediately requires stopping the intake of the responsible drugs, intravenous hydration and, eventually, furosemide to facilitate urinary calcium excretion. Symptoms generally disappear in a few days, but kidney injury may persist with kidney failure.[59,60]

CALCIUM SULFATE BEADS HYPERCALCEMIA

Calcium sulfate beads (CSBs) are biocompatible hydrophilic crystals, the use of which has increased in the last few years in orthopedic surgery complications such as peri-prosthetic joint infections, osteomyelitis, and open fractures.[61,62] CSBs are completely absorbable and act as antibiotics carrier material to deliver and release antibiotics directly in the infection site or as bone void filler.[63] Hypercalcemia has been described as a rare complication of CSB use and was firstly demonstrated in an animal dog model.[64] A recent systematic review on the complications of CSB procedures evaluated 5 studies and 770 patients; in 44 of them, moderate transient hypercalcemia was reported (mean total serum calcium 11.7 mg/dL) and spontaneously resolved after a maximum of 5 days after CSB implantation.[65–67] In 2 patients, hypercalcemia was symptomatic and required hydration with saline and iv bisphosphonates; 1 patient had severe hypercalcemia (total serum calcium 14.2 mg/dL) and was treated in intensive care.[66,67] In this series, hypercalcemia was related to the volume of injected CSBs, and the authors concluded that patients who receive CSBs should be monitored for serum calcium after administration, particularly patients who are at risk for hypercalcemia, including those with renal insufficiency, immobilization, and history of calcium metabolism disorders.[68,69]

MANGANESE INTOXICATION

Manganese exposition poisoning appears as a Parkinson-like neurologic syndrome accompanied by a rare form of hypercalcemia.[70] In experimental model, in the 1970s, Chandra and colleagues[71] demonstrated that rabbits treated with manganese dioxide developed alteration in serum calcium, phosphate, and ALP levels. Subsequently, hypercalcemia was demonstrated also in patients exposed to manganese intoxication, and it seems to develop gradually after poisoning;[72] however, the physiopathological mechanism still needs to be completely elucidated.

POSTACUTE KIDNEY FAILURE HYPERCALCEMIA

Hypercalcemia may occur during the recovery phase after an acute kidney failure/injury (AKI) and it is due to secondary hyperparathyroidism caused by hyperphosphatemia and hypocalcemia during the oliguric initial phase.[73]

Some rare cases of hypercalcemia have been described during the recovery phase of AKI caused by rhabdomyolysis, a condition resulting from severe muscle trauma or myotoxins and hesitating in AKI in 10% to 65% of cases.[74] In the initial phase of rhabdomyolysis-related AKI calcium phosphate deposits are formed in the injured muscles.[75] During the recovery from the diuretic phase of AKI, the dissolution of calcium-phosphate deposits causes hypercalcemia.[76] Hypercalcemia may be severe (in some clinical cases total serum calcium was up to 20 mg/dL) and can last up to 10 days in most cases.[77]

HYPERCALCEMIA IN PAGET'S DISEASE

Hypercalcemia rarely occurs rarely in patients with Paget disease as a consequence of immobilization and/or in association with malignancy.[78] Moreover, hypercalcemia has been reported in 73 patients who had Paget disease associated with Primary Hyperparathyroidism (PHPT). This association is likely because of the coexistence of two common diseases of the elderly, rather than being inter-related.[79] In these cases, clinical features and treatment of hypercalcemia are the same as in patients with isolated PHPT.[80]

CLINICS CARE POINTS

- In immobilization hypercalcemia, treatment options to be considered are rehabilitation and/or remobilization when possible, hydration with caution in patients with kidney failure, loop diuretics, and bisphosphonates.
- In children, hypercalcemia occurs less frequently than in adults, but it is needed to pay attention to some rare heritable diseases, which are associated with hypercalcemia in the first years of life.
- Because of increasing spreading of cosmetic surgery worldwide, hypercalcemia associated with cosmetic injections should be taken in account in hypercalcemia differential diagnosis.

DISCLOSURE

The authors have nothing to disclose.

REFERENCES

1. Albright F, Burnett CH, Cope O, et al. Acute atrophy of bone (osteoporosis) simulating hyperparathyroidism. J Clin Endocrinol Metab 1941. https://doi.org/10.1210/jcem-1-9-711.
2. Tsai WC, Wang WJ, Chen WL, et al. Surviving a crisis of immobilization hypercalcemia. J Am Geriatr Soc 2012. https://doi.org/10.1111/j.1532-5415.2012.04129.x.
3. Maynard FM. Immobilization hypercalcemia following spinal cord injury. Arch Phys Med Rehabil 1986. https://doi.org/10.5555/uri:pii:0003999386905034.
4. Benjamin RW, Moats-Staats BM, Calikoglu's A, et al. Hypercalcemia in children. Pediatr Endocrinol Rev 2008. https://doi.org/10.36485/1561-6274-2020-24-2-42-51.
5. Linstow M v, Biering-Sørensen F. Immobilisation-induced hypercalcemia following spinal cord injury affecting the kidney function in two young native Greenlanders. Spinal Cord Ser Cases 2017. https://doi.org/10.1038/scsandc.2017.10.
6. Cano-Torres EA, González-Cantú A, Hinojosa-Garza G, et al. Immobilization induced hypercalcemia. Clin Cases Miner Bone Metab 2016. https://doi.org/10.11138/ccmbm/2016.13.1.046.
7. Battaglino RA, Sudhakar S, Lazzari AA, et al. Circulating sclerostin is elevated in short-term and reduced in long-term SCI. Bone 2012. https://doi.org/10.1016/j.bone.2012.04.019.
8. Stewart AF, Adler M, Byers CM, et al. Calcium homeostasis in immobilization: an example of resorptive hypercalciuria. N Engl J Med 1982. https://doi.org/10.1056/nejm198205133061903.
9. Carroll MF, Schade DS. A practical approach to hypercalcemia. Am Fam Physician 2003. https://doi.org/10.1117/12.644391.
10. Malberti F. Treatment of immobilization-related hypercalcaemia with denosumab. Clin Kidney J 2012. https://doi.org/10.1093/ckj/sfs133.
11. De Beus E, Boer WH. Denosumab for treatment of immobilization-related hypercalcaemia in a patient with advanced renal failure. Clin Kidney J 2012. https://doi.org/10.1093/ckj/sfs116.
12. Uehara A, Yazawa M, Kawata A, et al. Denosumab for treatment of immobilization-related hypercalcemia in a patient with end-stage renal disease. CEN Case Rep 2017. https://doi.org/10.1007/s13730-017-0254-5.
13. Pober BR. Williams–beuren syndrome. N Engl J Med 2010. https://doi.org/10.1056/nejmra0903074.

14. Sammour ZM, Gomes CM, De Bessa J, et al. Congenital genitourinary abnormalities in children with Williams-Beuren syndrome. J Pediatr Urol 2014. https://doi.org/10.1016/j.jpurol.2014.01.013.
15. Strømme P, Bjømstad PG, Ramstad K. Prevalence estimation of Williams syndrome. J Child Neurol 2002. https://doi.org/10.1177/088307380201700406.
16. Martens MA, Wilson SJ, Reutens DC. Research review: Williams syndrome: a critical review of the cognitive, behavioral, and neuroanatomical phenotype. J Child Psychol Psychiatry Allied Discip 2008. https://doi.org/10.1111/j.1469-7610.2008.01887.x.
17. Leyfer OT, Woodruff-Borden J, Klein-Tasman BP, et al. Prevalence of psychiatric disorders in 4 to 16-year-olds with Williams syndrome. Am J Med Genet B Neuropsychiatr Genet 2006. https://doi.org/10.1002/ajmg.b.30344.
18. Stokes VJ, Nielsen MF, Hannan FM, et al. Hypercalcemic disorders in children. J Bone Miner Res 2017. https://doi.org/10.1002/jbmr.3296.
19. Twite MD, Stenquist S, Ing RJ. Williams syndrome. Paediatr Anaesth 2019. https://doi.org/10.1111/pan.13620.
20. Thomas Collins R. Cardiovascular disease in Williams syndrome. Curr Opin Pediatr 2018. https://doi.org/10.1097/MOP.0000000000000664.
21. Amenta S, Sofocleous C, Kolialexi A, et al. Clinical manifestations and molecular investigation of 50 patients with Williams syndrome in the Greek population. Pediatr Res 2005. https://doi.org/10.1203/01.PDR.0000157675.06850.68.
22. Sforzini C, Milani D, Fossali E, et al. Renal tract ultrasonography and calcium homeostasis in Williams-Beuren syndrome. Pediatr Nephrol 2002. https://doi.org/10.1007/s00467-002-0889-z.
23. Sindhar S, Lugo M, Levin MD, et al. Hypercalcemia in patients with Williams-Beuren Syndrome. J Pediatr 2016. https://doi.org/10.1016/j.jpeds.2016.08.027.
24. Morris CA, Braddock SR, Chen E, et al. Health care supervision for children with Williams syndrome. Pediatrics 2020. https://doi.org/10.1542/peds.2019-3761.
25. Lameris ALL, Geesing CLM, Hoenderop JGJ, et al. Importance of dietary calcium and vitamin D in the treatment of hypercalcaemia in Williams-Beuren syndrome. J Pediatr Endocrinol Metab 2014. https://doi.org/10.1515/jpem-2013-0229.
26. Linglart A, Biosse-Duplan M. Hypophosphatasia. Curr Osteoporos Rep 2016. https://doi.org/10.1007/s11914-016-0309-0.
27. Mornet E, Yvard A, Taillandier A, et al. A molecular-based estimation of the prevalence of hypophosphatasia in the European population. Ann Hum Genet 2011. https://doi.org/10.1111/j.1469-1809.2011.00642.x.
28. McKiernan FE, Berg RL, Fuehrer J. Clinical and radiographic findings in adults with persistent hypophosphatasemia. J Bone Miner Res 2014. https://doi.org/10.1002/jbmr.2178.
29. McKiernan FE, Dong J, Berg RL, et al. Mutational and biochemical findings in adults with persistent hypophosphatasemia. Osteoporos Int 2017. https://doi.org/10.1007/s00198-017-4035-y.
30. Weiss MJ, Cole DEC, Ray K, et al. A missense mutation in the human liver/bone/kidney alkaline phosphatase gene causing a lethal form of hypophosphatasia. Proc Natl Acad Sci U S A 1988. https://doi.org/10.1073/pnas.85.20.7666.
31. Watanabe A, Satoh S, Fujita A, et al. Perinatal hypophosphatasia caused by uniparental isodisomy. Bone 2014. https://doi.org/10.1016/j.bone.2013.12.009.
32. Lia-Baldini AS, Muller F, Taillandier A, et al. A molecular approach to dominance in hypophosphatasia. Hum Genet 2001. https://doi.org/10.1007/s004390100546.
33. Taillandier A, Lia-Baldini AS, Mouchard M, et al. Twelve novel mutations in the tissue-nonspecific alkaline phosphatase gene (ALPL) in patients with various

forms of hypophosphatasia. Hum Mutat 2001. https://doi.org/10.1002/humu. 1154.

34. del Angel G, Reynders J, Negron C, et al. Large-scale in vitro functional testing and novel variant scoring via protein modeling provide insights into alkaline phosphatase activity in hypophosphatasia. Hum Mutat 2020. https://doi.org/10.1002/humu.24010.

35. Whyte MP. Physiological role of alkaline phosphatase explored in hypophosphatasia. Ann N Y Acad Sci 2010. https://doi.org/10.1111/j.1749-6632.2010.05387.x.

36. Sebastián-Serrano Á, De Diego-García L, Martínez-Frailes C, et al. Tissue-nonspecific alkaline phosphatase regulates purinergic transmission in the central nervous system during development and disease. Comput Struct Biotechnol J 2015. https://doi.org/10.1016/j.csbj.2014.12.004.

37. Baujat G, Michot C, Le Quan Sang KH, et al. Perinatal and infantile hypophosphatasia: clinical features and treatment. Arch Pediatr 2017. https://doi.org/10.1016/S0929-693X(18)30016-2.

38. Fallon MD, Teitelbaum SL, Weinstein RS, et al. Hypophosphatasia: clinicopathologic comparison of the infantile, childhood, and adult forms. Medicine (Baltimore) 1984. https://doi.org/10.1097/00005792-198401000-00002.

39. Girschick HJ, Schneider P, Kruse K, et al. Bone metabolism and bone mineral density in childhood hypophosphatasia. Bone 1999. https://doi.org/10.1016/S8756-3282(99)00164-7.

40. Kocijan R, Haschka J, Feurstein J, et al. New therapeutic options for bone diseases. Wiener Medizinische Wochenschrift 2021. https://doi.org/10.1007/s10354-020-00810-w.

41. Whyte MP, Greenberg CR, Salman NJ, et al. Enzyme-replacement therapy in life-threatening hypophosphatasia. N Engl J Med 2012. https://doi.org/10.1056/nejmoa1106173.

42. Nampoothiri S, Fernández-Rebollo E, Yesodharan D, et al. Jansen metaphyseal chondrodysplasia due to heterozygous H223R-PTH1R mutations with or without overt hypercalcemia. J Clin Endocrinol Metab 2016. https://doi.org/10.1210/jc.2016-2054.

43. Holthusen W, Holt JF, Stoeckenius M. The skull in metaphyseal chondrodysplasia type Jansen. Pediatr Radiol 1975. https://doi.org/10.1007/BF01006898.

44. Khan R, Oakes P, Fisahn C, et al. Skull base and cervical spine involvement in Jansen Syndrome: case report. Pediatr Neurosurg 2017. https://doi.org/10.1159/000455924.

45. Funt D, Pavicic T. Dermal fillers in aesthetics: an overview of adverse events and treatment approaches. Clin Cosmet Investig Dermatol 2013. https://doi.org/10.2147/CCID.S50546.

46. Lemperle G, Gauthier-Hazan N, Wolters M, et al. Foreign body granulomas after all injectable dermal fillers: Part 1. possible causes. Plast Reconstr Surg 2009. https://doi.org/10.1097/PRS.0b013e31818236d7.

47. Visnyei K, Samuel M, Heacock L, et al. Hypercalcemia in a male-to-female transgender patient after body contouring injections: a case report. J Med Case Rep 2014. https://doi.org/10.1186/1752-1947-8-71.

48. Saponaro F, Saba A, Zucchi R. An update on vitamin d metabolism. Int J Mol Sci 2020;21(18):1–19. https://doi.org/10.3390/ijms21186573.

49. Kozeny GA, Barbato AL, Bansal VK, et al. Hypercalcemia associated with silicone-induced granulomas. N Engl J Med 1984. https://doi.org/10.1056/nejm198410253111707.

50. Tachamo N, Donato A, Timilsina B, et al. Hypercalcemia associated with cosmetic injections: a systematic review. Eur J Endocrinol 2018;178(4):425–30.
51. Khan O, Sim JJ. Silicone-induced granulomas and renal failure. Dial Transpl 2010. https://doi.org/10.1002/dat.20448.
52. Dangol GMS, Negrete H. Silicone-induced granulomatous reaction causing severe hypercalcemia: case report and literature review. Case Rep Nephrol 2019. https://doi.org/10.1155/2019/9126172.
53. Edwards BJ, Saraykar S, Sun M, et al. Resection of granulomatous tissue resolves silicone induced hypercalcemia. Bone Rep 2016. https://doi.org/10.1016/j.bonr.2015.07.001.
54. Picolos MK, Lavis VR, Orlander PR. Milk-alkali syndrome is a major cause of hypercalcaemia among non-end-stage renal disease (non-ESRD) inpatients. Clin Endocrinol (Oxf) 2005. https://doi.org/10.1111/j.1365-2265.2005.02383.x.
55. Minisola S, Pepe J, Piemonte S, et al. The diagnosis and management of hypercalcaemia. BMJ 2015. https://doi.org/10.1136/bmj.h2723.
56. Cooke AM. Alkalosis occurring in the alkaline treatment of peptic ulcers. QJM 1932. https://doi.org/10.1093/oxfordjournals.qjmed.a066602.
57. Medarov BI. Milk-alkali syndrome. Mayo Clin Proc 2009. https://doi.org/10.4065/84.3.261.
58. Felsenfeld AJ, Levine BS. Milk alkali syndrome and the dynamics of calcium homeostasis. Clin J Am Soc Nephrol 2006. https://doi.org/10.2215/CJN.01451005.
59. Patel V, Mehra D, Ramirez B, et al. Milk-alkali syndrome as a cause of hypercalcemia in a gentleman with acute kidney injury and excessive antacid intake. Cureus 2021. https://doi.org/10.7759/cureus.13056.
60. Haubrich WS. Burnett of Burnett's syndrome. Gastroenterology 2000. https://doi.org/10.1016/s0016-5085(00)70314-3.
61. Helgeson MD, Potter BK, Tucker CJ, et al. Antibiotic-impregnated calcium sulfate use in combat-related open fractures. Orthopedics 2009. https://doi.org/10.3928/01477447-20090501-03.
62. Cooper JJ, Florance H, McKinnon JL, et al. Elution profiles of tobramycin and vancomycin from high-purity calcium sulphate beads incubated in a range of simulated body fluids. J Biomater Appl 2016. https://doi.org/10.1177/0885328216663392.
63. Wahl P, Livio F, Jacobi M, et al. Systemic exposure to tobramycin after local antibiotic treatment with calcium sulphate as carrier material. Arch Orthop Trauma Surg 2011. https://doi.org/10.1007/s00402-010-1192-2.
64. Peltier LF. The use of plaster of paris to fill large defects in bone. A preliminary report. Am J Surg 1959. https://doi.org/10.1016/0002-9610(59)90305-8.
65. Abosala A, Ali M. The use of calcium sulphate beads in periprosthetic joint infection, a systematic review. J Bone Jt Infect 2020. https://doi.org/10.7150/jbji.41743.
66. Kallala R, Haddad FS. Hypercalcaemia following the use of antibiotic-eluting absorbable calcium sulphate beads in revision arthroplasty for infection. Bone Joint J 2015. https://doi.org/10.1302/0301-620X.97B9.34532.
67. Kallala R, Harris WE, Ibrahim M, et al. Use of Stimulan absorbable calcium sulphate beads in revision lower limb arthroplasty: safety profile and complication rates. Bone Joint Res 2018;7(10):570–9. https://doi.org/10.1302/2046-3758.710.BJR-2017-0319.R1.
68. Vora A, Ali S. Prolonged hypercalcemia from antibiotic-eluting calcium sulfate beads. AACE Clin Case Rep 2019. https://doi.org/10.4158/accr-2019-0194.

69. Lane K, Kim S, Grock S, et al. MON-345 hypercalcemia after placement of antibiotic-loaded calcium sulfate beads. J Endocr Soc 2020. https://doi.org/10.1210/jendso/bvaa046.1173.
70. Jacobs TP, Bilezikian JP. Clinical review: rare causes of hypercalcemia. J Clin Endocrinol Metab 2005. https://doi.org/10.1210/jc.2005-0675.
71. Chandra SV, Imam Z, Nagar N. Significance of serum calcium, inorganic phosphates and alkaline phosphatase in experimental manganese toxicity. Ind Health 1973. https://doi.org/10.2486/indhealth.11.43.
72. Chandra SV, Seth PK, Mankeshwar JK. Manganese poisoning: clinical and biochemical observations. Environ Res 1974. https://doi.org/10.1016/0013-9351(74)90038-3.
73. Kelly KJ. Acute kidney injury. In: Comprehensive toxicology. 3rd edition; 2017. https://doi.org/10.1016/B978-0-12-801238-3.95645-9.
74. Holt SG, Moore KP. Pathogenesis and treatment of renal dysfunction in rhabdomyolysis. Intensive Care Med 2001. https://doi.org/10.1007/s001340100878.
75. Vanholder R, Sever MS, Erek E, et al. Rhabdomyolysis. J Am Soc Nephrol 2000; 11(8):1553–61. https://doi.org/10.1681/ASN.V1181553.
76. Shrestha SM, Berry JL, Davies M, et al. Biphasic hypercalcemia in severe rhabdomyolysis: serial analysis of PTH and vitamin D metabolites. A case report and literature review. Am J Kidney Dis 2004. https://doi.org/10.1053/j.ajkd.2003.10.045.
77. Hechanova LA, Sadjadi SA. Severe hypercalcemia complicating recovery of acute kidney injury due to rhabdomyolysis. Am J Case Rep 2014. https://doi.org/10.12659/AJCR.891046.
78. Reifenstein EC, Albright F. Paget's disease: its pathologic physiology and the importance of this in the complications arising from fracture and immobilization. N Engl J Med 1944. https://doi.org/10.1056/nejm194409072311001.
79. Pino Rivero V, Trinidad Ruiz G, Pardo Romero G, et al. Association between primary hyperparathyroidism and Paget's disease. Report of a case. An Otorrinolaringol Ibero Am 2005;32(4):317–22.
80. Brandi ML, Falchetti A. What is the relationship between Paget's disease of bone and hyperparathyroidism? J Bone Miner Res 2007. https://doi.org/10.1359/JBMR.06S213.

Treatment of Hypercalcemia of Malignancy

Marlene Chakhtoura, MD, MSc, Ghada El-Hajj Fuleihan, MD, MPH, FRCP*

KEYWORDS

- Cancer • Hypercalcemia of malignancy • Fluids • Furosemide
- Antiresorptive therapy • Bisphosphonates • Denosumab • Refractory

KEY POINTS

- Osteoclast-mediated bone resorption is the final common pathway in hypercalcemia of malignancy.
- Therapies consist of restoring intravascular volume, increasing renal calcium excretion, and decreasing bone resorption.
- The effect of hydration and calcitonin occurs within hours, whereas that of zoledronic acid and denosumab occurs in 2 to 3 days, and lasts few weeks.
- Intravenous zoledronic acid constitutes the first-line therapy.
- Denosumab is the alternative treatment of refractory cases or those with renal failure.

INTRODUCTION

Cancer is among the leading causes of death from noncommunicable diseases worldwide. Based on 2015 to 2017 data, approximately 39.5% of men and women will be diagnosed with cancer at some point during their lifetime.[1] Hypercalcemia of malignancy (HCM) was first described in 1921 and occurs in 20% to 30% of patients with advanced cancer at some point during the clinical course.[2,3] The most common solid cancers associated with HCM are breast cancer, renal cell carcinoma, and all types of squamous cell cancer. For liquid tumors, multiple myeloma takes the lead; the others are leukemias and non-Hodgkin lymphomas.[4,5] Humoral HCM, mediated by parathyroid hormone-related protein (PTHrP), constitutes most cases (>80%), in cancers of the breast, lung, and kidney, followed by direct bone involvement/metastases (multiple myeloma, breast cancer), calcitriol-mediated hypercalcemia (lymphomas and leukemias), and rarely parathyroid carcinoma or ectopic secretion of PTH by some cancers (ovarian, lung, gastric, pancreatic, and neuroectodermal tumors). Osteoclastic bone resorption is the final common pathway for the development

Calcium Metabolism and Osteoporosis Program, Division of Endocrinology, WHO Collaborating Center for Metabolic Bone Disorders, American University of Beirut, PO Box 11-236, Riad El-Solh, Beirut 1107 2020, Lebanon
* Corresponding author.
E-mail address: gf01@aub.edu.lb

Endocrinol Metab Clin N Am 50 (2021) 781–792
https://doi.org/10.1016/j.ecl.2021.08.002   endo.theclinics.com
0889-8529/21/© 2021 Elsevier Inc. All rights reserved.

of HCM in all cases, which in the case of bone metastases involves other bone-resorbing cytokines,[6] and thus the central role of antiresorptive drugs in its treatment. The receptor activator of nuclear factor kappa-B (RANK)-RANK ligand (RANKL) system plays a central role in the pathophysiology of HCM.

HCM is usually considered a poor prognostic sign, with an estimated median survival rate between 30 days and 2 to 3 months, regardless of the active treatment in older studies.[7,8] Survival in patents with HCM may have improved with advanced antineoplastic, adjuvant, and immune therapy, and thus the need for safe and effective treatment. The clinical manifestations of HCM are nonspecific, and symptoms are closely related to the serum absolute calcium level (SCa), and the rapidity with which it was reached.[9] The severity of hypercalcemia can be defined as mild (SCa < 12 mg/dL or 3 mmol/L), moderate (SCa 12–14 mg/dL that is 3–3.5 mmol/L), or severe (>14 mg/dL that is 3.5 mmol/L). The grading of hypercalcemia can also be defined according to the Common Terminology Criteria for Adverse Events[10] as grade 1: corrected SCa between upper limits of normal, 11.5 mg/dL (up to 2.9 mmol/L); grade 2: corrected SCa greater than 11.5 to 12.5 mg/dL (>2.9–3.1 mmol/L); grade 3: corrected SCa greater than 12.5 to 13.5 mg/dL (>3.1–3.4 mmol/L); and grade 4: corrected SCa greater than 13.5 mg/dL (>3.4 mmol/L).[10] Total SCa often reflects serum ionized calcium levels, with the exception of conditions that affect serum albumin or protein levels, or abnormalities in serum pH, in such a manner that total calcium may be high or low but ionized calcium may be normal. Notoriously, high protein levels such as seen in multiple myeloma, a condition known to be associated with HCM, results in pseudohypercalcemia.[11] Symptoms are rarely seen in patients with mild hypercalcemia and can be absent in patients with moderate elevation if the progression is slow. Symptoms are usually present in severe hypercalcemia.[9] Renal failure and coma are dreaded complications rendering this condition an oncologic emergency.

Therapeutic interventions for HCM are based on correction of hypovolemia, enhancing calcium excretion with fluids and occasionally loop diuretics, and decreasing bone resorption with antiresorptive drugs.[6,12] Fluid hydration constitutes the earliest treatment because of the rapidity of therapeutic effect, occasionally with the addition of furosemide as loop diuretic, calcitonin for its equally fast onset of action, in combination with potent antiresorptive drugs such as bisphosphonates (BP) or denosumab (Dmab) (**Table 1**). The therapeutic strategy may combine antiresorptive drugs with glucocorticoids in cases caused by elevated calcitriol levels, or calcimimetics in cases of parathyroid carcinoma or ectopic PTH secretion.[9] The mode of action, doses, route of administration, onset, and duration of therapeutic effect of the various drugs used in HCM are outlined in **Table 1**. The treatment of vitamin D-mediated hypercalcemia, and of HCM from PTH hypersecretion are discussed in detail in the articles Karl Peter Schlingmann article, "Vitamin D-Dependent Hypercalcemia" and Filomena Cetani, and colleagues' article, "Parathyroid Carcinoma and Ectopic Secretion of PTH" in this issue. In rare cases of very severe hypercalcemia (SCa greater than 17–18 mg/dL [4.25–4.5 mmol/L]), with symptomatic HCM and neurologic symptoms, or severe renal failure, hemodialysis is an option provided the patient is hemodynamically stable.[13–15] HCM usually represents aggressive, advanced, or progressive disease, and thus the need to concomitantly treat the underlying cancer, to prevent recurrence.

FLUIDS, LASIX, CALCITONIN
Fluids

Hydration constitutes the first step in the management of HCM. One small interventional study (N = 16 patients, majority with breast or lung cancer, SCa greater than

Table 1
Treatment regimens for hypercalcemia of malignancy[a]

Intervention Dose and Frequency	Mode of Action	Onset of Action	Duration of Action
Isotonic saline hydration Bolus of 1-2 L then 200–500 mL/h to maintain urine output at 100–150 mL/h	Restores depleted intravascular volume Enhances urinary calcium excretion	Immediate	During infusion
Loop diuretics[b] 160 mg/d–100 mg/h intravenously, or 40–60 mg/d orally	Increase urinary calcium excretion by inhibiting renal calcium reabsorption in the thick ascending loop of Henle and proximal and distal renal tubules Interferes with the chloride cotransport system	Within 3–60 min	2 h if bolus During therapy if IV drip
CT 4–8 units/kg SQ q 6–12 h	Inhibits bone resorption by interfering with osteoclast function Promotes urinary calcium excretion, as well as that of magnesium, sodium, potassium, and phosphate	4–6 h	IM and SC 6–8 h Tachyphylaxis at 48–72 h
BPs APD 60–90 mg IV over 2–6 h ZLN 3–4 mg IV over 15–30 min	APD and zoledronic acid are nitrogen-containing BPs Inhibit bone resorption by inhibiting FPPS within osteoclasts and causing osteoclast apoptosis. They also interfere with osteoclast recruitment and function	24–72 h	7–14 d May last 2–4 wk
Glucocorticoids Hydrocortisone 200-400 mg IV/d for 3-5 days Prednisone 60 mg/d for 10 d, or 10–20 mg/d for 7 d	Decrease intestinal calcium absorption Decrease 1,25-dihydroxyvitamin D production by activated mononuclear cells in patients with granulomatous diseases or lymphoma	2–5 d	As long as on therapy

(*continued on next page*)

Table 1 (continued)			
Intervention Dose and Frequency	**Mode of Action**	**Onset of Action**	**Duration of Action**
Dmab 120 mg SQ, repeat 1, 2, and 4 wk later, then monthly thereafter	Inhibits bone resorption via inhibition of RANKL. Dmab is an antibody to nuclear factor-kappa ligand (RANKL). Upon binding to RANKL, Dmab blocks the interaction between RANKL and RANKK (receptor on osteoclast surfaces) and prevents osteoclast formation and thus bone resorption	3–10 d	Time to complete response 23 d; median duration response 104 d
Oral calcimimetics: 30 mg twice daily; increase dose incrementally every 2–4 wk (to 60 mg twice daily, 90 mg twice daily, and 90 mg 3–4 times daily) as necessary to normalize serum calcium levels	Calcium-sensing receptor agonist, reduce PTH secretion	2–3 d	During therapy

Abbreviations: APD, pamidronate; CT, calcitonin; FPPS, farnesyl pyrophosphate synthase; IM, intramuscular; IV, intravenous; SC, subcutaneous; SQ, subcutaneous; ZLN, zoledronic acid.

[a] Information on mode of action, onset of action, and duration of effect obtained in part from Lexicomp Copyright 1978 to 2021, or relevant papers cited in this article.

[b] Loop diuretics should not be used routinely. However, in patients with renal insufficiency or heart failure, judicious use of loop diuretics may be required to prevent fluid overload during saline hydration.

13 mg/dL [3.25 mmol/L]) administered 0.9% NaCl, at the rate of 1 L every 6 hours for the first 48 hours, followed by 2 L daily until achieving the lowest SCa, and reported volume reexpansion within the first 48 hours.[16] With the lack of randomized controlled trials (RCTs) comparing various hydration protocols in patients with HCM, experts recommend isotonic fluid at the rate of 200 to 500 mL/h, possibly preceded by a bolus of 1 to 2 L, to maintain a urine output of 100 to 150 mL/h, taking into consideration the patient's renal and cardiac function.[2,17]

Furosemide

Old case reports and case series (N = 3–11 patients), published before 1983, described the use of furosemide in the treatment of HCM.[18] The doses used ranged between 160 mg/d and 100 mg/h intravenously (IV), or 40 and 60 mg/d orally, with concomitant fluid replacement, which reached in one case 40 L/d.[18] Although calcium levels dropped in all cases, there was a wide variability in the response between patients.[18] Therefore, furosemide may only be considered in patients prone to fluid overload and only after appropriate hydration.[18]

Calcitonin

Calcitonin has been traditionally considered as one of the initial treatment options of HCM. Calcitonin reduces serum calcium by suppressing bone resorption and by increasing calciuresis.[17] Calcitonin is an attractive option given its immediate effect, starting within the first 24 hours of treatment initiation, allowing a drop in SCa of 1.1 mg/dL (0.275 mmol/L) on day 1.[19,20] However, the efficacy of calcitonin weans off after 48 to 72 hours, possibly due to the development of antibodies.[19–21] Although calcitonin is typically given subcutaneously for the treatment of HCM, intramuscular[20] and intranasal preparations[22] have been used. An observational study, derived from a nationwide database in North Carolina, enrolled 4874 patients with HCM.[8] Calcitonin use was reported in 27% of cases, more so in patients with bone metastases, multiple myeloma, and renal injury,[8] and was not associated with any change in the length of hospital stay or mortality.[8] A recent retrospective study compared the use of BP (pamidronate [APD] or zoledronic acid [ZLN]) alone (n = 94) to BP with calcitonin (n = 46) in patients with HCM, most with a solid tumor.[23] Although the decrease in serum calcium at 48 hours favored the combination group, with a difference in the mean SCa of 1.4 (95% confidence interval [CI], 0.8–2.0) mg/dL (0.35 [0.2–0.5] mmol/L) between groups at 72 hours, time to normocalcemia, length of hospital stay, and mortality did not differ.[23] Furthermore, the investigators conducted a cost analysis and concluded that providers might consider restraining from prescribing it, in view of the high cost of calcitonin coupled with limited clinical benefit.[23] Serious hypersensitivity reactions including anaphylaxis have been reported, and a test dose should therefore be considered before treatment. Milder side effects include nausea (with or without vomiting, 10%), infection at the injection site (10%), and flushing of the face and hands (2%–5%).[24]

Following a signal for an increased risk of prostate cancer with the use of oral calcitonin, the US Food and Drug Administration (FDA) conducted a systematic review and meta-analysis of 21 RCTs and concluded that there was an increased risk of malignancy with calcitonin compared with placebo.[24,25] Therefore, the FDA indications for use include the treatment of Paget disease of bone, of postmenopausal osteoporosis, and of HCM. In the first 2 instances, it specifies use only in the event of contraindications, lack of tolerance, or response to established alternative treatments.[24] Calcitonin is indicated for the early treatment of hypercalcemic emergencies, along with other drugs.[24]

BISPHOSPHONATES AND DENOSUMAB

The main treatment of HCM consists of potent, long-lasting, antiresorptive drugs, such as IV BPs, still considered first-line cornerstone therapy to date. Subcutaneous Dmab is an alternative that is indicated in cases of refractory hypercalcemia or if renal function is severely compromised.[26] Nitrogen-containing BPs, such as alendronate, risedronate, and ZLN, but not clodronate, act through the mevalonate pathway and selectively inhibit farnesyl pyrophosphate synthase (FPPS) within osteoclasts. Osteoclast endocytosis of BP from the bone surface leads to FPPS inhibition and osteoclast apoptosis.[26] Dmab is a monoclonal antibody that works as a potent inhibitor of RANK ligand (RANKL).[26] BPs and Dmab are also approved by the FDA for the treatment of bone complications in patients with multiple myeloma and patients with solid tumors, in conjunction with standard antineoplastic therapy.[27,28] BPs and Dmab have been shown to decrease the skeletal complications in patients with multiple myeloma and the following solid tumors, prostate cancer, lung cancer, and breast cancer.

Bisphosphonates

Early RCTs have established the efficacy of IV BPs etidronate and clodronate, but these were rapidly superseded by the most potent and effective IV BPs APD and ZLN.[12] The onset of action occurs between 1 and 3 days, the nadir of SCa is achieved between days 4 and 7, and the response can last for 1 to 3 weeks (see **Table 1**).[29] Several small RCTs (total N = 32–86) compared the efficacy of older BP (clodronate, etidronate, APD), with each other[30–33] or with ZLN,[34,35] in the treatment of HCM. Before the year 2000, the most widely studied BP was APD, at a dose of 60 to 90 mg once. Compared with clodronate and etidronate, APD resulted in a lower SCa,[30,31] higher complete response rate,[33] and a longer time to relapse (10–14 days with clodronate and etidronate, and 28 days with APD).[30,32] Compared with ibandronate, APD was as efficacious in dropping the SCa, but it seemed less potent in patients with serum calcium levels greater than 14 mg/dL (3.5 mmol/L).[36] A network meta-analysis of a recent Cochrane systematic review identified 5 RCTs (total N = 1349 participants) evaluating the risk of HCM in patients with prostate cancer and skeletal metastasis, receiving BP therapy.[37] There was no significant reduction in the risk of developing HCM with the use of any BP (ZLN, APD, clodronate) compared with placebo/control, and there was no significant difference between individual BPs.[37] Another systematic review and meta-analysis targeted patients with biopsy-proven myeloma with bone involvement and identified 10 RCTs evaluating the risk of HCM (defined as an SCa $\geq$10.6 mg/dL [2.65 mmol/L]). The total N was 1349, with 3 RCTs for each clodronate and APD, 2 RCTs on ZLN, and 1 RCT on each etidronate and ibandronate.[38] There was no significant risk reduction with the use of BP compared with placebo/control.[38] One RCT compared etidronate (n = 25) with placebo (n = 37), given orally daily for 6 months in patients with solid or hematologic malignancy, who had been successfully treated for HCM.[39] There was no significant difference in mean serum calcium or in the time to recurrence of hypercalcemia between groups.[39]

Both APD and ZLN drugs are approved by the FDA for the treatment of HCM. However, ZLN remains the preferred therapy because of the ease of its use, as a 15-min infusion, as opposed to 2 hours with APD, and its superior efficacy.[34] Two identical, concurrent, parallel, multicenter, randomized, double-blind double-dummy trials compared the efficacy and safety of ZLN (4 or 8 mg via a 5-minute infusion) and APD (90 mg via 2-hour infusion) for treating patients with moderate to severe HCM (corrected SCa$\geq$ 12.0 mg/dL [3 mmol/L]). Both doses of ZLN were clearly superior to APD. The complete response rates by day 10 were 88.4% (P = .002) for ZLN 4 mg, 86.7% (P = .015) for ZLN 8 mg, and 69.7% for APD 90 mg. Normalization of corrected SCa occurred by day 4 in around 50% of patients treated with ZLN and in only 33.3% of the APD-treated patients. The median duration of complete response favored ZLN 4 and 8 mg over APD 90 mg, with response durations of 32, 43, and 18 days, respectively.[34]

ZLN is indicated for the treatment of HCM, defined as an albumin-corrected calcium greater than 12 mg/dL (3 mmol/L), using the formula corrected SCa mg/dL = SCa mg/dL+ 0.8 (4 g/dL − patient's albumin in g/dL).[40] The approved dose is 4 mg as a single IV dose administered in no less than 15 minutes. Owing to the risk of clinically significant deterioration in renal function, which may progress to renal failure, this dose should not be exceeded and the duration of administration should not be shortened. Patients should be adequately hydrated, with a urine output of 2 L/d. Adequate calcium and vitamin D intake are important to avoid the development of hypocalcemia. Serum creatinine level should be available before the infusion, and renal function should be monitored in all patients on ZLN. Dose adjustments are not necessary in treating patients with HCM and moderate renal impairment (serum creatinine <4.5 mg/dL).[27] Re-treatment with 4 mg can be given after a minimum of 7 days if SCa does not normalize or remains elevated after the first dose. The most common adverse reactions (>25%) are those of an acute phase reaction, fever, bone and joint pains, possibly nausea, fatigue, anemia, vomiting, and dyspnea, which usually resolve within 24 to 48 hours.[27] This reaction is less severe with repeated injections. Severe incapacitating bone, joint, and/or muscle pain may rarely occur and last days or weeks. Osteonecrosis of the jaw has been reported, dental examinations should be performed before the administration of ZLN, and invasive procedures are to be avoided. Atypical subtrochanteric femoral fractures (AFF) have been reported after minimal or no trauma. Patients with thigh or groin pain should be evaluated to rule out AFF, and discontinuation of ZLN is advised in patients suspected to have AFF. Severe incapacitating joint and muscle aches may occur, and in such instances ZLN should be discontinued.[27]

Denosumab

Comparison between zol and denosumab

Two similar multicenter noninferiority RCTs compared Dmab 120 mg subcutaneous with ZLN 4 mg IV, every 4 weeks, for 34 months, on the time to first skeletal-related event (SRE) as a primary outcome, in patients with breast cancer metastatic to the bone (total N = 2049, NCT00321464)[40] or advanced solid tumor, excluding breast or prostate cancer, or myeloma (total N = 1779, NCT00330759).[41] Hypercalcemia was not a prespecified outcome (NCT00330759[41] and NCT00321464)[40]. An exploratory analysis combining data from both RCTs (mean age 58 years, 70% women) showed a 32% reduction in the risk of the first episode of HCM, defined as an SCa greater than 11.5 mg/dL (2.875 mmol/L) (hazard ratio [HR] 0.63 [0.41–0.98]), with Dmab compared with ZLN, in patients with SCa 8 to 11.5 mg/dL (2–2.875 mmol/L) at study entry.[42] The number needed to treat was 12.3 patient-years.[42] Similarly, the risk of recurrent HCM was reduced by 52% (HR 0.48 [0.29–0.81]) with Dmab compared with ZLN.[42] A third RCT with a similar design evaluated the same interventions and outcomes in patients with prostate cancer and skeletal metastasis.[43] However, the rate of HCM was very low (<1%) in the overall study population, a rate that did not allow any conclusion on the efficacy of Dmab compared with ZLN in preventing HCM in this specific population.[43]

Refractory hypercalcemia of malignancy

Dmab is used for the treatment of BP-refractory HCM.[28] The evidence was initially based on case reports and case series of patients with hypercalcemia secondary to solid or hematologic malignancies, with wide variability in the presence of refractory HCM, and no or inadequate response after one or more courses of IV hydration and ZLN (1–4 courses).[44–47] All reported higher potency and longer-lasting effect with Dmab (dose 60 or 120 mg once). One multicenter open-label single-arm study enrolled 33 patients (median age 63 years; 64% men; 73% with solid malignancy) with refractory hypercalcemia, defined as SCa greater than 12.5 mg/dL (3.125 mmol/L), and having received BPs, with or without chemotherapy and hydration, in the previous 7 to 30 days.[48] Dmab was given at a dose of 120 mg subcutaneously on day 1, at weeks 1, 2, and 4, and then every 4 weeks. At day 10, 64% and 33% of patients had SCa ≤11.5 mg/dL (2.875 mmol/L) (primary outcome) and ≤10.8 mg/dL (2.7 mmol/L) (complete response), respectively. By the end of the study, the rates of partial and complete response increased to 70% and 64%, respectively. The median time to response was

9 (95% CI, 5–19) days, and the median duration of complete response was 34 (95% CI, 1–134) days. The time to relapse after a complete response was 114 days.[48] The positive findings from this study led to the FDA approval of Dmab (XGEVA) at a dose of 120 mg monthly, with additional doses at weeks 1 and 2 after the first injection, for the treatment of BP-refractory HCM.[28] To note, the prescribing information of XGEVA does not include a clear definition of the number of BP cycles characterizing refractory HCM.

PARATHYROID CRISIS

Parathyroid crisis is a rare entity characterized by an acute severe elevation in serum calcium level, usually greater than 14 mg/dL (3.5 mmol/L), associated with multiorgan involvement and manifestations, of which the gastrointestinal symptoms are the most common.[49] The causes of hypercalcemic crisis are similar to conditions in the differential diagnosis of hypercalcemia. The most common cause is primary hyperparathyroidism with baseline mild hypercalcemia, decompensated by immobilization, high-dose vitamin D, medications, and others.[49] The treatment approach consists of hydration, calcitonin, and BP, in case of HCM, in addition to glucocorticoid therapy in multiple myeloma and lymphoma.[49] Dialysis is the last resort, when other therapies fail, especially in patients with renal failure.[15]

ALTERNATIVE THERAPIES AND RESEARCH DIRECTIONS

ZLN remains the cornerstone therapy for HCM in view of its established efficacy, enduring effect for weeks, and acceptable risk-benefit profile. The potency of ZLN coupled with the availability of Dmab for select or refractory cases may explain the scarcity of alternative therapies on the horizon. PTHrP being the main mediator of HCM led to the development of PTHrP antibodies in an attempt to treat HCM, efforts that have been stalled by poor bone concentrations and a short half-life (see the article Mimi I. Hu article, "Hypercalcemia of Malignancy" in this issue); this led to the development of novel PTHrP antagonists containing collagen-binding domains, which were tested in mice models of breast and colon cancer; data published as abstract in scientific meetings.[50,51] The authors are unaware of any additional publications in mice, and they did not identify any on their use in humans. Other targets that address the pathophysiology of HCM are the PTH1 receptor or RANKL antagonists.

Cinacalcet is the only oral therapy available to date, and although only approved for parathyroid carcinoma, it could be used for other rare PTH-secreting tumors. Cinacalcet was also recently proposed as a potential treatment modality for HCM refractory to antiresorptive therapy, including BP and Dmab.[52] Several case reports from the United States, Europe, and New Zealand, in patients with solid tumors, and PTHrP-mediated HCM, showed a significant and sustainable drop and normalization of serum calcium level for up to 18 months, with cinacalcet at a dose of 60 to 120 mg/d.[52–54] The mechanism of action is not clear, although antagonizing the effect of the calcium receptor in bone and kidney is one possibility.

Searching ClinicalTrials.Gov for studies investigating therapies for refractory HCM reveals 2 trials. The first entitled "A Clinical Trial to Assess the Efficacy and Safety of JMT103 in Patients With Refractory HCM," NCT04198480, is a phase 1/2, single-arm, open-label, multicenter clinical trial that is anticipated to recruit 17 individuals and is sponsored by Shanghai JMT-Bio Inc and CSPC ZhongQi Pharmaceutical Technology Co, Ltd. Eligible subjects are to receive JMT103 at a dose of 2 mg/kg subcutaneously (SC) every 4 weeks with a loading dose of 2 mg/kg SC on study days 8 and 15.[55] JMT103 is a novel, full human IgG4 monoclonal antibody targeting RANKL. In preclinical studies, JMT103 demonstrated strong activity by blocking RANKL receptor, RANK on the surface of osteoclasts, leading to inhibition of osteoclast differentiation, activation, and maturation and reduction of bone resorption. The trial status is not yet recruiting, yet the completion date is anticipated by December 31, 2021. The second entitled "An Intra-individual Titration Study of KRN1493 for the Treatment of Hypercalcemia in Patients With Parathyroid Carcinoma or Intractable Primary Hyperparathyroidism," NCT01460030, is a phase 3 open-label trial investigating cinacalcet, posted as completed.[56] The study report includes 5 Japanese patients with parathyroid carcinoma and 2 with intractable PHPT enrolled in an open-label, single-arm study consisting of titration and maintenance phases. At the end of the titration phase, 1 mg/dL (0.25 mmol/L) minimal reduction in SCa concentration from the baseline was observed in 5 patients (3 with carcinoma and 2 with PHPT) and SCa decreased to the normocalcemic range in 5 patients (3 with carcinoma and 2 with PHPT).[56,57]

CLINICS CARE POINTS

- Fluid hydration with isotonic saline is the initial and most pressing treatment of HCM, keeping urine output at 150 to 200 mL/h, within the first 24 to 48 hours.
- Calcitonin is considered a bridging therapy with an onset of action within the first day and that lasts 2 to 3 days.
- IV BPs in general, and ZLN in particular, are considered cornerstone therapy with onset of action by 48 to 72 hours; they have a long-lasting effect for moderate and severe HCM. Redosing is indicated if the response is inappropriate after 7 days. Pretreatment creatinine level and monitoring thereafter are recommended.
- Dmab is the second-line treatment, indicated for BP-refractory HCM, based on an open-label single-arm study defining refractory HCM as a serum calcium level greater than 12.5 mg/dL in a patient who has received BPs in the previous 7 to 30 days.
- Findings from 2 systematic reviews and meta-analyses of RCTs in patients with prostate cancer or multiple myeloma showed there is no evidence that BPs prevent the occurrence of HCM.
- Dmab, compared with ZLN, is associated with a lower risk of HCM, both first episode and recurrence, in patients with breast cancer and multiple myeloma. Data on prostate cancer are inconclusive.

DISCLOSURE

Nothing to disclose.

REFERENCES

1. National Cancer Institute-Cancer Statistics. Available at: https://www.cancer.gov/about-cancer/understanding/statistics. Accessed July 6, 2021.
2. Stewart AF. Hypercalcemia associated with cancer. N Engl J Med 2005;352(4): 373–9.
3. Lumachi F, Brunello A, Roma A, et al. Cancer-induced hypercalcemia. Anticancer Res 2009;29(5):1551–5.
4. Vassilopoulou-Sellin R, Newman BM, Taylor SH, et al. Incidence of hypercalcemia in patients with malignancy referred to a comprehensive cancer center. Cancer 1993;71(4):1309–12.

5. Rosner MH, Dalkin AC. Onco-nephrology: the pathophysiology and treatment of malignancy-associated hypercalcemia. Clin J Am Soc Nephrol 2012;7(10): 1722–9.

6. Goldner W. Cancer-related hypercalcemia. J Oncol Pract 2016;12(5):426–32.

7. Ralston SH, Gallacher SJ, Patel U, et al. Cancer-associated hypercalcemia: morbidity and mortality. Clinical experience in 126 treated patients. Ann Intern Med 1990;112(7):499–504.

8. Wright JD, Tergas AI, Ananth CV, et al. Quality and outcomes of treatment of hypercalcemia of malignancy. Cancer Invest 2015;33(8):331–9.

9. Asonitis N, Angelousi A, Zafeiris C, et al. Diagnosis, pathophysiology and management of hypercalcemia in malignancy: a review of the literature. Horm Metab Res 2019;51(12):770–8.

10. Common terminology criteria for adverse events National Cancer Institute. Available at: https://ctep.cancer.gov/protocoldevelopment/electronic_applications/ctc.htm. Accessed July 6, 2021.

11. king RI, Florkowski CM. How paraproteins can affect laboratory assays: spurious results and biological effects. Pathology 2010;42(5):397–401.

12. Zagzag J, Hu MI, Fisher SB, et al. Hypercalcemia and cancer: differential diagnosis and treatment. CA Cancer J Clin 2018;68(5):377–86.

13. Koo WS, Jeon DS, Ahn SJ, et al. Calcium-free hemodialysis for the management of hypercalcemia. Nephron 1996;72(3):424–8.

14. Leehey DJ, Ing TS. Correction of hypercalcemia and hypophosphatemia by hemodialysis using a conventional, calcium-containing dialysis solution enriched with phosphorus. Am J Kidney Dis 1997;29(2):288–90.

15. Basok AB, Rogachev B, Haviv YS, et al. Treatment of extreme hypercalcaemia: the role of haemodialysis. BMJ Case Rep 2018;2018. bcr2017223772.

16. Hosking DJ, Cowley A, Bucknall CA. Rehydration in the treatment of severe hypercalcaemia. J Assoc Physicians 1981;50(4):473–81.

17. Dellay B, Groth M. Emergency management of malignancy-associated hypercalcemia. Adv Emerg Nurs J 2016;38(1):15–25 [quiz E1].

18. Legrand SB, Leskuski D, Zama I. Narrative review: furosemide for hypercalcemia: an unproven yet common practice. Ann Intern Med 2008;149(4):259–63.

19. Thiébaud D, Jacquet AF, Burckhardt P. Fast and effective treatment of malignant hypercalcemia: combination of suppositories of calcitonin and a single infusion of 3-Amino 1-Hydroxypropylidene-1-. Arch Intern Med 1990;150(10):2125–8.

20. Matsumoto T, Nagata N, Horikoshi N, et al. Comparative study of incadronate and elcatonin in patients with malignancy-associated hypercalcaemia. J Int Med Res 2002;30(3):230–43.

21. Fatemi S, Singer FR, Rude RK. Effect of salmon calcitonin and etidronate on hypercalcemia of malignancy. Calcified Tissue Int 1992;50(2):107–9.

22. Dumon JC, Magritte A, Body JJ. Nasal human calcitonin for tumor-induced hypercalcemia. Calcif Tissue Int 1992;51(1):18–9.

23. Khan AA, Gurnani PK, Peksa GD, et al. Bisphosphonate versus bisphosphonate and calcitonin for the treatment of moderate to severe hypercalcemia of malignancy. Ann Pharmacother 2021;55(3):277–85.

24. Highlights of Prescribing Information These highlights do not include all the information needed to use MIACALCIN injection safely and effectively. Initial U.S. Approval: 1975. Available at: https://www.accessdata.fda.gov/drugsatfda_docs/label/2014/017808s035lbl.pdf. Accessed July 9, 2021.

25. Wells G, Chernoff J, Gilligan JP, et al. Does salmon calcitonin cause cancer? A review meta-analysis. Osteoporos Int 2016;27(1):13–9.

26. Russell RG. Pharmacological diversity among drugs that inhibit bone resorption. Curr Opin Pharmacol 2015;22:115–30.

27. Highlights of Prescribing information these highlights do not include all the information needed to use Zoledronic Acid Injection safely and effectively. Initial U.S. Approval: 2001. Available at: https://www.accessdata.fda.gov/drugsatfda_docs/label/2016/203231s011lbl.pdf. Accessed July 9, 2021.

28. Highlights of Prescribing Information These highlights do not include all the information needed to use XGEVA® safely and effectively. Initial U.S. Approval: 2010. Available at: https://www.accessdata.fda.gov/drugsatfda_docs/label/2013/125320s094lbl.pdf. Accessed July 9, 2021.

29. Camozzi V, Luisetto G, Basso SM, et al. Treatment of chronic hypercalcemia. Med Chem 2012;8(4):556–63.

30. Vinholes J, Guo CY, Purohit OP, et al. Evaluation of new bone resorption markers in a randomized comparison of pamidronate or clodronate for hypercalcemia of malignancy. J Clin Oncol 1997;15(1):131–8.

31. Ralston SH, Dryburgh FJ, Cowan RA, et al. Comparison of aminohydroxypropylidene diphosphonate, mithramycin, and corticosteroidsicalcitonin in treatment of cancer-associated hypercalcaemia. Lancet 1985;326(8461):907–10.

32. Purohit OP, Radstone CR, Anthony C, et al. A randomised double-blind comparison of intravenous pamidronate and clodronate in the hypercalcaemia of malignancy. Br J Cancer 1995;72(5):1289–93.

33. Gucalp R, Ritch P, Vandepol CJ, et al. Comparative study of pamidronate disodium and etidronate disodium in the treatment of cancer-related hypercalcemia. J Clin Oncol 1992;10(1):134–42.

34. Major P, Lortholary A, Seaman J, et al. Zoledronic acid is superior to pamidronate in the treatment of hypercalcemia of malignancy: a pooled analysis of two randomized, controlled clinical trials. J Clin Oncol 2001;19(2):558–67.

35. Sabry NA, Habib EE. Zoledronic acid and clodronate in the treatment of malignant bone metastases with hypercalcaemia; efficacy and safety comparative study. Med Oncol 2011;28(2):584–90.

36. Pecherstorfer M, Steinhauer EU, Rizzoli R, et al. Efficacy and safety of ibandronate in the treatment of hypercalcemia of malignancy: a randomized multicentric comparison to pamidronate. Support Care Cancer 2003;11(8):539–47.

37. Jakob T, Tesfamariam YM, Macherey S, et al. Bisphosphonates or RANK-ligand-inhibitors for men with prostate cancer and bone metastases: a network meta-analysis. Cochrane Database Syst Rev 2020;(12):CD013020.

38. Mhaskar R, Kumar A, Miladinovic B, et al. Bisphosphonates in multiple myeloma: an updated network meta-analysis. Cochrane Database Syst Rev 2017;(12):CD003188.

39. Schiller JH, Rasmussen P, Benson AB, et al. Maintenance etidronate in the prevention of malignancy-associated hypercalcemia. Arch Intern Med 1987;147(5):963–6.

40. A study comparing denosumab vs. zoledronic acid for the treatment of bone metastases in breast cancer subjects. NCT00321464. Available at: https://clinicaltrials.gov/ct2/show/NCT00321464. Accessed July 9, 2021.

41. Sudy of denosumab vs. zoledronic acid to treat bone metastases in subjects with advanced cancer or multiple myeloma. NCT00330759. Available at: https://clinicaltrials.gov/ct2/show/NCT00330759. Accessed July 9, 2021.

42. Diel IJ, Body J-J, Stopeck AT, et al. The role of denosumab in the prevention of hypercalcaemia of malignancy in cancer patients with metastatic bone disease. Eur J Cancer 2015;51(11):1467–75.

43. Fizazi KP, Carducci MMD, Smith MMD, et al. Denosumab versus zoledronic acid for treatment of bone metastases in men with castration-resistant prostate cancer: a randomised, double-blind study. Lancet 2011;377(9768):813–22.
44. Adhikaree J, Newby Y, Sundar S. Denosumab should be the treatment of choice for bisphosphonate refractory hypercalcaemia of malignancy. BMJ Case Rep 2014;2014. bcr2013202861-bcr.
45. Dietzek A, Connelly K, Cotugno M, et al. Denosumab in hypercalcemia of malignancy: a case series. J Oncol Pharm Pract 2015;21(2):143–7.
46. Salahudeen AA, Gupta A, Jones JC, et al. PTHrP-induced refractory malignant hypercalcemia in a patient with chronic lymphocytic leukemia responding to denosumab. Clin Lymphoma Myeloma Leuk 2015;15(9):e137–40.
47. Ashihara N, Nakajima K, Nakamura Y, et al. Denosumab is effective for controlling serum calcium levels in patients with humoral hypercalcemia of malignancy syndrome: a case report on parathyroid hormone-related protein-producing cholangiocarcinoma. Intern Med 2016;55(23):3453–7.
48. Hu MI, Glezerman IG, Leboulleux S, et al. Denosumab for treatment of hypercalcemia of malignancy. J Clin Endocrinol Metab 2014;99(9):3144–52.
49. Ahmad S, Kuraganti G, Steenkamp D. Hypercalcemic crisis: a clinical review. Am J Med 2015;128(3):239–45.
50. Ponnapakkam T, Anbalagan M, Stratford RE Jr, et al. Novel bone-targeted parathyroid hormone-related peptide antagonists inhibit breast cancer bone metastases. Anticancer Drugs 2021;32(4):365–75.
51. Choppin A, Bedinger D, Hunt R, et al. A Novel anti-PTH1R receptor antagonist monoclonal antibody reverses hypercalcemia induced by PTH or PTHrP: a potential treatment of primary hyperparathyroidism and humoral hypercalcemia of malignancy. ENDO, Annual Meeting SAT 399, USA.
52. O'Callaghan S, Yau H. Treatment of malignancy-associated hypercalcemia with cinacalcet: a paradigm shift. Endocr Connect 2021;10(1):R13–24.
53. Sternlicht H, Glezerman IG. Hypercalcemia of malignancy and new treatment options. Ther Clin Risk Manag 2015;11:1779–88.
54. Asonitis E, Kassi M, Kokkinos I, et al. Hypercalcemia of malignancy treated with cinacalcet. Endocrinol Diabetes Metab Case Rep 2017;2017(1).
55. A clinical trial to assess the efficacy and safety of JMT103 in patients with refractory HCM. NCT04198480. Available at: https://clinicaltrials.gov/ct2/show/NCT04198480. Accessed July 9, 2021.
56. An intra-individual titration study of KRN1493 for the treatment of hypercalcemia in patients with parathyroid carcinoma or intractable primary hyperparathyroidism NCT01460030. Available at: https://clinicaltrials.gov/ct2/show/NCT01460030. Accessed July 9, 2021.
57. Takeuchi Y, Takahashi S, Miura D, et al. Cinacalcet hydrochloride relieves hypercalcemia in Japanese patients with parathyroid cancer and intractable primary hyperparathyroidism. J Bone Miner Metab 2017;35(6):616–22.

Moving?

Make sure your subscription moves with you!

To notify us of your new address, find your **Clinics Account Number** (located on your mailing label above your name), and contact customer service at:

Email: journalscustomerservice-usa@elsevier.com

800-654-2452 (subscribers in the U.S. & Canada)
314-447-8871 (subscribers outside of the U.S. & Canada)

Fax number: 314-447-8029

Elsevier Health Sciences Division
Subscription Customer Service
3251 Riverport Lane
Maryland Heights, MO 63043

*To ensure uninterrupted delivery of your subscription, please notify us at least 4 weeks in advance of move.